This book is dedicated to my father Bernard,

a holocaust survivor,

for his love,

honesty,

modesty,

dedication,

and wonderful humor

which enabled me to fulfill my and his dreams and wishes.

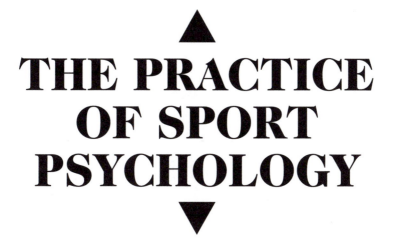

THE PRACTICE OF SPORT PSYCHOLOGY

GERSHON TENENBAUM

Editor

FLORIDA STATE UNIVERSITY

A Project of the International Society of Sport Psychology (ISSP)

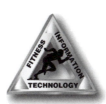

Fitness Information Technology, Inc. • P.O. Box 4425
Morgantown, WV 26504-4425 • USA

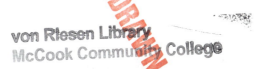

Library of Congress Card Catalog Number: 01-126255

ISBN: 1-885693-30-3

Copyeditor: Sandra Woods, Candace Jordan, Geoff Fuller
Cover Design: Krafty Kat Designs
Managing Editor: Geoffrey C. Fuller
Production Editor: Craig Hines
Proofreader: Maria denBoer
Indexer: Maria denBoer
Printed by Data Reproductions, Inc.
10 9 8 7 6 5 4 3 2 1

Fitness Information Technology, Inc.
P.O. Box 4425, University Avenue
Morgantown, WV 26504 USA
800.477.4348
304.599.3483 phone
304.599.3482 fax
Email: fit@fitinfotech.com
Website: www.fitinfotech.com

Contents

Contents

An Introduction to the Book: From Personal Reflections to the Practice of Sport Psychology

Gershon Tenenbaum

When I completed my graduate studies at the University of Chicago, sport and exercise psychology was a very young domain of practice and inquiry. While some psychologists in America, Europe, and Asia were introducing this new domain, it was not well established. After graduating, I retired from competitive sports, but I was very much aware of the important role my mental-emotional state had played in determining my performance quality. During my long athletic career, however, nobody taught me how to regulate my emotions and thoughts so that I might optimize my performance. Instead, practice sessions were devoted entirely to the development of physical fitness, motor skills, tactics, strategies, and team technique.

At that time, there were only two journals in the field: *The International Journal of Sport Psychology* and *The Journal of Sport Psychology* (it was not until later that the word *Exercise* was added to the title). These two journals published articles on both research/theory and practical issues. Since then, the field of sport and exercise psychology has accelerated in its development. Over time, more journals and books were published, more national and international societies were established, and eventually I realized that sport psychology was the domain in which I desired to study and to teach.

I thought then that my greatest contribution to this fascinating new domain would be the development of new methods of measuring the psychological traits and states crucial to the athlete's performance. At that time, Benjamin Bloom was collecting the data on multidomain expertise that he later published in 1985. I was his PhD student and his assistant. As a young psychometrician, I believed I could first determine the variables that influence performance (e.g., motor skills, mental skills, and quality of practice), operationalize them in terms of measurement devices, and determine their individual and interactive effect via some function.

The idea was to measure how these components *change* during the careers of athletes. The measures of change were a major challenge because these variables failed to share common scales or units of measurement, and were not standardized. I thought that maybe it was too ambitious a task for me, and that there might be a better way to postulate the model and then to examine it piece by piece. The model consists of Bloom's (1976) conceptualization of educational achievements. It is the simplest and most convenient way to show how the *quality of practice* is the primary *mediator* between present motor, physical, and mental skills and future performance quality. The

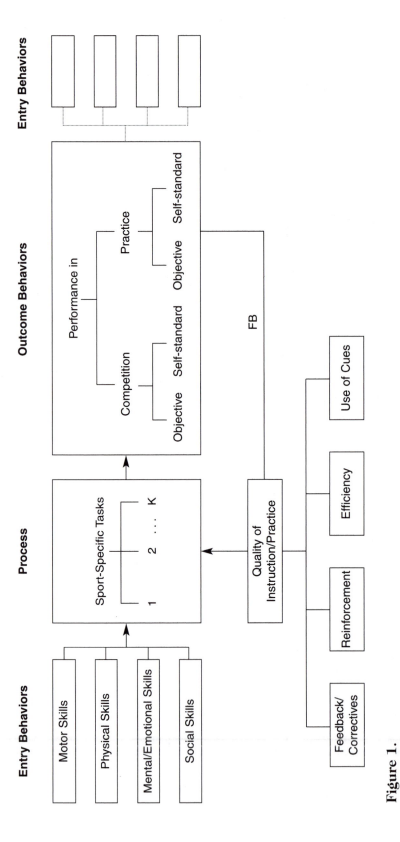

Figure 1.
A model that postulates the relationship between entry behaviors and outcome behaviors mediated by the quality of instruction/practice

model has a dynamical nature; i.e., the performance components at each time are perceived as *entry behaviors* for the subsequent developmental stages (see Figure 1).

We sport psychologists are believed to be the professionals who contribute primarily to the mental and emotional states of the athlete in his or her attempt to reach full potential. The underlying assumption is that once the athlete achieves an optimal emotional or mental state, that individual can indeed focus, concentrate, and be at his or her best. My main concern as a sport psychologist is to determine the method that will increase the probability of successful outcomes. Is there one way of working with athletes, coaches, and organizations that is preferable to others? Are there many methods of work that secure successful outcomes? If so, do these methods have anything in common?

I ask these questions because during my 12 years at the Center for Research and Sport Medicine Sciences at the Wingate Institute, Israel, I was approached by sport psychology practitioners who argued that what we teach and research is *not* what the field requires, nor is it what is actually done in practice. At that time I believed that the disputes between the scientists and the practitioners, typical to most disciplines, stemmed from conceptual and personal misunderstandings. The scientist strives for objective measures, controlled environments, well-defined variables, and statistical features that represent the *central* and *dispersion* trends of his or her data. The practitioner, on the other hand, works in a dynamical and alterable environment, not perfectly controllable, and his or her primary concern is the *individual* athlete or the *team* rather than a mean or a variation estimate. It was evident to me that the *concerns*, the *language,* and, consequently, the *methods* became distinct from one another. I strongly believed, at that time, that the gap between concerns and methods

could be narrowed if scientists were asked to adopt an *action methodology*—to become part of the sport scene by involving themselves in the process of athletic practices. I also believed that enhanced communications between scientists and practitioners would give rise to new, shared concerns and would inspire the development of a *field-driven* theory. Unfortunately, such developments did not begin until recently. Some positive signs lie on the horizon, however.

During the last 6 years, as I have prepared graduate students in psychology to become professional sport psychologists, I have continued to experience this same disparity between science and practice. My students at the University of Southern Queensland in Australia have all been well educated, both in psychology and in sport and exercise sciences. They have been very enthusiastic about studying sport psychology for 2–4 years and then practicing in that relatively new, and promising, profession. A committee established by the Australian Psychological Society (APS) postulated the *competencies,* the *course contents,* and the *practicum/placement requirements* that are supposed to transform a psychologist into a proficient sport psychologist. My students learned the required theories, research methods, individual and team interventions, individual assessment procedures, program-evaluation techniques, and principles of applied work and practice. Then, at the end of the first year, they practiced their competencies in the field, meeting with athletes, coaches, administrators, organizers, and other scientists and professionals from related fields. It did not take long for them to come back to me and say, politely, "Gershon, you know, the issues we learned in psychology and sport psychology are very interesting, and they enhanced our declarative and procedural knowledge, but the problems we encounter in the field are not the same as you taught us in class." Here, again, I faced the disparity between what we teach, research, and publish and the multifaceted issues practitioners encounter in their work with coaches, athletes, and administrators.

In light of this, I thought the time had come for me to put aside (for a while) my academic concerns—that is, my attempts to find better methods of measurement in sport psychology—and to devote more time to the study of *real practice*. By real practice I mean the real issues that concern sport psychologists and the methods sport psychologists employ in dealing with those issues. To accomplish this, I approached several *expert practitioners,* people with vast experience in fieldwork, and shared my concerns with them. I asked each of them to write a chapter for a book I was editing that featured sport psychologists' reflections on their work. I supplied them with the following guidelines:

> As a co-coordinator and editor of this project I do not wish to put ANY constraints on your writing. Each of the contributors to this project has complete freedom to determine the outline he/she wishes to follow. It is, however, recommended to follow a logical sequence and to support your arguments with your own reflections and your athletes' behavior, thoughts, feelings, and outcomes. If you wish to offer a model, which supports your arguments, feel free to do so. Do not limit yourself to problems associated only with the sport. Expand it to other aspects of life. A holistic approach is very much recommended.

When I read their chapters, I was more convinced than ever that (a) their concerns and methods are not adequately represented in the published literature, and that (b) we lack sufficient knowledge to educate and prepare students who wish to become proficient in the practice of sport psychology. The aim of this book is to raise these issues and to learn from the expert practitioners how to deal with them in an efficient, professional manner. It is my hope that new directions will promote practitioner-scientist collaboration and will give rise to new topics for systematic investigation, so that sport psychology will become a well-established discipline with sound, field-driven theory.

The expert practitioners address a variety of issues and concerns and come from different backgrounds, institutes, and programs. They differ from one another in their personalities and attitudes, and they have different philosophies and concepts about the manner in which sport psychological services should be provided. Each perceives his or her work from a different perspective: is it clinical, health oriented, community oriented, feminist, social, practical, or any other; and each has developed his or her unique methods of practice. However, all of the expert practitioners are similar in their intent to optimize mental and emotional conditions so that the athletes and teams with whom they work will meet their desired goals.

The keys for successful practice seem to be related to a deep understanding of the conditions under which performance can be optimized. These conditions take into account the individual's desires, level of skill, and emotional and cognitive development, as well as the type of task and the environment (e.g., facilities, coaches, etc.) in which the task is performed. The practitioners perceive the athlete in a holistic way. A successful athlete is one who *enjoys challenges* and strives to develop his or her *general self* through positive, challenging sport experiences. Successful practice is about exploring all the resources necessary for a successful performance, whether they be internal coping strategies or external sources of social, emotional, medical, or personal support. It is also about *trial and error,* especially when circumstances do not match expectations. The practitioner is the one who has the *knowledge* not only to suggest but also to explore new methods of coping with success, as well as with failure and its consequences. It is about the *flexibility* of *options* rather than about a narrow, unidirectional line of treating problems and ensuring effective coping and outcomes.

Effective sport psychology practice also involves *knowing oneself* and one's *role* within the team and the organization. It involves knowing what is allowed and what is forbidden when one is on a short or a long tour with athletes. It involves knowing about injuries and frustrations, about sexual and emotional harassment, about young athletes who miss their families and have other priorities and personal needs, about young adults and adults who sacrifice their youth for what they love most. Effective sport psychology practice requires knowledge of how to communicate with coaches, athletes, politicians, and other scientists and professionals (i.e., physicians, physiotherapists, biotechnicians, physiologists, etc.).

The process of talent discovery, development, and refinement, as I postulate it in Figure 2, is well addressed in the various chapters of this book. At each stage, it is important to remember that excellence and expertise—in any field—do not compensate for all the other needs that people have. The practice and attention athletes receive in their areas of expertise should be balanced with attention to their needs as human beings. In some chapters this quest for balance is soundly expressed, while in others it can be read between the lines. The aim of psychological services in sport is to prepare the athlete to cope efficiently with stressful and demanding situations. At the same time, psy-

chological services should enable the athlete to keep a balance between sport and other life events so that transitions from one stage to the other will be as smooth as possible. Moreover, effective psychological services should ensure that the athlete's transition to another phase of life upon career termination will not be traumatic, whether that transition is expected or unexpected. Sport, when well balanced, can be a tool for creating good citizens and happy individuals.

Various aspects of the work of the sport psychologists documented in this book can be clustered as follows:

- Ongoing, periodic psychological service;
- Periodic meetings;
- Single meeting;
- Team issues and activities;
- Individual issues and interventions;
- Coach/athlete-related issues;
- Private counseling;
- Formal/institutionalized counseling;
- Coach-centered concept;
- Athlete-centered concept;
- Interactional approach;
- Activities in the club/on the field/at practice/on tours;
- Activities in the clinic;
- Sport-specific issues; and
- General (life) issues.

Also discussed are the various roles of the psychologist as

- a professional consultant,
- a provider of performance-enhancement services,
- an entertainer and an arbiter of disputes,
- a friend (When? Under what circumstances?),
- a confidante, and
- a mediator for ethical disputes and issues of misconduct.

The book then addresses important issues

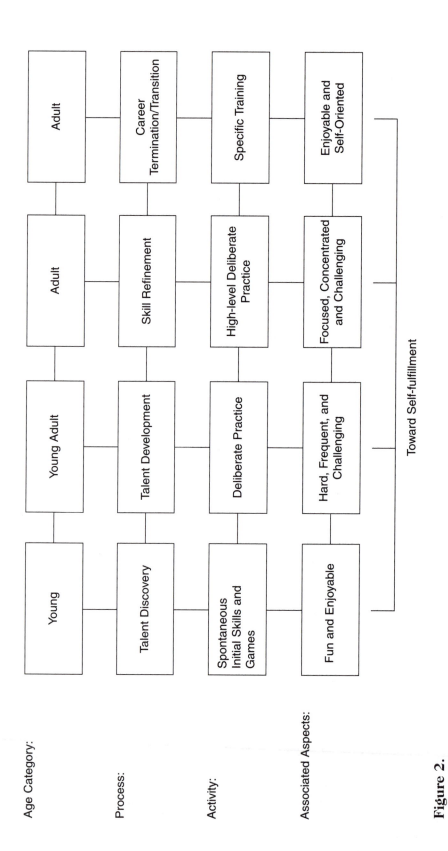

Figure 2.
A developmental process in sport as a basis for delivery of psychological services

that further relate to how psychologists choose to work, including:

- Diagnosis-dominated interventions,
- Theory-based interventions,
- Common-sense interventions,
- Performance-enhancement interventions, and
- Clinical interventions.

Before I close this introduction, here is a review of each chapter of the book and a brief outline of the various concerns addressed by the expert practitioners. Their contributions reveal the variety of approaches and techniques they use to enhance athletes' well-being and to prepare them for personal challenges.

Sandy Gordon provides his insight regarding the use of the operational philosophy with professional cricket teams and their respective sport organizations to facilitate and establish a "culture of success." According to Gordon, who perceives himself as a "mental skills trainer," one should concentrate on three types of functions: results, individual, and team. *Results functions* relate to setting long-term goals and to making all individuals who are involved with the team—trainers, athletes, support staff, athletes' spouses or life partners—aware of those goals (thereby creating a "vision"). *Individual functions* relate to achieving personal growth and to making worthwhile contributions to the team. *Team functions* involve developing a "shared purpose" (i.e., "Together Each Achieve More"; TEAM). Gordon describes the fundamentals of his professional work with the cricket players, and he explains how he applies the cognitive-affective and educational approaches in real-life situations so that the players "play smart." Any player and/or coach can use his ideas about mental skills training for cricket in any team sport. To establish a culture of success, Gordon describes in detail the emphasis on competency profiling, individual and team performance profiles, personal success, and social support within the team. The techniques used to establish a "success culture" and the practitioner-scientist approach are illustrated clearly, so that many of them can be learned and applied.

Trisha Leahy introduces the feminist-practice approach. She presents her definition of *feminism* and describes its impact on her day-to-day practice as well as on her scientist-practitioner approach. Leahy believes the role of the sport psychologist to be different from the one adopted by AAASP in 1990. She is engaged more in therapeutic work than in educational and performance-enhancement activities. She sees many parallels between the work of a psychologist and the work of a sport psychologist; the contexts of the athletes' and other clients' lives may differ, but the therapeutic process remains the same. From Leahy's perspective, sport psychology practice is divided into three levels of intervention: *primary* (e.g., performance-related mental skills, organization and policy development); *psychoeducational* (e.g., eating disorders, sexual harassment awareness training, conflict resolution with a team, body-image enhancement, support groups, etc.); and *therapeutic* (e.g., individual concerns such as disordered eating, sexuality, and multisymptomatic sequelae of prolonged and repeated trauma). Leahy outlines the principles of the feminist theory and the ways they are reflected in sport psychology practice and intervention; she also describes a workshop/study in which these principles were applied. Finally, to encourage the establishment of practice and research within a feminist framework, she introduces her reflections on politics in sport and its impact on female athletes.

Dan Gould describes his 5-year experience as an "educational sport psychology consultant" with the U.S. freestyle mogul ski team in the Nagano Winter Olympic Games.

Gould outlines in detail his long-term involvement with the team and describes the psychological program, including preparation and the special issues that arise during the preparation period; intervention strategies; and program evaluation. According to Gould, his involvement in the athletes' preparation for the Olympics served three main purposes: (a) to help the athletes peak at the games and to provide assistance, (b) to provide informational and emotional support to the coaches and staff, and (c) to provide social support to the athletes (i.e., to act as an unbiased and objective source of support). The preparation of athletes for the Olympic Games is a unique, multifaceted opportunity and involves such aspects as understanding the nature of the sport; maintaining relations with coaches who differ in their views regarding the discipline of sport psychology; providing support during the selection of the athletes who will represent the nation in the games; designing the mental-training consulting schedule within a long time period; developing intervention strategies (group and team meetings, individual consultations, and coach briefing and debriefing); and making changes and alterations to the program. Gould describes these tasks in a diary format so that the reader can relive the sport psychologist's feelings, thoughts, and decision-making processes throughout the entire period. The work before and during the games is outlined in words and summarized in tables. The reflections of athletes and coaches lend a special flavor to Gould's work, and the lessons to be learned from his experiences are essential for everyone who wishes to work as a sport psychologist.

Keith Henschen relates his powerful experiences as a psychologist with an NBA team. Henschen works from a holistic perspective: The professional player is viewed as a friend, someone with whom the psychologist might dine, play golf, exchange ideas, and philoso-

phize. The client-athlete is not merely a performer; he or she is a unique person with special physical talents, a person with social, intellectual, spiritual, and performance needs. Of course, young performers deserve different treatment than do mature, elite athletes. A successful sport psychologist, Henschen believes it is imperative that practitioners understand the value systems, behavior patterns, reinforcement preferences, cultural pressures and expectations, and general life philosophies of the athletes with whom they work. In his chapter, he offers advice on how to choose appropriate language for communicating with athletes, how to overcome potential gender-related problems, how to know one's limitations, and how to exhibit one's competencies. Through his experiences, readers learn about becoming themselves, pleasing themselves, using healthy intuition, developing confidence and self-concept, using different tools with different athletes, becoming passionate and compassionate, establishing a systematic method, and developing counseling skills.

Dieter Hackfort, a scientist and practitioner, shows how a sound theory, such as the *Action Theory,* can prove the most practical tool for working with athletes. The Action Theory builds upon the *person,* the *environment,* and the *task.* Both objective and subjective factors play a role in making decisions and executing an action plan. Once a goal is defined, awareness of the person-environment-task connection is vital for making decisions and taking actions. Actions are perceived as goal-directed behaviors that are guided and purposeful for human beings. Athletes operate within their unique environments and choose strategies derived from their personal experiences and representative of their orientations. The sport psychologist must capture the subjective concepts and interpret them in order to plan his or her intervention. As the first step in the process of recovery from failure or injury or, alternatively, in the enhancement of their performance quality, athletes must reflect on their experiences. Hackfort substantiates his arguments by introducing his athletes' reflections on events they experienced, based on their recollections. Then, what the athlete feels integrates with reality, and subsequently leads the psychologist and the athlete to regulate the athlete's actions. Hackfort then outlines how sensitivity to athletes' feelings "makes it possible to initiate safety strategies in time, and to protect against threatening circumstance." He further elaborates on methods that can be applied in action regulation at various stages (anticipation, realization, and interpretation)—methods such as planning, calculating, tuning, processing, controlling, and evaluating. He goes on to discuss various issues relating to orientation regulation and to demonstrate his concepts as they relate to the sport of golf.

Sidónio Serpa and João Rodrigues collaborated to write the chapter on their experiences. Serpa is a sport psychologist, and Rodrigues is a top sailor. Their contribution to this book is unique not only in its presentation and its messages but especially in the authors' perception of experience in top sport as a means of achieving harmony as a human being. Their writings and views are influenced by Greg Louganis's book *Breaking the Surface* and by Victor Frankl's *Man's Search for Meaning*. The depth and insight that competitive sport can offer will impress the reader. The authors emphasize how much can be learned from frustration and from overwhelming experience, and how rewarding performance-oriented (in contrast to outcome-oriented) approaches to competitive sport can be. Serpa and Rodrigues recommend that both athlete and practitioner attempt to work in "harmony" rather than to "think winning"; according to the authors, this is the way to enjoy top sport and to de-

velop a positive and harmonic personality. In a question-and-answer format, Rodrigues describes the respect he felt for his competitors, his desire for self-discovery and perfection, the evolution of the athlete-person relationship, and his enjoyment of the sport environment. Serpa describes the *Integrated Model of Psychological Training*, which consists of active performance analysis by the athlete from the initial stages of talent development using self-reflections and in-depth thought about well-defined goals and objectives (similar to the approach mentioned by Hackfort). The *initiatory, developmental,* and *specialization* stages have their distinct characteristics, and the sport psychologist should take them into consideration when offering psychological services. Throughout the chapter, the authors stress the "need for self-fulfillment." Their concepts and reflections offer a great deal to practitioners in the field who believe in these messages.

Robert Nideffer, Mark-Simon Sagal, Mark Lowry, and Jeffrey Bond believe top sport performance to be similar to performance in business and in the military; all three arenas present similar challenges and pressures. In order to better cope with such demands, individuals must learn certain coping strategies and styles; these strategies must be taught, learned, and brought to maturity. The authors' approach consists of a detailed comparison between performers and managers/coaches in any field. Later in the chapter, they recommend ways to maintain effective communication, teamwork, and other elements important to psychological consultants. The authors are very pragmatic in their approach, asking questions regarding the athlete's ability to fit, to function, to cope, to be motivated and self-disciplined, and to master the skills required for optimal performance. Often, consultants are asked to help athletes perform their best despite emotional and physical sacrifices, as well as to help them make the appropriate transitions and adjustments. The authors offer a systematic approach for that purpose: an assessment procedure that they believe provides data regarding the information-processing capacity of the athlete; the degree of distraction generated by various environmental distractors; the athlete's ability to analyze information without feeling overloaded; the athlete's ability to concentrate and to focus; and a variety of intrapersonal, interpersonal, and emotional-stability characteristics, all of which are crucial for top performers. The TAIS is the tool they offer for assessment. They then substantiate their claims by analyzing these traits in top athletes and business managers, and go on to outline the implications their data have for psychological consultants.

Clark Perry expands the definition of the term *winning* to present his views about working with elite athletes. He argues that society views success in terms of outcomes, but that paradoxically, the more practitioners and athletes focus on winning, the less likely it is to occur. Winning, according to Perry, does not describe performance. He advocates a process-centered approach in working with extremely talented athletes, young and adult. Perry introduces several symptoms, which he terms *inhibitions* that may signify process problems. When athletes repeatedly avoid a desired activity, exhibit extreme self-consciousness, are consistently unlucky, are overly concerned with the environment, and report negative somatic symptoms just before competition, they need assistance in order to overcome these inhibitions. Perry's excellent examples make these arguments real and convenient for practitioners. Perry also outlines possible motives athletes might have for not trying hard enough, such as a fear of arousing envy, a fear of ultimate failure, a desire for independence, a fear of losing identity, or a fear

of falling short of goals. These may be expressed verbally or exhibited in practice and competition. The sport psychologist is responsible for assisting the athlete in overcoming his or her difficulties through the use of techniques that emphasize the *process,* as these symptoms result from the *outcome* orientation.

Barry Kerr brings community and education into the practice of sport psychology. His experiences of working with young child-athletes in the demanding and stressful environment of competitive sport have led him to develop important recommendations not only for the athletes, but also—primarily—for the coaches, the participating parents, and the sponsors of athletic programs. Kerr outlines the dangerous consequences a negative approach to child training may have on society and on the athlete's well-being. He suggests that sport psychologists facilitate scientific and educational programs addressing the issues of stress, expectations, and child development; and he recommends coping strategies to assist children in a proactive way prior to, during, and after competitions. Coaches should be educated to increase awareness of their coaching styles and of the positive and negative effects those styles may have on their young athletes. With adult athletes, Kerr suggests a counseling approach. He advocates a partnership between the athlete and the sport psychologist. This partnership begins with both parties negotiating on their expectations of one another and on what is required for a successful partnership. These negotiations determine the level of security or insecurity in the relationship. Once the partnership is agreed upon, an intervention program is designed and carried out. Kerr points out various issues that may arise during work with athletes and suggests cognitive and psychodynamic strategies for solving them. He illustrates his techniques with examples of actual cases so that sport psychologists can better visualize and, if necessary, apply those techniques to any similar cases they might encounter in their work.

Noam Eyal introduces a clinical approach in his work with athletes. He asks, "What is the Point of Archimedes from which the psychologist can, or is asked to, affect the psychology of the athlete?" He then discusses the dilemmas and the complexities presented by possible answers to this question. Eyal contrasts sport-specific psychoregulations with a more holistic, comprehensive psychological perspective. He also offers a variety of reasons why individuals and teams employ sport psychologists, and he addresses the psychologist's role within the team, with individual athletes, and with other sport scientists. Taking an ethical perspective, Eyal discusses in detail the types of communication that tend to develop between the athlete and the psychologist. To illustrate the countless number of cases and their complexity, he presents five actual cases. Each stands alone and is described comprehensively. These "mystery stories" and their unique solutions are fascinating, and each is a lesson with a message. The link between each "story" and its resolution is the most important message in Eyal's essay. Eyal demonstrates how athletes differ from one another and how much care should be given to them in order to avoid mistakes that cannot be reversed.

Kenneth Ravizza introduces a practical approach that integrates mental skills with the existing practice of performance procedures so that athletes can develop, refine, and practice various performance techniques in the midst of pressure situations. He emphasizes his own personal, holistic approach, developed during his last 25 years of working with athletes. From the outset, Ravizza emphasizes that he is not a psychologist and that he refers athletes with psychological problems (e.g., eating disorders, drug is-

sues, etc.) to professional psychologists. His domain is performance enhancement, and his methods involve the development and refinement of mental skills in a manner similar to the development and refinement of physical and motor skills. The educational approach Ravizza adopts consists of providing the athlete with accurate, relevant, and up-to-date information, the opportunity to practice skills, and daily support in learning those skills. According to him, practitioners should be realistic in providing the appropriate performance-enhancement techniques; as such techniques do not affect all athletes identically. Ravizza provides examples to illustrate how varied the communications and the work with different athletes can be. The principles of performance-enhancement, in conjunction with the support given to the athletes, are of utmost importance. Ravizza also emphasizes the importance of the preparation and ongoing, preseason mental preparation, and distinguishes it from the medical approach. He is continually aware of playing a "small though important" part in the whole scenario; thus, he recognizes how essential it is for him to establish a proactive approach to working with athletes. Ravizza also emphasizes his collaboration with coaching staff, his use of coaches' and athletes' knowledge in session, his techniques for team meetings, and his principles of work (e.g., know the sport, earn trust and respect, learn the context). Ravizza believes that "awareness" is essential in order for performers to make the adjustments required of elite-level athletes; he uses a metaphor of "brake control" to show how this concept can be learned and developed. He also introduces the *quality-of-practice* principles, which can be applied by practitioners in various sports. Finally, Ravizza generously offers young practitioners some helpful hints that may save them much agony in the beginning stages of their work with athletes.

Jeff Bond shares his experiences of and lessons regarding the services a sport psychologist provides to athletes, coaches, and the entire delegation during competition tours. He views his work as holistic, incorporating many facets of athlete preparation including technical, physical, and mental aspects. He believes that the athlete's performance outcome depends on a complex series of events—events that should be taken into consideration in planning intervention programs. The various emotional and mental states, which the athlete experiences at the moment, are fundamental for designing a psychological intervention. According to Bond, in order for psychological services to be successful they must be integrated with medical and other scientific services; additionally, and most importantly, the coaching staff must accept them. To illustrate his holistic views regarding the provision of psychological services to athletes, Bond presents the National Rowing Team Service-Provision Model. He describes the dynamics and the complexity of his work with the rowers, the coaches, and other team staff. The rigorous daily schedule of elite rowers and the systematic, difficult work in which they, their coaches, and their trainers engage will impress readers. Bond then outlines and elaborates on principles important for a touring sport psychologist. He discusses and illustrates topics such as practitioner responsibilities, interactions with coaches and athletes, needs analyses, adoption of a process focus, competitive performance requirements, "preparing for the worst," confidentiality, time and energy commitments, planned obsolescence, professional relationships, inclusiveness, and more. Bond's chapter deals with issues seldom addressed in the scholarly literature; thus, its importance and relevance to the profession is undeniable.

Boris Blumenstein shares his experiences of working in Russia and Israel. The social and cultural differences in these two countries are reflected in his work with young and Olympic athletes. The Russian era was dominated by systematic provision of personality inventories, as well as by specific questionnaires that were developed for specific sports. The resulting psychological profile of the athlete was used both for interventions and for the selection of the young athlete into the "appropriate" sport. Blumenstein also describes how individual regulation styles were used to enhance the quality of the athlete's performance. Of particular interest are his descriptions of the interactions between sport psychologists and the coaches and athletes of the former USSR. The immigration to Israel resulted in alterations in these interactions. It also led to the adoption of a different value system and of a westernized culture with substantially fewer athletes and resources for elite sport. Prestart diagnoses of the athlete's motivational state, goals, and levels of arousal, attention, concentration, focus, and self-regulation, using sophisticated and computerized biofeedback equipment, replaced the inventories and other techniques used in Russia. Blumenstein developed a 5-step approach, a method he used very successfully with top Olympic athletes who later became European and Olympic champions. Blumenstein shares the principles of this method and his experiences with those athletes so that readers might apply the principles in working with their own clients.

Grace Pretty describes the unique dynamics of the relationship between a horse and its rider. Competitive excellence demands that this relationship be a harmonious one. Pretty introduces methods that can help the equestrian resolve problems such as anxiety, fear, loss of confidence and concentration, and performance stress, which are transferred to the horse and result in performance decrements. Both rider and horse are sensitive to messages transmitted by touch, speech, and gesture; an understanding of this sensitivity is useful for intervention. When working with the equestrian, the sport psychologist deals with two clients: the rider and the horse. The horse is the performer, while the rider provides support; thus, their relationship is the key element to consider in the provision of psychological support. Pretty provides many case examples, as well as riders' reflections on their horses, to demonstrate the approaches psychologists should take when confronting problems between horse and rider. For example, how can the sport psychologist help the rider deal with frustration that arises when the rider's attempts to modify the horse's behavior are unsuccessful? Through Pretty's examples and suggestions, the reader becomes acquainted with procedures that may resolve such problems. The psychology of creating harmony between horse and rider is elaborated for what is perhaps the first time in sport psychology literature.

Patrick Thomas devoted much time and energy to the psychology of two sports: golf and orienteering. After many years of work, he developed a conceptual model to guide practitioners in their work with golfers and orienteers. The six-phase model consists of diagnostic procedures, psychological skill training procedures, implementation procedures, and evaluation procedures that sport psychologists should incorporate in their work with athletes. Thomas uses this conceptual framework to structure reflections on his own professional practice with athletes, particularly golfers. Additionally, he includes the reflections of athletes who participated in programs aimed at enhancing their mental skills. These reflections were used to extend the programs and to adjust them to the athletes' individual needs. Thomas presents a holistic approach to the practice and the enhancement of golf and

orienteering skills. He appreciates the mental aspects of developing physical, technical, tactical, and life skills; and he uses those aspects to establish current and target profiles for each athlete. His systematic, holistic methodology is very impressive.

The final chapter of the book, written by Steven Christensen, is devoted to the *process* of becoming a sport psychologist. Christensen offers the analogy of a journey—a journey that begins with the individual's interest in sport psychology and ends with the individual becoming a sport psychologist. The journey begins with many dreams, ambitions, and hopes, as well as some degree of apprehension and uncertainty. It ends with the acquisition of professional competencies, which introduce the person to practice, and the psychological services he/she might provide the athletes. To make the journey (i.e., specialist training) successful and enjoyable, Christensen draws a conceptual map for the aspiring sport psychologist. He describes the stages of the journey, including the planning. According to Christensen, one should plan the journey by asking oneself "Where am I now?" One should then plan the destination by asking, "Where do I want to go?" Christensen introduces four dimensions (*content, energy, space,* and *time*) to guide the young, ambitious sport psychologist toward his or her destination. He also draws attention to issues of ethical and professional conduct that arise throughout the journey, and he addresses the question, "How do I get there?" This is a key question for those who wish to partake of experiences like the ones described throughout this book.

The stories and reflections of the sport psychologists who have contributed to this book represent, to me, an important step toward (a) enhancing the discipline of sport psychology; (b) bridging the gap between practice and science, thereby raising new issues relevant to the field; and (c) allowing students to learn more about the field and to develop their skills through exposure to the best and most experienced practitioners in the world. Additionally, for those who prepare the new sport psychology cadets, the last chapter provides an overview of the guiding principles of teaching sport psychology.

Each chapter in this book reveals the personal experiences of a different sport psychologist. The reader will find that the methods suggested are as diverse as the discipline itself. Each practitioner brings his or her own flavor to the field; therefore, those who educate and prepare students for careers in sport psychology should perhaps bear in mind the lyrics of Harry Chapin's song, "Flowers Are Red." Indeed, flowers are of many colors.

The little boy went first day of school
He got some crayons and started to draw
He put colors all over the paper
For colors was what he saw
And the teacher said . . . What you doin' young man
I'm paintin' flowers he said
She said . . . It's not the time for art young man
And anyway flowers are green and red
There's a time for everything young man
And a way it should be done
You've got to show concern for everyone else
For you're not the only one

And she said . . .
Flowers are red young man
Green leaves are green
There's no need to see flowers any other way
Than the way they have always been seen

But the little boy said . . .
There are so many colors in the rainbow
So many colors in the morning sun
So many colors in the flower and I see every one

Well the teacher said . . . You're sassy
There's ways that things should be
And you'll paint flowers the way they are
So repeat after me . . .

And she said . . .
Flowers are red young man
Green leaves are green
There's no need to see flowers any other way
Than the way they always have been seen

But the little boy said . . .
There are so many colors in the rainbow
So many colors in the morning sun
So many colors in the flower and I see every one

The teacher put him in a corner
She said . . . It's for your own good
And you won't come out 'til you get it right
And all responding like you should
Well finally he got lonely

Frightened thoughts filled his head
And he went up to the teacher
And this is what he said . . . and he said

Flowers are red, green leaves are green
There's no need to see flowers any other way
Than the way they always have been seen

Time went by like it always does
And they moved to another town
And the little boy went to another school
And this is what he found
The teacher there was smiling
She said . . . Painting should be fun
And there are so many colors in a flower
So let's use every one

But that little boy painted flowers
In neat rows of green and red
And when the teacher asked him why
This is what he said . . . and he said

Flowers are red, green leaves are green
There's no need to see flowers any other way
Than the way they always have been seen.

—1978

FLOWERS ARE RED by Harry Chapin
© 1978 Five J's Songs
All Rights Reserved   Used by Permission
WARNER BROS. PUBLICATIONS U.S. INC., Miami, FL 33014

sport psychology should perhaps bear in mind the lyrics of Harry Chapin's song, "Flowers Are Red." Indeed, flowers are of many colors.

References

Bloom, B. S. (1976). Human characteristics and school learning. New York: McGraw-Hill.

Chapin, H. (1978). Flowers Are Red. www.littlejason.com/chapin/songs/flowers.html. Site visited on December 10, 2000.

Reflections on Providing Sport Psychology Services in Professional Cricket

Sandy Gordon

Introduction

Cricket is played by females and males worldwide, but for those readers unfamiliar with the rules of the game perhaps this riddle can help: "You have two sides, one out in the field and one in. Each player that's in the side that's in goes out, and when he's out, he comes in, and the next player comes in until he's out. When all players get out, the side that's out comes in, and the side that's been in goes out and tries to get those coming in, out. Sometimes you get players still in and not out. When both sides have been in and out, including the not outs, that's the end of the game" (Whimpress, 1985).

The intention of this chapter is not to unravel meaning from the above but to reflect on my experiences working as a sport psychologist with two professional cricket teams, Western Australia's State team, the Western Warriors, and Australia's National Test and One-Day teams.[1] More specifically, I hope to provide some insight on my operational philosophy that seems to work with both these professional teams and their respective sport organizations. Second, I will describe how I try to look at the bigger picture and facilitate "cultures of success" and excellence for both individuals and teams in both organizations. Third, I will explain how I have evaluated what I do by describing the methods, procedures, and results of a study I conducted among six players during a winter training school. Finally, I will comment on how I contributed to the preparation of both the Western Warriors for their successful defense of the Sheffield Shield (national title) and the Australian One-Day Team, which won the 1999 Cricket World Cup in England.

Operational Philosophy

Since March 1987, the Western Australian Cricket Association (WACA) has retained me as mental-skills coach. As I have explained elsewhere (Gordon, 1990), I was initially appointed to the WACA Coaching Panel to serve the Western Warriors (male state team); however, my role has expanded considerably over the years. I now teach

---

1. The Western Warriors (Western Australian state team) annually competes in Australia's Pura Cup (formerly Sheffield Shield) competition, which involves 10 home and away 4-day games against five other state teams—New South Wales, Queensland, South Australia, Victoria, and Tasmania. The Warriors also compete against the same States in the Mercantile Mutual Cup, which involves 10 home and away One-Day games (October–March). The Australian National Teams compete internationally and year-round in both Test (5-day games) and One-Day (limited overs) competitions against several other national teams such as South Africa, West Indies, Pakistan, India, New Zealand, England, Zimbabwe, and Sri Lanka.

mental skills to Under 13-, 15-, and 16-year-old squads (n=60/squad), and to Under 17- and Under 19-year-old representative teams and to a Colts (Second XI) team (n=18/team). Upon request, I have also worked with the Western Australian Country XI (n=18) and with the Western Fury (women's state team; n=18). In addition to my WACA responsibilities, I was formally contracted by the Australian Cricket Board (ACB) in September 1998 to the appointment of sport psychologist to both the Test and One-Day National Teams (n=25 contracted players).

I think it is essential that sport psychologists develop and refine a working philosophy that is both practical and comprehensible. It is also important that this philosophy be articulated clearly in the form of an employment contract and explained in lay terms to both coaches and players. In this section, therefore, I would like to share my understanding of my job description, the key performance attributes I think professional cricketers must possess to be successful, some assumptions I have for players, which I refer to as FUNdaMENTALS, and my psychological platform, which refers to the perspective I have adopted as a psychologist working in sport.

Job Description

Over 14 consecutive years working with part-time and full-time professional cricketers, I have come to understand that my job as a mental-skills coach is to be effective at three interrelated levels: results, individual, and team. To perform the *results* function, I help coaches develop a long-term vision and direction for their teams and set group goals and action plans to achieve that vision. Top coaches in cricket (and any sport) should have a 3- to 5-year plan for their teams and for the style of cricket and cricketer they want to produce. I try to ensure that each member of the group (players, coaches, sup-port staff, wives, and partners) is aware of that vision and of the role each plays in achieving goals and plans. I also assist coaches in monitoring and evaluating progress towards their vision.

To perform the *individual* function, I try to ensure that each player gets a sense of personal growth and achievement out of playing his role in a team. I want to help players feel they are making a worthwhile contribution to Western Australian and Australian cricket, and to do this, I assist coaches in setting challenges appropriate to each player's individual needs and abilities. Veteran players who may be close to retirement through to first-year squad members just starting their careers should all be aspiring to achieve challenging and personally meaningful goals in a variety of areas (physical, technical, tactical, mental, behavioral, noncricket career, etc.) each season. I can also assist coaches in giving feedback, recognizing and rewarding achievements, and building each player's self-esteem, social skills, and noncricket lifestyle.

To perform the *team* function, I assist coaches in developing a shared purpose and communicating this regularly with the group. For example, the Western Warriors' motto is TEAM, which is an acronym for *Together Each Achieves More*. I try to promote a team spirit that encourages all team and support staff members to identify themselves strongly with their respective teams. I also help build team cohesion and commitment such that all team members share group failures as well as both individual and group successes.

Key Performance Attributes

From close observation of professional cricket at state, national, and international levels, I have come to realize that truly great cricketers can be characterized by at least five key attributes:

- First, they possess considerable physical ability and natural talent.
- Second, they have an enormous work ethic referring to a desire, motivation, passion, and commitment to both training and competing.
- Third, they have a healthy and balanced lifestyle, which includes cultivating a career "outside" cricket as well as self-regulation of both diet and sleep.
- Fourth, they expose themselves (or are exposed) to simulated competitive pressure regularly.
- Finally, they have a strong mental approach to their game.

Although the players who make it to either the Warriors or ACB teams may all be more or less physically and/or technically gifted, some seem to lack the desire and discipline necessary to reach their full potential. Some also seem to lack the mental tools necessary to play their best on a consistent basis. Although I may not be able to change inborn natural physical talent and technical ability, I have come to realize that I can certainly assist both players and coaches in the other areas. Specifically, I can modify an individual's work ethic, discipline, level of commitment, attitude to health and postcricket career, and of course, I can help the individual develop a strong mental approach to professional cricket. Effecting "intentional change" within an individual, however, as opposed to change that may occur naturally due to maturation, development, or external factors often requires considerable effort and patience. Unfortunately, I have found that some exceptionally talented cricketers who possess the first attribute (natural talent) plateau very early in their careers. They do not reach their ultimate potential either because they do not have one (or any) of the other four attributes or because they are simply not "ready" for change.

FUNdaMENTALS

Over the years, I have also developed (or collected) some assumptions for working with players and coaches that I sometimes need to share in order to get players, coaches, and myself on the "same page." I agree with Ravizza and Hanson (1995) and Rotella (1995), who believe it is important that sport psychologists create and declare ground rules for working with prospective clients, but until very recently, I have been reluctant to share these publicly. My current list of assumptions of professional cricketers I work with:

1. You choose to have fun—no matter what—and to enjoy Warriors/ACB cricket. As with most achievement areas, cricketers have to enjoy what they are doing in order to be good at it.
2. You have been selected to play because you are the best, you want to represent WA/Australia, and you want to be part of a winning team.
3. You will try to learn each day and to keep things simple. Cricketers who think they know everything or begin to complicate what is a simple game may not achieve their potential.
4. All that you do daily (training, on, and off-field) is compatible with your own and the team's mission. The 1% of things that professional athletes do or avoid doing "accumulate" over time. This refers to cognitive and behavioral factors that must be consistent with pursuing excellence.
5. You will realize that although you cannot control all that happens around you, you *can* control your response(s) to it. Cricketers also need to learn early in their careers that to control their performance, they must first learn to control themselves.
6. You will accept responsibility for the

consequences of your thoughts and behavior. How you "think" is how you "feel" is how you "behave."

7. You have "something to go to" when adversity occurs. Adversity will occur, so this is not negative planning—it's planning proactively.

8. You mentally practice what you are going to do in games regularly.

9. You absorb yourself in the moment and have a present focus. This is a critical skill in cricket.

10. You have a game plan, comprising both individual and team performance goals, and you commit yourself totally to executing that plan.

11. You give every delivery your best effort using predelivery routines, and you play the game patiently, ball by ball.

12. You are decisive in all you do, accept all challenges, regard each as opportunities, take positive risks, play to win, and never ever quit.

Psychological Platform

As a sport psychologist, my platform, or working perspective, remains the same as it was when I was first appointed to the WACA in 1987, and that is cognitive-affective and educational. Thinking, therefore, is understood to be the main source of feelings or emotions, which, in turn, are important links between thoughts and behavior. Consequently, I believe that the key to producing best cricket performances on a consistent basis is through education and awareness of thoughts or appraisal processes players have in situations they find themselves. In the

Table 1. PLAY SMART: WACA Mental Skills Program

Message	Mental Skill and Content	Junior Warriors			Youth-Senior Warriors	
		U/13	U/15	U/16	U/17	U/19 and Colts
Plan	Goal Setting Diaries	✔	✔	✔	✔	✔
Lock-in	Concentration Skills Pre-delivery Routines	✔	✔	✔	✔	✔
Attitude	Self-Confidence and Dealing with Pressure	✔	✔	✔	✔	✔
Your feel	Creating Individual Zones of Optimal Functioning		✔	✔	✔	✔
See yourself	Visualization			✔	✔	✔
March Ready	Game Readiness and Ideal Performance States			✔	✔	✔
Aroused	Managing Emotional Energy under Adversity				✔	✔
Round-off	Coping Processes: Injury, Travel, Media				✔	✔
Toughness	Balance and Perspective Play/Work Hard				✔	✔

Table 2. Mental Skills Drill: Visualization

Learning Objective(s): To introduce visualization to outswing bowling

Total time:　　　10–15 minutes

Explanation(s): Following a period of technical instruction and short practice, ask the cricketers to "get a ball each and gather round quietly. Close your eyes and turn your attention inwards. Take 4 or 5 deep breaths and pay attention to the feelings in your body. We're going to learn the skill of visualization." Be patient and tolerant as the group settles and calms down.

Key Teaching Point(s): beginning/middle/end
Beginning: "Now, while you are relaxed, imagine you are over there at the nets bowling, just as you were a few moments ago. See if you can remember what outswing bowling FEELS like . . . what is involved? Pretend in your mind that you are bowling again. Bowl six deliveries."

Middle: "It's a bit strange isn't it? Let's try it again, and see if you can get it to work a little better this time." (Repeat above instructions.) "FEEL yourself as well as SEE yourself bowling six outswing deliveries."

End: Summarize by explaining "visualization is practicing or rehearsing in your mind, or picturing yourself in your minds-eye performing. It will help you learn skills more thoroughly. We'll do this again next practice."

Equipment and/or Space Required: Normal net practice area; cricket ball each.

Progressions: Once (in their own judgment), athletes can visualize while walking around relaxed, ask them to repeat the exercise once or twice an over, then prior to each successive delivery; finally, have them transfer the exercise to games.

Comments:
Look for:　nonverbal indices of confusion among individual players.
Expect:　some negative reactions—but don't dwell on those
Tell them:　"Try to be patient. Learning some mental skills will take time."

next section, I hope to illustrate how I structure the educational aspect of my work across all age-groups at the WACA using PLAY SMART.

PLAY SMART Cricket

In 1994, the WACA Director of Coaching, Graham House, and I came up with the PLAY SMART acronym that represents all the mental skills I teach cricketers. Table 1 illustrates what each of these skills is and when, approximately, in a cricketer's career they are introduced. More detail of these skills is provided for readers in an earlier description of the services I offer at the WACA (Gordon, 1990). About this time, the ACB

sport psychology consultant, Graham Winter, also produced an excellent Junior (Under 13 years), Intermediate (Under 17 years), and Under 19 years PSYCHskills program (Winter, 1995). The content from each program roughly complemented each other, and I have now integrated both within PLAY SMART, which I refine each year by asking both under-age-group players and their coaches for their opinions.

Although PLAY SMART is well received by players, parents, and coaches, the latter are particularly impressed with the Mental-skills Drills concept I have also introduced in the Level 2 Coaching Course: Mental Skills Training for Cricket. Both Winter (in

PSYCHskills) and I have developed a means of helping coaches introduce and develop mental-skills training during practices, and an example of how to introduce visualization at net practice is provided in Table 2. Note that the words used are the coach's words (not a sport psychologist's), and like a typical teaching lesson plan, progressions are provided. At the WACA, we now have introductory, intermediate, and advanced level mental skill drills for each PLAY SMART "message." By encouraging Level 2 WACA coaches to both devise and use mental-skills drills within their normal net sessions, I believe sport psychology in cricket can finally get out of the "classroom" and into the game. Cricket coaches will readily admit that the time (priority) spent on mental skills at practice rarely, if ever, reflects the considerable mental demands of the game. Top cricket coaches and players have told me that up to 95% of the game is mental, and yet few coaches would ever claim that they spent even close to 10% of training time on mental skills. PLAY SMART and mental skill drills in particular, therefore, provide an effective coach-friendly and coach-driven educational curriculum across a lifespan. By using this curriculum and method of coaching, all cricket coaches should be able to reduce the discrepancy between the mental demands of the game and the time they currently do *not* spend in teaching mental skills.

Creating Cultures of Success

Although the challenges and demands of providing educational services at the WACA have been very rewarding, I am very aware that the bottom line for any professional sport organization is "success." Although "winning" is never mentioned in my contract with either the WACA or ACB, it would be naive to rationalize my contribution to both teams purely on the basis of educational and developmental benefits to all. In this section, therefore, I hope to describe how I have aligned myself with success and winning through educational means.

Competency Profiling

At the WACA (1996) and more recently with the ACB (1998), I have introduced the need for identifying performance competencies among all players (individuals) and teams (units). To achieve overall organizational effectiveness in any corporate structure requires an alignment of leadership strategies, which basically refers to the process of identifying and defining core values, functions, goals, and processes for both individuals and teams within the organization. I focus only on cricket operations at the WACA and ACB—cricket department, manager, coaching, and development. I do not operate within the realms of finance, administration, sales, marketing, sponsorship, and communication; and under the current terms of respective contracts, I am unlikely to do so in the near future.

Individual Performance Profiles

In keeping with performance-profiling principles (Butler, 1996), I have facilitated the identification of key qualities for performing respective tasks by both individuals and teams. At the WACA, criteria or "qualities" have been developed for individual performance evaluations of physical performance, fast bowling, swing bowling, and mental skills. With the ACB, only a mental-skills profiling instrument has been produced after recent discussions with the national team coach. Once the criteria for specific profiles were agreed upon, players were simply asked to rate themselves on each performance criterion (1 = very poor; 10 = ideal). Their responses were subsequently contrasted on a pie chart (or bar graph) with the evaluations of an assessor, usually their coach, who knows them best.

A fictitious example of a mental skills performance profile for an Australian National Team member is provided in Table 3 and, based on the assessor's evaluations, the priorities for training for this player are also listed at the bottom. Where there is no differentiation in shading on any criterion, the coach and player ratings were the same.

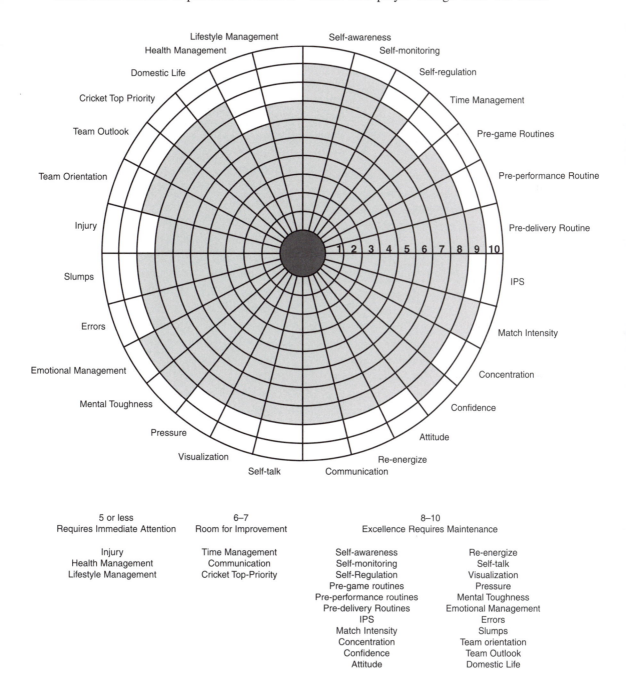

5 or less Requires Immediate Attention	6–7 Room for Improvement	8–10 Excellence Requires Maintenance	
Injury Health Management Lifestyle Management	Time Management Communication Cricket Top-Priority	Self-awareness Self-monitoring Self-Regulation Pre-game routines Pre-performance routines Pre-delivery Routines IPS Match Intensity Concentration Confidence Attitude	Re-energize Self-talk Visualization Pressure Mental Toughness Emotional Management Errors Slumps Team orientation Team Outlook Domestic Life

Table 3. Example of a Mental Skills Performance Profile

Once profiling and pictorial representations are complete and copies of the data are distributed to both player and assessor/coach, I suggest that the coach and player meet privately to discuss the results in a responsible and Socratic manner. Then I ask players to discuss with me how I can help move them from a self-evaluation of 5, 6, or 7 to 8. My goal is for all Warriors and National team players to rate themselves 8 or above on each criterion. All mental-skills performance criteria are, of course, defined more explicitly on an inventory I have created—only single-word descriptors appear in Table 3—and include nonperformance issues, to which I will refer later.

The development of mental-skills performance criteria, or what I refer to as mental correlates of excellence, was based on the psychological skills I have taught first class cricketers over the last 14 years. However, the items are also based on considerable firsthand experience observing and working closely with very successful players, teams, and coaches during that period. Although the process of creating mental-skills criteria was relatively easy for me, I should point out that the development of criteria for physical performance, fast bowling, and swing bowling profiles at the WACA, proved to be much more difficult. This was because coaches simply could not reach a consensus agreement very easily. A general agreement among five coaches and trainers has resulted (in 1997) in a 20-item instrument for evaluating physical performance (10 items for general conditioning and fielding, 3 for batsmen, 3 for medium/fast bowling, 2 for spin bowling, and 2 for wicket keepers). However, the process took almost 18 months. At the time of writing (after 28 months), coaches are still undecided on suitable criteria for fast bowling and swing bowling!

I believe profiling provides a more useful current assessment of what coaches and players consider are strengths and weaknesses on any aspect of performing (mental, technical, tactical, physical), at any given point in a season or career than does any other assessment system available (e. g., physiological or psychometric tests). As a consultant working with adult part-time or full-time professional cricketers, therefore, I consider performance-profiling techniques both extremely practical and useful.

Team Performance Profiles

Currently, I am also assisting both the Warriors and National team coaches in creating and refining criteria or qualities for team performance evaluations in their respective competitions. Since execution of individual and team game plans (performance goals) is essential for competitive consistency and success in any professional sport, performance-profiling can again provide a useful means of getting all individuals within a team on the "same page."

The procedure was quite simple. Key players (2–3) from each team were invited to facilitate a meeting on team performance goals in three performance-related areas (batting, bowling, and fielding) and two nonperformance areas (training and social). From their meeting, the Western Warriors produced a document entitled "The Warrior Way" (August, 1998) although the Australian Test and One Day Teams produced similar blue prints for success entitled respectively "The Aussie Way" (September, 1998) and "The Road to Lords" (January, 1999). Each player, coach, and member of support staff received a copy of each document, which remains the intellectual property of each team and, therefore, cannot be illustrated here. Subsequently, my role has been to periodically refer everyone back to these performance goals, at both team and individual meetings, and to discuss self and coach ratings of each performance criterion.

Personal Success

In addition to on-field performance goals, I have also stressed with both coaches and players the importance of personal success in other areas and setting and maintaining lifestyle, balance, and perspective goals. To promote a more holistic focus of personal success, I helped initiate a WACA Player Welfare Committee in 1993. Membership comprises our club doctor, physiotherapist, podiatrist, trainer, coach (as chair), cricket manager (and his secretary), and myself. We meet monthly to discuss each squad member's general health and employment status as well as his performance. Since 1996, following consultations with the local Athlete Career and Education (ACE) program manager, who is based full-time at the Western Australian Institute of Sport (WAIS), all WACA coaches and players also have weekly access to professional advice on career planning and development. In the 1999/2000 season the ACE manager was included in the WACA player welfare committee meetings.

Social Support:
The "Team Within a Team"

Following the first ACB camp (September 1998) where I introduced myself to players, coaches, and support staff, I decided to convene a meeting with the players' wives and/or partners—labeled Australia's "Second XI" by the National Team coach. I wanted to assist partners in their valued role within the ACB organization by simply affording them an opportunity to pool their resources and experiences. Several senior players thought that this was a good idea, and one observed that perhaps they could learn how to support each other more as well as support us. An inventory was sent to each ACB contracted player's wife or partner requesting responses to several open-ended questions. Items related to ways of coping with both controllable and uncontrollable factors in the life of a professional cricketer, suggestions or advice they had on dealing with the least pleasant aspects of their role, and what kind of advice they would offer others such as newcomers.

Results were collated and redistributed to all partners of contracted players (May 1999), who subsequently decided to convene another meeting later in the 1999–2000 season. The unanimous appreciation for this exercise by survey respondents confirms that this Second XI is an untapped source of strength and social support that has been relatively ignored to date. Improvements in both intrateam (Second XI) and interteam (players and partners) social support are anticipated.

Evaluation

In May 1994, the Western Australian Cricket Association (WACA) appointed Mike Veletta as coach of their inaugural cricket academy, now known as the "Warriors Cricket Academy." The program philosophy was "to physically, technically and mentally prepare a select group of six potential Sheffield Shield cricketers for the 1994–1995 season 'at home' in Perth, rather than having them leave to play or coach overseas" (Graham House, WACA Director of Coaching, personal communication, 1994). In this section, I will briefly describe the results of a formal evaluation of the mental-skills training component of the program that I presented over a 5-month period (May–October).

A program evaluation inventory, similar to that used by Brewer and Shillinglaw (1992) and Gould, Petlichkoff, Hodge, and Simons (1990) was administered to the six male players at four time periods: May (Week 1 of the mental-skills program), October (end of Academy program), December (halfway through the season), and March (end of season). The inventory consisted of 18 items assessing the players' "knowledge of," "importance placed on," and "use of" each of the six mental skills presented in the program. Ratings for all items were recorded on 7-point scales with anchors of 1=*very low* and 7=*very high*.

The mental-skills training program consisted of six core skill areas: goal setting, concentration, arousal control, imagery, confidence, and creating and maintaining the Ideal Performance State (IPS). In addition to this material, however, it was decided to issue each of the six players (mean age = 20 years; range 19–24 years) a copy of Winter's (1992) text *The Psychology of Cricket* as further required reading. Over a period of 8 weeks, each of the six skills was presented in separate 60- to 90-minute workshops. Week 1 was set aside for an overview of the significance of mental skills in cricket, assignment of reading and presentation material for the following week, and completion of the evaluation inventory. Week 8 activity consisted of a one-hour written exam that the players elected to complete under formal examination conditions (no notes). The 15 questions used in the exam are illustrated in Table 4; they reflect some of the content of each mental-skills workshop, which included examinations of injury and media-management strategies taught during the arousal-control workshop.

Each mental-skill workshop (Workshops 2–7) began with one player summarizing, in 15 to 20 minutes, the appropriate previously assigned chapter from Winter's text (e. g., chapter 3, "Motivation and goal setting") and the most relevant information to him personally (as batsman, bowler, wicket keeper, or fielder). Exercises on the same topic, both during and following group discussions, and audio and videotape material were also used. Finally, written homework exercises were assigned over a 4-day period for each mental-skill area and were marked by myself and returned to each player at the beginning of

the next workshop.

This style of program presentation deliberately obliged players to take responsibility for both reading and talking about material that *they* decided was relevant and practicable and to discuss, in a collegial spirit, its significance in enhancing cricket performance. By having to prepare to teach others, players benefited enormously from presentation experiences and later reported a sense of ownership of both the content of each workshop and the pace of delivery. The homework exercises, which resembled workshop activities, were usually scenarios in which players had to simply apply what was learned to their own current understanding of the game. Minimal writing was involved.

Mean scores for each mental skill area across four time periods are illustrated in Figure 1. Dependent t-tests, performed to investigate differences in "knowledge of," "importance of," and "use of" each skill between Time 1 (May 1994) and Time 4 (March 1995), indicated a significant increase in knowledge of five mental skills: goal setting, concentration, arousal control, imagery, and ideal performance state. No significant differences, however, were observed for knowledge of confidence or for any of the importance or use of ratings.

Anticipated trends in the self-report data confirmed that knowledge of all skills improved over time, and each mental skill was considered "very important." However, from an applied perspective, trends in the use of skills were disappointing. In general, the cricketers did not increase their use of mental skills to a desirable level across time periods. One notable exception, however, was Player 1, whose data are illustrated in Figure 2. This batsman/spin bowler started in the Warriors Shield team in the 1994 to 1995 season, was dropped three games later, but returned to play pivotal roles in the last three games of that season. Figure 2 indicates that

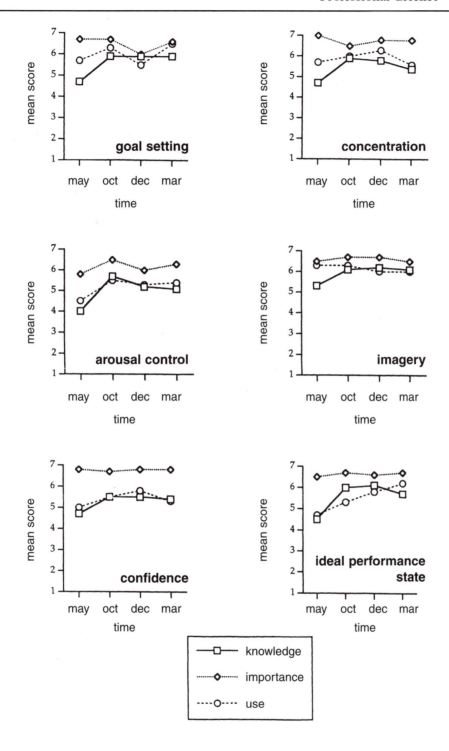

Figure 1.
Mean scores for the six mental skill areas

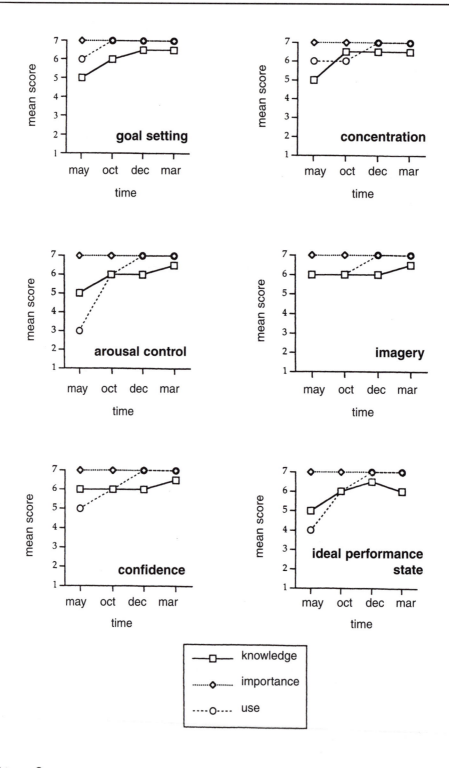

Figure 2.
Scores for the six mental skill areas for Player 1

his self-reported use of all mental skills, particularly arousal control and ideal performance state, increased markedly from Time 1 (May). Furthermore, post-Academy program interviews with the coach confirmed that this player's intentions were to continue to work on improving these skills. The player believed these skills significantly helped him maintain his form and intensity during grade cricket and to break back into the Sheffield Shield team and, later that year, the National team.

This evaluation of the "Warriors Cricket Academy" indicates improved ratings of knowledge of mental skills among six talented young players who, in addition, consistently rated these skills over a 10-month period as "very important." For concomitant improvements in performance, however, results also suggest that players must both increase and sustain their use of these skills. Simply knowing more about these skills and acknowledging their importance in cricket may not be enough to enhance performance. Cricketers, therefore, must be encouraged to regularly use and improve their mental skills at practice. As mentioned previously, only when mental skills are integrated within normal practice net sessions can coaches claim their training practices accurately reflect the demands of the game.

Preparation for a National Title and World Cup Campaign

Western Warriors' Defense of the Sheffield Shield

Regardless of how hard I work with individuals and teams and how much I may privately rate my own significance and self-importance to organizations, I have always understood and believed that *players win games*. In this section, however, I will describe and try to explain how I contributed to both (a) the Western Warriors' preparation for their successful defense of the Sheffield Shield (National Title) in Brisbane, March 1999, and (b) the National Team's success at the World Cup in England, May/June 1999.

Leading into the Sheffield Shield Final between the top two teams in Australia, the Queensland Bulls were playing well and were regarded as strong favorites especially having earned the right to play the game at home courtesy of finishing top of the table. On the other hand, the form of the Western Warriors had been patchy, and only a few players were performing consistently well. In the last regular season game against Victoria in Melbourne, the Warriors barely managed a draw to secure a place in their fourth consecutive Shield Final. Consequently, when I joined the team in Brisbane four days prior to the Final, I found an emotionally drained and physically exhausted team that had already been written off by both the media and several expert cricket commentators. Despite this, however, the Warriors went on to beat the Bulls quite comprehensively by an innings and 31 runs and with more than 11 hours to spare.

Tuesday. To prepare for the first day of the Final on Friday, the first port of call upon my arrival was, of course, the coach's room where, with the captain, vice-captain, and support staff (trainer, physiotherapist, and myself), a schedule of training and both team and individual meetings was mapped out.

Wednesday. Poolside at the hotel the next morning, I spoke briefly to the team and asked each player to complete the sheet illustrated in Table 5 and make arrangements to meet with me in my room later that morning or afternoon. No physical training was planned for this day apart from treatment to certain players and a team morning/evening pool workout, followed by a casual team dinner. Our focus at this stage was on complete rest, reenergizing, and recuperation.

During the meetings, I listened carefully

Table 4. Warrior Cricket Academy Mental-Skills Exam

1. Why is goal setting such an important mental skill for cricketers?
2. What are the main guidelines for setting goals?
3. What are some of the common mistakes and problems in goal setting?
4. What are the characteristics of cricketers who are fully concentrating?
5. What are the most obvious symptoms of poor concentration during a game?
6. Describe your predelivery routines for bowling, batting, and fielding.
7. Explain and illustrate the relationship between arousal and cricket performance.
8. List two things you can do when underaroused and overaroused during a match.
9. Provide an example of using "thought stoppage" to deal with an adverse situation in batting, bowling, and fielding.
10. Provide three stressful situations you encounter regularly in competitive cricket and appropriate mental and physical coping responses you can use.
11. When and how can imagery help you as a cricketer?
12. Self-efficacy or self-confidence is an elusive and much coveted mental skill. How would you set about enhancing or maintaining your confidence, particularly during a perceived performance slump?
13. Explain the IPS concept and 4Rs in postgame analysis. How would you create and maintain your IPS mentally, physically, and emotionally?
14. List some coping strategies you could use upon serious injury and during prolonged periods of rehabilitation.
15. List some guidelines you might adopt for dealing with the mass media.

as each player outlined how he was going to play against Queensland on their wicket and in Brisbane conditions (very hot and humid). As each player described his personal performance goals, I could sense confidence growing, and I simply suggested that these plans be put into practice at each net practice and warm-up leading up to and during the game itself, and mentally rehearsed (visualized) regularly for the entire Final campaign. The purpose in having players write performance goals and verbalize them with me was to ensure that each individual was focussing on and committed to the "controllables" (his own performance) and, therefore, the "process" of winning the game as opposed to the outcome itself. I believe in the adage that "the probability of getting the outcome you want increases when you let go of the *need* to have it." In other words, the

more important winning the Shield is to players 3 days from the game, the less likely they are to get it because the *requirement* to win actually interferes with the process of success. The Warriors have learned over the years that if they control the "controllables" (their individual performances), the outcome (winning) looks after itself.

Discussing plans for adversity also boosted confidence. Because the Warriors and Bulls knew each other intimately, each player had a very good idea of what the opposition's game plan would be for him when batting and bowling. My role was to focus again on what the Warriors had control over when under pressure (their response plan) and to encourage practice and visualization of the same at every opportunity. I have noticed that, when under pressure or in adverse circumstances, some inexperienced players become either "other aware" and focus on what others are doing (e. g., the opposition players, umpires, other team mates) or "self-aware" and focus on their inadequacies (e. g., *my* poor technique, fatigue, nervousness). Neither focus is appropriate. The key to managing adversity and pressure is to stay "task aware" and to focus only on responses to the simple question "What is it I have to do right now?" I believe that "where your mind goes, everything else will follow" and that cricketers who earn the reputation of being "mentally tough" under pressure are simply those who are task aware under adversity.

Thursday. Following a full morning training session at the ground and pool session at the hotel, we had a lunchtime team meeting in the coach's room to discuss our overall game plan for the 5 days of scheduled play starting the next day. This included a detailed discussion, led by the coach, captain, and vice-captain, of the tactics we would apply to each Bulls batsmen and bowler. As usual, each Warriors player contributed freely to this 60-minute discussion, which included play-

ers' reflections on the key behaviors and attitudes we needed in order to execute our individual and team game plans. The latter can be summed up by the following words, which we had used all year and which were written up on a white board and transferred later to our changing-room wall: ENCOURAGEMENT, BODY LANGUAGE, COMMITMENT, DESIRE, DISCIPLINE, and the four Ps—PRESSURE, PARTNERSHIPS, PERSISTENCE, and PATIENCE. That afternoon we all went to see the movie *Payback*, only because Queensland had beaten the Warriors 2 years previously in Perth, and after a casual team meal in the evening, the players retired early to their hotel rooms.

Friday. To emphasize a present focus during the entire Final, the coach and I posted a grid on a wall next to the words listed above, something we do before every Shield game. Illustrated in Figure 3, the grid explains how we segmented a 5-day event into manageable chunks of play. Our game plan was simply to outplay the opposition each hour each day knowing that if we ended up

Time	Friday	Saturday	Sunday	Monday	Tuesday
10AM–11AM	—	✓	✓	✓	
11AM–12PM	✓	✓	✓	✓	
12.40PM–1.40PM	✓	Rain	—	✓	
1.40PM–2.40PM	✗	Rain	✗	Warriors win	
3PM–4PM	✓	Rain	✓		
4PM–5PM	—	Rain	✓		

Figure 3.
Western Warriors process of winning the Sheffield Shield Final 1999

with more check marks on the grid than crosses we would ultimately achieve the outcome we wanted. Each day at formal breaks in play (lunch and tea), I asked different players to rate our efforts for each hour of play with a check mark, dash, or cross. Then, at the resumption of play after each break, the captain simply reminded the team of the tactics for the next segment of play. This strategy from Friday to Monday effectively kept all the Warriors absorbed in the moment with a present focus despite several potentially distracting controversies during the game and long rain delays. We executed this plan so well we outplayed the opposition each day and ended up worthy winners. Although several outstanding individual performances (batting and bowling) were posted, I was especially proud of the Warriors' discipline over 4 days, which was undoubtedly a critical factor in a decisive victory.

The World Cup

The 1999 World Cup was hosted by the England and Wales Cricket Board from May 14 to June 20 and involved 12 teams (Australia, Bangladesh, England, India, Kenya, New Zealand, Pakistan, Scotland, South Africa, Sri Lanka, West Indies, and Zimbabwe), 42 matches at 21 venues. I met up with the National squad ($n=15$), which had just toured the West Indies, and their partners, in London (May 2, 1999) and traveled separately with the latter in a bus to our base camp in Cardiff. The 3-hour journey afforded me with a valuable opportunity to chat informally with several partners about various observations they had made during the recent Caribbean tour.

After almost 2 days of official media and World Cup functions, I was finally able to meet privately with each player to discuss his responses to two exercises. First, I asked each player to reflect on the following "personal development exercise":

Aside from your cricket commitments, what personal priorities and goals have you set for yourself during the 1999 World Cup? In your own words, describe what you would like to get out of this tour in England, for yourself (e. g., places and friends to visit, things to do, new people to meet).

Players listed several responses to this exercise and remarked how positive an experience (exercise) it had been. They had clearly not anticipated being asked to consider anything other than cricket or performance-related questions. The second exercise was similar to the questions listed in Table 5, adapted to the National team. It was immediately evident that players anticipated different pressure situations for both batting and bowling that were specific to One-Day cricket as opposed to the longer 4- or 5-day format of the game.

At the first team meeting, I shared some observations, illustrated in Figure 4, which I had previously discussed with both the coach and captain. I explained how, as a highly ranked team in the competition, *complacency* appeared to be our greatest threat and, therefore, our greatest challenge ahead ("our" = each individual, the team/squad, and support staff). Consequently, our mental mission to the end of the 1999 World Cup, to combat complacency was to pursue *consistency, discipline, patience,* and *passion*. This mission was achievable by (a) players' creating and recreating their *ideal performance state* (IPS or "zone"), (b) players' maintaining *positive mental momentum* regardless of personal or team form, and (c) players' remaining *task aware,* particularly during adversity. I further suggested that *consistency* comes from discipline, which ought not be regarded as narrow-minded joylessness. Rather, the processes and outcomes from discipline ought to be approached as challenges

Table 5. Western Warriors Sheffield Shield Final 1999 team sheet

Please write your responses to the following statements in the spaces provided. Thank you.

1. Performance goals.

   "When batting or bowling or wicket keeping or fielding, what I need to do play well is . . .?"

Batting	Bowling	WK/Fielding
_____	_____	_____
_____	_____	_____
_____	_____	_____
_____	_____	_____
_____	_____	_____
_____	_____	_____

2. Dealing with adversity and pressure.

   Identify an anxiety- and/or pressure-laden situation and remedy it by being task aware.

   "So, if . . . (this happens)"   "I will . . . (do this) "

   1. _____   1. _____
   2. _____   2. _____
   3. _____   3. _____
   4. _____   4. _____

Please bring your responses to our meeting. Thank you.

Time	Friday	Saturday	Sunday	Monday	Tuesday
10AM–11AM	—	✓	✓	✓	
11AM–12PM	✓	✓	✓	✓	
12.40PM–1.40PM	✓	Rain	—	✓	
1.40PM–2.40PM	✕	Rain	✕	Warriors win	
3PM–4PM	✓	Rain	✓		
4PM–5PM	—	Rain	✓		

✕ = hour won by Western Warriors

✓= hour won by Queensland Bulls

— = even

WORLD CUP: MENTAL MISSION to JUNE 20, 1999

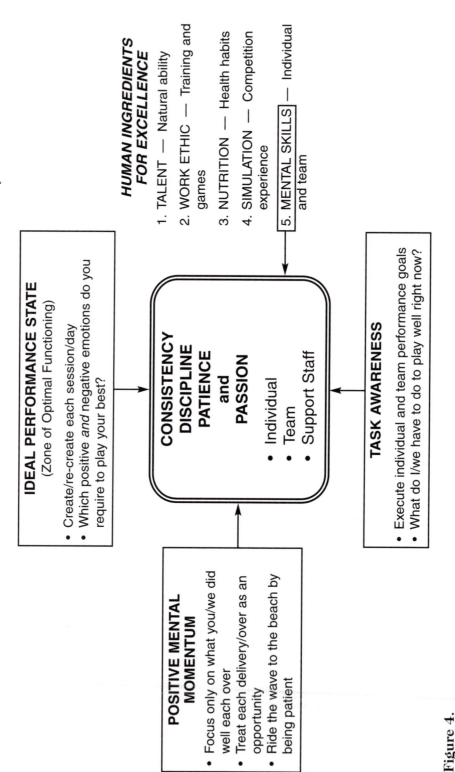

HUMAN INGREDIENTS FOR EXCELLENCE

1. TALENT — Natural ability
2. WORK ETHIC — Training and games
3. NUTRITION — Health habits
4. SIMULATION — Competition experience
5. MENTAL SKILLS — Individual and team

IDEAL PERFORMANCE STATE
(Zone of Optimal Functioning)

- Create/re-create each session/day
- Which positive *and* negative emotions do you require to play your best?

CONSISTENCY DISCIPLINE PATIENCE and PASSION

- Individual
- Team
- Support Staff

POSITIVE MENTAL MOMENTUM

- Focus only on what you/we did well each over
- Treat each delivery/over as an opportunity
- Ride the wave to the beach by being patient

TASK AWARENESS

- Execute individual and team performance goals
- What do I/we have to do to play well right now?

Figure 4.
World Cup team mental mission

and opportunities for personal and team growth. *Discipline*, of course, does not guarantee winning all the time, or even achieving a team's performance goals, but its absence certainly assures falling short of what is possible with the potential the 1999 Australian team had. *Patience*, simply, is about accepting results and staying in the present. *Passion* comes from total absorption in the tasks at hand, with *heart and soul*.

Limited space precludes an in-depth account of interactions I had with players, reserves, captain, and vice-captain; however, my main role was to keep everyone focused on the mental mission. At team meetings the night before each game (immediately preceding a team meal), the coach announced the team for the next day. Next, he clarified his expectations of the team in relation to five areas: focus and concentration, discipline, patience, spirit and support, and determination. He focused first on what the team was doing well in each area (why we kept winning) and then on where and how individuals and the team could improve. Each player was then asked to summarize his opinions of a selected player from the opposition; that is, strengths, weaknesses, how to play him. The group also contributed to this analysis, which generated a fascinating in-depth profile of all opposition players and teams. The captain and vice-captain then commented briefly on what the game plan was likely to be and what was expected of each player. Finally, the coach and both captains conveyed a clear message of belief and confidence in each player and the team.

Among several observations and learning experiences too numerous to mention here, the factors that contributed most to the World Cup success, in my opinion, were:

1. The consolidated commitment to, and execution of, a mental mission.
2. The coach's emphasis on why the team was winning and a collective will and encouragement to improve.
3. The mental toughness and outstanding form of key role players; that is, captain and vice-captain.
4. A much-coveted "Aussie bloody-mindedness" and formidable culture of determination to win.

I respectfully salute each member of the team and team management for their deserved success. Fond memories and learning experiences of the 1999 World Cup will remain a career highlight—until the next time!

Summary

In this chapter, I have tried to describe some of the things I have learned over 14 years as a sport psychologist working with professional cricket teams. By using and adapting certain techniques, I believe I have coped fairly well with the different demands from both educational and performance (outcome) expectations, and the increasing pressures from commercial influences on both the players and the game itself. No doubt I still have plenty to learn, and I will have to periodically refine my operational style, without compromising the integrity of my training, in order to develop and sustain a holistic focus on both the person and the cricketer. Facilitating "good thinking" in such a mental game as cricket will always be an engaging task; however, I eagerly look forward to all the personal and professional challenges ahead. In the meantime, I sincerely hope the reader has benefited in some way from my reflections.

Perhaps the following address from Lord Harris, former Captain of Kent and England on his 80th birthday is a fitting closure to what is a very intimate contribution both to the applied sport psychology literature and to the wonderful game of cricket itself. The reader is left to consider his or her reactions to the message's sobering appeal, which is directed at the caretakers (including sport psychologists) as well as the participants of any sport, played in the modern era.

> You do well to love cricket for it is more free from anything sordid, anything dishonourable than any game in the world. To play it keenly, generously, self-sacrificingly is a moral lesson in itself, and the classroom is God's air and sunshine. Foster it my brothers, so that it may attract all who find the time to play it, protect it from anything that would sully it, so that it may grow in favour with all men. (Wynne, P. E. [Producer]. [1996]. Sir Don Bradman—97. Not out. Sydney: Channel Nine Network)

References

Brewer, B. W., & Shillinglaw, R. (1992). Evaluation of a psychological skills training workshop for male intercollegiate lacrosse players. *The Sport Psychologist, 6*, 139–147.

Butler, R. (1996). *Performance profiling*. Leeds: National Coaching Foundation.

Gordon, S. (1990). A mental skills training program for the Western Australian state cricket team., *The Sport Psychologist, 4*, 386–399.

Gould, D., Petlichkoff, L., Hodge, K., & Simons, J. (1990). Evaluating the effectiveness of a psychological skills educational workshop. *The Sport Psychologist, 4*, 249–260.

Ravizza, K., & Hanson, T. (1995). *Heads-up baseball: Playing the game one pitch at a time*. Indianapolis: Masters Press.

Rotella, R. (1995). *Golf is not a game of perfect*. Sydney: Simon & Schuster.

Whimpress, B. (1985). *Understanding cricket*. Chatswood, NSW: Rigby.

Winter, G. (1992). *The psychology of cricket: How to play the inner game of cricket*. Sydney: Sun.

Winter, G. (1995). *Cricket psychskills*. Jolimont, VIC: Australian Cricket Board.

(Wynne, P. E. [Producer]. [1996]. Sir Don Bradman—97. Not out. Sydney: Channel Nine Network)

Reflections of a Feminist Sport Psychologist

Trisha Leahy

Introduction

Feminism is a word with many connotations and associations. In this article, I discuss my own definition of feminism and the impact feminism has on my day-to-day practice. I begin by offering a definition of sport psychology practice that reflects my experience of working on two continents, Asia and Australia; it also reflects my adherence to the scientist-practitioner model, which understands *practice* as simultaneously constituting both clinical and research work.

I present my interpretation of the term feminism and describe how feminist values inform the way I practice psychology in the elite sports environment. In the final segment I outline how my research, which I see as an essential component of psychology practice, fits in with feminist values and with my clinical practice.

Defining Sport Psychology Practice

Before specifying what feminist sport psychology practice might be, it is perhaps appropriate to identify what sport psychology practice entails. The Association for the Advancement of Applied Sport Psychology (AAASP) model of sport psychology practice defines practitioners as "consultants" and the work they do as "an educational enterprise involving the communication of principles of sport psychology to participants in sports training and competition, exercise and physical activity" (AAASP, 1990). As a psychologist working full-time in an elite sport context, I find that this definition covers only a minor part of the work that I do on a daily basis. I would describe my work as being primarily therapeutic, thereby including, of course, some educational components. To me, the sport psychology practitioner is not an educational consultant but a psychologist. A more appropriate definition of sport psychology practice, therefore, is one that stresses the psychology, or therapeutic nature of the interaction between the practitioner and the client, be the client athlete or coach. The therapeutic skills required to work with a client group of elite athletes are the same as those required for any other client group who may seek psychological help. The context of their lives may differ, but the therapeutic process remains the same.

In my experience, sport psychology practice involves three levels of intervention. The first is *primary prevention* (to borrow from health psychology models). This is the primarily educational component, similar to the description of practice included in AAASP definition. Primary prevention targets all those involved in sport, such as coaches, athletes, officials, and administrators. It functions, as the label implies, to prevent problems. Typical interventions at this level might be, for example, performance-related mental skills training, stress management skills, conflict management, and negotiation skills. Related interventions might reflect organizational psychology input, advocacy work, and participation in policy development.

The second level of intervention requires a more therapeutic approach, and I describe this type of intervention as *psychoeducational*. Typically, this type of intervention is with groups or teams in sport, and might include sessions relating to eating disorders, sexual harassment awareness training, conflict resolution within teams, body-image enhancement, and support groups.

The third, most intensively *therapeutic*, level of intervention occurs at the individual level. This level demands the most of the practitioner's psychological knowledge and therapeutic skills. Over the years, athletes with whom I have come in contact have worked on issues ranging from relationship management, disordered eating, and sexuality to the multisymptomatic sequelae of prolonged and repeated trauma.

Overlying these various levels of applied intervention is the scientist-practitioner paradigm to which I adhere. Within this framework, both clinical and research work constitute practice, each informed by the other. However, as I later describe, my understanding of this concept differs from the traditional, positivist meaning generally associated with the word *scientist*—that of an objective, socially neutral investigator.

Feminism

Feminism is a perspective that acknowledges that women's experiences differ from men's (Krane, 1994). It also acknowledges the existence of a sexist bias in the knowledge base due to androcentric epistemologies. This bias requires that knowledge be reassessed and reexamined through the ex-periences of women. Feminism thus places gender at the center of analysis. Within the context of sport, a feminist approach recognizes the marginalization of women in this domain and strives to understand sport through this perspective.

My personal perspective, however, is not synonymous with an exclusive and restricted focus on gender or on women. Gender-exclusive definitions and practices in elite sport, as in any sector of the community, can be understood in terms of power processes at work. Just as with other cultural forms that become institutionalized, sport is affected by, and, in turn, affects existing structures of power and inequality in society (Hall, 1993, 1996). Power and powerlessness do not relate to gender alone, but also intersect with race, socioeconomic status, ethnicity, sexuality, and (dis)ability. My feminism is concerned with gendered or powered social behavior and the impact of gendered and powered social structures on both women and men.

Feminism and Psychology

Issues of gender, power, and social inequality have always been peripheral to the mainstream of applied psychology theory and practice (Boyle, 1997). Feminist critiques of applied clinical psychology point out that the development of a gender-aware (and, to me, power-aware), applied clinical psychology may present a considerable challenge to existing theory and practice in mainstream psychology. For example, clinical psychology service structures are designed to focus on pathological individuals rather than on pathological social structures (Boyle, 1997). The idea that people possess problematic attributes and that the aim of services is to change these remains fundamental to much clinical practice.

Similar criticisms can be applied to the practice of sport psychology. The ethos of individual pathology as opposed to systemic pathology has been especially prevalent in sport psychology, articulated through the concept of "mental toughness." Inherently dysfunctional traditions and systems have been perpetuated through this culture.

An athlete came to see me soon after winning his gold medal. He threw the medal on the table and declared, "Tell me why this is worth it. Tell me how to value it. It's been too hard. I can only remember the pain of it all." The athlete went on to describe how his coach emotionally abused and manipulated him throughout a number of years of preparation for this medal. The coach felt that creating this hostile, "challenging" environment would enable this athlete to excel, that it would make him "mentally tough." No one in the athlete's environment seemed to question these coaching methods.

The athlete did excel, but the whole experience had been so traumatizing that he was now experiencing diagnosable symptoms of post-traumatic stress. He had spent so much time repressing and disassociating from his feelings as a way of coping—of being "mentally tough"—that when the competition was over, he found himself vacillating wildly between periods of complete emotional numbness and periods of extreme emotional distress. As I affirmed this athlete's feelings and validated his pain, he sat back in surprise.

"What is it?" I asked.

He said, "You are the first person who has ever said that my feelings are OK. I was so afraid to talk about this, in case you would just tell me more strategies on how to be mentally tough. That's all I've heard in the last few years. What a great coach this person is. How I need to be tougher."

The sporting support structure around this athlete had failed him. His experience had been invalidated, any discussion of his distress neatly depoliticized and intervention diverted from the systemic dysfunction that allowed the acceptance of abusive coaching behaviors. This was done by claiming that the problem lay with the athlete, who was, supposedly, not "mentally tough" enough.

We worked together for an intensive six months before this talented athlete was able to regain his sense of himself as a worthwhile, empowered person—six months, before he was able to reclaim even a portion of the joy in achievement that should have been his on the medal podium. He still has no plans to compete again.

The Sport Psychologist: Practicing Within a Feminist Framework

My personal model of feminist psychology includes a number of principles, or values, based within feminist theory. In this section, I first discuss my understanding of these principles as they relate to psychology practice. I then offer examples of my work in elite sport that I believe reflect such principles.

Valuing the Female Perspective

Valuing the female perspective does not entail devaluing the male perspective. Rather, it recognizes that women's experiences and knowledge have often been marginalized or ignored, sometimes at great cost. The historical study of the traumatic sequelae of child sexual abuse in psychology and psychiatry provides a poignant example of this. At the turn of the century, Freud wrote, " . . . sexual abuse committed by another person" was the specific cause of the complex symptoms manifested by his patients (Freud, 1896/1962, p.152). Unfortunately, possibly due to the political climate of the time (Herman, 1992), Freud subsequently repudiated this hypothesis, stating that his patients' reports of childhood sexual abuse were nothing more than their "fantasies" (Freud, 1925/1959, p.34). Psychoanalysis, one of the most influential theories of 20th century psychiatry and psychology, was thereby built on the denial of the real-life trauma experienced by women, favoring male-constructed fantasy and fantasy-related, intrapsychic conflicts (Herman, 1992; Masson, 1984; van der Kolk, Weisaeth, & van der Hart, 1996). It took most of the rest of the century to break the silence on the reality of sexual violence in the lives of women and children and to reintegrate and value this female perspective in psychology practice and research.

Valuing the Female Perspective in Sport Psychology Practice

A colleague and I recently designed and ran a psychoeducational group intervention project on body-image awareness for a team of elite female athletes. The impetus for the project came from our individual work with female athletes who were battling negative body image and unhealthy weight-control behaviors arising from those negative images. The overall goal of the program was to facilitate the development of a positive body image.

In sport, there is an increasing awareness of the complex and contradictory influences on young people regarding body image. Recent research has shown that body-image dissatisfaction is a better predictor of eating attitudes, eating behaviors, and eating pathology than other variables such as self-esteem, depression, and social anxiety combined (Gross & Rosen, 1988). Similarly, Wardle and Foley (1989) have shown that body-image disturbance is one of the main areas of maladjustment in individuals with eating disorders.

Three process goals were identified, reflecting the particular therapeutic approach that informed the design of our program. That approach, known as *narrative therapy*, assumes that people experience problems in their lives when the dominant stories or narratives that they or others have constructed

of their lives do not sufficiently represent their lived experience. For example, for the female athletes who were speaking to me of their difficulties with body image, their lived experience of being in their bodies as strong muscular athletes contrasted with the dominant story about "ideal" body shape that exists in popular youth culture in Australia.

Narrative therapy provides a forum in which individuals with problem-saturated stories of their lives can "re-author" their lives and relationships (White & Epston, 1990). Thus, the process goals of the body-image intervention project were (a) to identify dominant stories (myths) that exist in our culture about young women and how they look; (b) to identify when, even in a small way, individual challenges were mounted against these stories (myths); and (c) to create new stories for and about ourselves as young women and how we look.

We gathered both quantitative and qualitative data to evaluate the program. Whether or not we succeeded in having a long-term, positive impact on the body image of this group of female athletes is uncertain. The measures did indicate positive changes between pre- and post testing and, on some measures, between the control group and the intervention group. At follow-up, 6 months later, this positive change was already declining.

The qualitative data reflected some success in achieving the process goals. Comments from the athletes regarding what they felt they had gained from the intervention included "I learned about the many issues influencing females in today's society" and "I became aware about where the influences come from that give us perceptions of body image." We understood statements like this to reflect awareness of the dominant cultural stories (myths) about young women. Other statements, such as "I felt pleased that I can actively be a nonconformist in other ways" and "If people don't like me—stuff them!"

and "I learned to stand up for myself and what I believe in," reflected successful challenges to the dominant, problematic, cultural stories about young women.

An example of how these athletes engaged in the creation of new stories for and about themselves was most movingly displayed in the final session. In that session we addressed the complex area of sexual body image. We prepared a gallery of pages from an up-market fashion magazine that contained photographs of young fashion models in overtly sexualized poses. The task for the athletes was to discuss the following questions: How is young women's sexuality and body image portrayed in these media pictures? Is there anything problematic in such images? What are they telling young women and young men about women's bodies, attractiveness, and sexuality? What would the group like other young women and young men to realize about female bodies, attractiveness, and sexuality?

The athletes were then invited to construct their own gallery by making graffiti posters publishing their stories about female bodies, attractiveness, and sexuality—stories about themselves that they wanted to share with their peers. In a symbolic performance of these new stories, the athletes hung their posters over the magazine pictures as they spoke about their creations. Statements such as "We R what we R!!!" and "We'll do what we want!!! And be who we want!!!" and "Big is beautiful too!" and "We will not be used and abused" provided moving testament to the powerful new stories these athletes had created for and about themselves.

I have offered this snapshot of the body-image project as an example of an attempt to practice valuing female experiences in sport. The project provided a forum in which young, female athletes could articulate their unique experiences and be heard, respected, and empowered. It also provided an environment constructed to challenge the notion of body-image concerns as an individual, female pathology by facilitating discussion and naming the dysfunctional cultural and social scripts of the "ideal" female body.

The generation of data on the body-image issues of elite athletes had further, broader implications for elite sport in Australia. It was used to educate coaches on sensitivity and on best-practice issues relating to monitoring and maintaining healthy weight control behaviors for elite female athletes. It was further used to inform the development of a national position statement on the apparent systemic sexualization of women's sport in Australia, a phenomenon that has recently emerged.

Sensitivity to Diversity

There is no homogeneous women's or men's experience. The sports world, theoretically, comprises the whole planet, yet the English-language, academic world of sport psychology often generalizes from a Western—usually Caucasian—view of women and men. This is also true of many Western psychological methods of healing or helping.

Being sensitive to diversity means expecting and respecting difference. Cultural differences have been considered to be the "covert" partner in any therapeutic relationship, helping to shape the definitions of problems, the processes of therapy and the choice of solutions (Leung & Lee, 1996). I would argue that these differences should be made overt in the therapeutic relationship. Any therapeutic interaction is essentially a cross-cultural one. Cultural practices, beliefs, and value systems do not occur only in the context of ethnicity and race (Corey, Corey, & Callanan, 1993). Gender, religion, economic status, sexuality, and physical capacity are all associated with such differences. A basic assumption for me is that each athlete I work with has had a history different from my mine, has had different experiences, and has different ways of making meaning of the world and his or her position in it.

Diversity in Sport
Psychology Practice

While I was working in Asia, a Western coach approached me and expressed great concern and frustration that his athletes did not appear to be motivated when competing against one another in various tests throughout the training season. To him, it seemed that either they did not care about improving, or that they were lazy, or that they lacked "fighting spirit." However, when it came to team selection trials, they would compete fiercely. This frustrated the coach even more, because he felt that they were unwilling to put in the hard work unless it was absolutely necessary.

While meeting with the athletes, I discovered a difference in interpretation of the training tests by the Asian athletes and the Western coach. From the coach's cultural perspective, individual success within any contest was highly valued regardless of whether the opponents were teammates and friends. In the athletes' Asian culture, harmonious social relations within the team were highly valued. Therefore, if a team member was leading a training test in which selection was not at stake, excessively challenging the leading athlete, and perhaps winning, would disrupt the harmony of the group and cause unnecessary loss of face. The athletes were not lacking motivation; they were simply placing more value on team relationships.

The solution lay in explicitly reframing the activity from a perspective of individual competition to one of team advancement. As each athlete took individual responsibility for pushing the others at each training test, the overall team standard would rise. The success of the selected team in the international arena would then be shared by all.

A young woman in some distress came to see me. A series of incidents had resulted in her deciding to seek some help. She informed me that she was a lesbian. She had told no one else. She had a strong sense that it would not be accepted by her peers, nor by her coaches in the elite sport environment where she lived and trained. She felt silenced, isolated, and depressed.

Some of her experiences reflected elite sport's insensitivity, by omission, to diversity. Others reflected the more familiar commission of homophobic behaviors. An example of the former occurred at a team meeting during which one of the female coaches addressed issues related to life upon retirement from elite sports. As part of the educational input, the coach mentioned that marrying and having children would be one of the most rewarding experiences the young women on the team would have to look forward to at the end of their sport careers. The athlete said to me, "I felt so left out by this. Did she not think that maybe some of us were not heterosexual?"

At another time, the athlete had overheard a coach referring to another (lesbian) coach's sexuality in a derogatory manner. She also overheard her peers' derogatory remarks about other openly lesbian athletes. She felt so intimidated by the prevailing negative attitudes toward homosexuality that she felt unable to approach the openly lesbian athletes, who may have been able to provide a supportive peer group for her.

She had chosen to talk to me about this, she said, because she had spoken to me previously about difficulties she was having in a relationship. At that time she had not known whether it was safe to tell me that she was a lesbian, so she had been careful to refer her girlfriend in a gender-neutral way ("my partner"), without using pronouns. She said she appreciated the fact that I had followed her lead in doing this and had not imposed "she" or "he" pronouns on the conversation. From my point of view, that had been my way of showing her that it was safe to tell me as much or as little as she wished and that I would respect her boundaries around this. I had not known she was a lesbian at that time, but it is important to me not to make assumptions about an individual's sexuality, and I take care to let clients identify the gender of their partners where they wish. This is my way of valuing diversity.

The Personal Is Political

Gill (1994) interprets this well-known feminist "dictum" to mean that psychologists working in sport must employ a social perspective when seeking to understand individual behavior. Understanding the immediate sport environment as well as the larger societal context is important in understanding the difficulties athletes experience. This is particularly true of elite sport, which is itself a unique subculture within the broader subculture of sport and recreation.

In line with traditional feminist thinking, my understanding of the "personal is political" principle incorporates more than just a consideration of social context. It involves advocacy and political action on behalf of the clients with whom I work. This may mean writing reports or letters on behalf of athletes and coaches, providing support in meetings, or facilitating meetings and liaising with organizational bodies. I also choose to be involved in committees working on policy development in areas such as harassment, sexual abuse, and issues affecting female athletes.

Political Sport Psychology Practice

An athlete came to see me soon after returning from a major international competition. This was an elite female athlete, not only ex-

tremely successful in her sport but also in her career and in other aspects of her life. She had been known as an extremely confident, outgoing woman. When I met her, she was very depressed and felt that she had lost her sense of self, both as an elite athlete and as a woman.

This athlete had been the only female member of the national team to travel overseas. The coaching and management staffs were all male. The experiences that had resulted in such distress reflected not only individual but also systemic harassment of the severest kind. Team management had not considered the needs of a lone female team member in even the most basic sense. Consequently, a separate room was neither budgeted for nor arranged. With no discussions, no choice, and no options, this female athlete was instructed not only to share a room with a male member of the team, but also to share the only bed in that room.

On the third evening, a "team" activity was arranged. The coach informed the female athlete, "The boys are going to buy me a drink, please don't cook anything. We won't be long." They returned in the early hours of the morning, and the coach brought a woman back to the apartment with him. Having refused to share a bedroom, the coach used the sofa in the lounge area as a bed, where he had sex with the woman. In the morning, the athletes had to ask him to stop having sex so that they could get to the bathroom and to the kitchen to start breakfast. During breakfast, there was a detailed discussion of the woman and her sexual abilities.

On many occasions, the male team members watched pornographic movies. Again there was extensive, loud, detailed discussion. This female athlete could not leave her room during these episodes. She felt completely intimidated and threatened by the group, listening to their constant, hostile comments about women. These comments continued in public. Any time an "attractive" woman walked by, the team would discuss in detail what she might be like as a sexual partner. As this athlete said to me, "I felt like I was in prison, totally trapped with no one to talk to and no way out. . . . I felt like a nonhuman."

She had sacrificed many years of her life to prepare for that major event. For me, it is impossible to hear of such abuse and not engage in political action and advocacy to ensure that the system protects and facilitates all athletes in their endeavors to excel.

Egalitarian Psychologist-Client Relationships

One of the basic assumptions I hold about the therapeutic relationship is that the client is the expert in his or her own life, not I. Therefore, I assume that I am unlikely to know the answer to the client's difficulties. Rather, we are, together, collaboraters in the process of finding those answers. I believe that each person, no matter how distressed at the time of seeking help, has resources and strengths. My role is to help the individual access these resources, to roll obstacles out of the way—not to point out the path which I believe should be followed.

However, I do have certain skills that may be helpful to the client. First, as someone who is not "in" the client's life, I am in a position to reflect an overview or metaperspective. Jones (1991) describes this very well. She says,

> . . . my technical skills (e.g., in asking circular or hypothetical questions), my respectful search for their own skills and resources, my widening of the area of inquiry to include wider contexts that may previously have been left out of account, my challenge to set ways of thinking, and my attempt to create a safe and containing space in which the

unthinkable and unsayable can be expressed, will have the effect of freeing up the client's own ability to explore, to grow, and to resolve dilemmas. (p. 7)

My interpretation of the maintenance of an egalitarian therapeutic relationship involves informing clients of the processes of the therapeutic work as they occur. Thus, at the end of the therapeutic relationship, when clients have successfully moved on in the context of their lives to the places they want to be, they know exactly how they did so.

Egalitarian Sport Psychology Practice

I provide the following vignette as an example of how one can so easily impede the therapeutic process by falling into the trap of "knowing" more about the client than the client does. This incident occurred four sessions into a therapeutic relationship with a male athlete. This athlete traveled a great distance to attend the sessions, and it became clear that our work together would be irregular because of this. It was also becoming clear to me that his life was dominated by very deep pain and his courageous struggles to contain it.

It was our last session before an unavoidable break of several weeks. I was concerned that he needed more regular contact and support than I could provide, given the difficulties with travel. As we prepared to finish the session, what I should have done was to affirm the commitment shown by this athlete to the difficult healing work he had undertaken. I should have spoken of my respect for his courage in finally speaking of what, for so many years, had seemed to him to be unspeakable. Instead, I effectively challenged that commitment and courage. I expressed concern that because of the irregularity of our sessions, it would be difficult to make real progress. I said, "Have you considered that by choosing a psychologist so far away from where you live, you may in fact be trying to avoid dealing with all this?"

The athlete interpreted this as a hostile rejection of his attempts to seek help. Not surprisingly, he immediately retreated from the therapeutic process. (We did schedule one further meeting before he left, and we resolved things and continued to work together for a long time.) What is important about this example is my assumption that I knew what was best for him. I *thought* he would make better progress with someone who could provide more frequent contact. He *knew* that he had chosen this particular arrangement because he could pace his healing more appropriately.

He was right.

Researching in Sport From Within a Feminist Framework

Some feminist thinkers have proposed that the rhetoric of "science," which is so ingrained in academic and professional psychology, is incompatible with the rhetoric of feminism, which has political ambitions (e.g., Holloway, 1989; Parker, 1993). I disagree, if only because, as mentioned earlier, my definition of the scientist-practitioner differs from the traditional, positivist one. The feminist framework within which I work requires adherence to two principles. The first is that of *reflexivity*, which involves the constant reflection on, and the critical questioning of, the values and assumptions that underlie all research endeavors. Values and assumptions are implicit in every stage of the research process, from the choice of research question to the way data are presented and interpreted. What must be done is to make these values and assumptions explicit. We can minimize unnecessary bias through this process, which must involve interdisciplinary discourses and discourses

with colleagues who do not work within a feminist framework.

The second principle is that of *praxis*. Praxis is the linking of theory, politics, and practice. As eminent sports sociologist M. Ann Hall describes it, praxis means that "those working in academe, whose focus is on research and scholarship, must work with those on the front line—athletes, teachers, coaches, policy makers or activists, so that together, we are doing critical political work to bring about change" (Hall, 1996). I work toward change in the forms and practices of power and inequality in sport. This influences the research questions I pose, the methodology I use, and my interpretation of data. Since I am in the unique position of working in a multidisciplinary elite sports facility, I find that I am both on the front line, in terms of my applied work, *and* involved in research and scholarship.

Feminist Research in Action— Sexual Abuse in the Lives of Athletes

Currently, I am conducting an investigation of sexual abuse experiences in the lives of elite athletes. I offer this research as an example of praxis. As I mentioned earlier, I work on the "front line," and in my work with athletes over the years it has become apparent to me that sexual abuse is no less common in athletes' lives than it is in the general community. Nor is it any less harmful.

It has been well documented internationally that approximately 20–30% of females and 10–20% of males experienced sexual victimization at some point during childhood (Brown, 1993; Finkelhor, Hotaling, Lewis, & Smith, 1989; Oates, 1996). An extensive literature also exists on the differential, traumatic effects of child and adult sexual abuse (e.g., Rowan, Foy, & Ryan, 1994).

My therapeutic work with athletes guides the two main goals of this research project.

The first goal of the research program is to investigate the effects of sexual abuse in a population of nonpsychiatric, adult Australian athletes. An extensive literature exists on the differential, traumatic effects of sexual abuse. However, it is apparent that there are two significant deficits in this otherwise valuable knowledge base. The first concerns the absence of coherent frameworks to explain the range of traumatization responses, which occur, and to identify potential mediators of traumatization responses (Baum et al., 1993; Foa & Riggs, 1993; Higgins, 1995; Jones & Barlow, 1990). The second deficit is the lack of investigation of traumatization in nonpsychiatric populations (van der Kolk & McFarlane, 1996). The sexual abuse research program is attempting to answer some of these deficits from within the context of a population of adult Australian athletes.

The second goal is to investigate a number of issues related to the occurrence of sexual abuse within sport. Using the knowledge of athletes who have suffered sexual abuse in sport, the study is providing information on how these athletes are recruited into sexually abusive situations within the sport environment and how power relations affect this process.

The objectives and research questions applied to the research program are informed not only by current psychological theory and research on trauma and sexual abuse, but also by feminist sociological perspectives. The design includes both quantitative and qualitative methodologies. The questions posed in the study address systemic and individual factors associated with sexual abuse in sport. This information is necessary for the formation of effective intervention programs within sport. Identification of warning signs, or indicators, of traumatization within an athlete population is an important component of this study. This information is of paramount importance to psychologists working with elite athletes, because effective intervention cannot take place without it. Similarly, questions on systemic response factors have important implications for the development of effective service-provision programs, including personnel training, effective intervention and prevention programs, and policy development. This, I believe, is praxis.

Conclusion

In this discussion, I have attempted to outline my views and values as a feminist psychologist working in elite sport. I have indicated that feminism, for me, involves analyses of power and powerlessness and the impact of such systems on women and men in the elite sports world. I have tried to discuss issues in a way that neither pathologizes women's distress nor colludes in the cultural silencing of men's distress that is so prevalent in our society. I acknowledge that my worldview is limited by my privileged, White, middle-class background, and I am happy to be made aware if I have been exclusionary in any part of this discussion.

References

AAASP. (1990). AAASP passes certification criteria. *AAASP Newsletter, 5*(1), 3–8.

Baum, A., Solomon, S. D., Ursano, R. J., Bickman, L., Blanchard, E., Green, B. L., Keane, T. E., Laufer, R., Norris, F., Reid, J., Smith, E. M., & Steinglass, P. (1993). Emergency/disaster studies: Practical, conceptual and methodological issues. In J. P. Wilson & B. Raphael (Eds.), *International handbook of traumatic stress syndromes* (pp. 125–133). New York: Plenum Press.

Boyle, M. (1997). Making gender visible in clinical psychology. *Feminism and Psychology, 7*(2), 231–238.

Brown, H. (1993). *Shadows and whispers: Sexual abuse and social problems among young people.* Melbourne: Youth Affairs Council of Victoria.

Corey, G., Corey, M., & Callanan, P. (1993). *Issues and ethics in the helping professions* (4th ed.). Pacific Grove, CA: Brooks-Cole.

Finkelhor, D., Hotaling, G., Lewis, I. A., & Smith, C. (1989). Sexual abuse and its relationship to later sexual satisfaction, marital status, religion, and attitudes. *Journal of Interpersonal Violence, 4,* 279–399.

Foa, E. B., & Riggs, D. S. (1993) Post traumatic stress disorder in rape victims. In J. M. Holdham, M. B. Riba, & A. Tasman (Eds.), *American Psychiatric Press Review of Psychiatry* (Vol. 12, pp. 273–303). Washington, DC: American Psychiatric Press.

Freud, S. (1959). An autobiographical study. In J. Strachey (Ed. and Trans.), *The standard edition of the complete works of Sigmund Freud* (Vol. 20, pp. 3–74). London: Hogarth Press. (Original work published 1925)

Freud, S. (1962). The aetiology of hysteria. In J. Strachey (Ed. and Trans.), *The standard edition of the complete works of Sigmund Freud* (Vol. 3, pp. 189–221). London: Hogarth Press. (Original work published 1896)

Gill, D. L. (1994). A feminist perspective on sport psychology practice. *The Sport Psychologist, 8,* 411–426.

Gross, J., & Rosen, J. C. (1988). Bulimia in adolescents: Prevalence and psychological correlates. *International Journal of Eating Disorders, 7,* 51–61.

Hall, M. A. (1993). Gender and sport in the 1990s: Feminism, culture and politics. *Sport Science Review, 2*(1), 48–68.

Hall, M. A. (1996). *Feminism and sporting bodies: Essays on theory and practice.* Champaign, IL: Human Kinetics.

Herman, J. L. (1992). *Trauma and recovery: From domestic abuse to political terror.* New York: Basic Books.

Higgins, J. (1995). *Traumatic stress reactions in police.* Unpublished doctoral dissertation, University of Wollongong, NSW Australia.

Holloway, W. (1989). *Subjectivity and method in psychology: Gender, meaning and science.* London: Routledge.

Jones, E. (1991). Working with adult survivors of child sexual abuse. *Systemic thinking and practice series Nos. 7–8.* New York: Karnac Books.

Jones, J. C., & Barlow, D. H. (1990). The etiology of posttraumatic stress disorder. *Clinical Psychology Review, 10,* 229–328.

Krane, V. (1994). A feminist perspective on sport psychology research. *The Sport Psychologist, 8,* 393–410.

Leung, P. W. L., & Lee, P. W. H. (1996). Psychotherapy with the Chinese. In M. Bond (Ed.), *The handbook of Chinese psychology* (pp. 441–456). New York: Oxford University Press.

Masson, J. (1984). *The assault on truth.* New York: Farrar, Straus & Giroux.

Oates, R. K. (1996). *The spectrum of child abuse: Assessment, treatment and prevention.* New York: Brunner/ Mazel.

Parker, I. (1993). *Discourse dynamics: Cultural analysis for social and individual psychology.* London: Routledge.

Rowan, A. B., Foy, D. W., Rodriguez, N., & Ryan, S. (1994). Posttraumatic stress disorder in a clinical sample of adults sexually abused as children. *Child Abuse and Neglect, 18,* 51–61.

van der Kolk, B. A., & McFarlane, A. C. (1996). The black hole of trauma. In B. A. van der Kolk, A. C. McFarlane, & L. Weisaeth (Eds.) *Traumatic Stress: The effects of overwhelming experience on mind, body, and society.* (pp. 3–23) New York: The Guilford Press.

van der Kolk, B. A., Weisath, L., & van der Hart, O. (1996). History of trauma in psychiatry. In B. A. van der Kolk, A. C. McFarlane, & L. Weisaeth (Eds.), *Traumatic stress: The effects of overwhelming experience on mind, body, and society* (pp. 47–76). New York: The Guilford Press.

Wardle, J., & Foley, E. (1989). Body image: Stability and sensitivity of body satisfaction and body size estimation. *The International Journal of Eating Disorders, 8,* 55–62.

White, M., & Epston, D. (1990). *Narrative means to therapeutic ends.* New York: W. W. Norton & Company.

Sport Psychology and the Nagano Olympic Games: The Case of the U.S. Freestyle Ski Team

Daniel Gould

The Olympic Games are one of the most significant athletic events in the World. Olympic athletes and coaches report that the Games are "bigger" and even more "pressure packed" than the other events in which they participate (Gould et al., 1998). It is no surprise, then, that more and more sport psychology consultants are involved in helping athletes and coaches prepare for the Olympic experience. However, students studying applied sport psychology and practicing sport psychology consultants have few resources to help them prepare for the Olympic consulting experience.

This article describes my experience as an educational sport psychology consultant who helped the U.S. freestyle mogul ski team prepare for the 1998 Nagano Olympic Games. The role I played as a sport psychology consultant at the Games themselves is also discussed. Specifically, my long-term involvement with the team is described with particular emphasis placed on the year leading up to the Nagano Games. Topics discussed include the purposes of the mental training program, the people involved, the Olympic-year mental training schedule, group and individual athlete intervention strategies, my role at the Games, issues that arose at the Games, and program evaluation. Recommendations and consulting lessons that I learned conclude the article.

Finally, it is important to recognize that a planned, long-term approach was taken with the consultation described. It involved a 5-year process that culminated in the Olympic Games experience. So I did not just arrive at the Games and actively mentally prepare the athletes and "fix" the competitors when things did not go right. In contrast, the coaches and I took a planned long-term approach to our mental training work. In many ways, this process is analogous to farming, where seeds were planted (e.g., I provided psychological skills training to the athletes), water was added on a consistent basis (e.g., coaches reinforced mental skills taught), and the garden was weeded and fertilized as needed (e.g., individual concerns were addressed in consultation sessions with the athletes) in hopes of bearing a superior crop when it counted (e.g., creating the best athletic performances at the Olympics).

Program Overview

History

My involvement with the mogul ski team can

Note: An earlier version of manuscript was presented at Second International Conference in Sport Psychology, Braga, Portugal, July 25–29, 1998.

best be thought of in two phases. The first phase occurred from 1991 to 1995. I worked with the mogul ski team, a specific discipline of freestyle skiing. A break in my consulting work occurred in 1995 to 1996 as U.S. Skiing faced severe financial difficulties and dismissed many coaches and staff and eliminated programs such as sport psychology.

Phase 2 involved the period from January 1997 to March 1998. Because of their performance potential, the mogul team received U.S. Olympic funding to help with their Olympic effort.[1] The mental training and preparation work in this phase will be the focus of this manuscript.

The first phase is important, however, because most of the athletes with whom I worked during the Olympic year and at the Olympic Games were individuals who had been involved in Phase 1. The Phase 2 work built on the Phase 1 efforts. So it would be misleading to discuss only the second phase.

Purposes

The program had three purposes. First, the coaches and administrators wanted an educational consultant to help the athletes prepare for peak performance. The U.S. Mogul team had been one of the most successful teams in the world and wanted to maintain their standing. They had an off year in 1995–1996, and they wanted to get back to winning medals in 1998. Moreover, they were expected to win, and they wanted to make sure that they delivered the goods. My role was to give advice as to how to help achieve that objective.

The second role I played was to provide assistance and support to the coaches and staff. So, in addition to my role as a peak-performance consultant for the athletes, I

provided both informational and emotional social support to the coaches. An example of this role occurred one week before the Olympics at the last World Cup event. The coaches were under tremendous pressure because two athletes who were not selected to make the Olympic team disagreed with this decision and filed a lawsuit against the team and U.S. Skiing. There was considerable tension between the athletes and coaches involved, and non-ski team members were actually yelling derogatory remarks at the coaches from the side of the course during practices and competition. It made for a distracting and disturbing environment for all those involved. Consequently, when I came in to meet with the team, everyone was very happy to see me. Although I could not solve any of the problems, I did provide an outlet for coaches to vent their emotions and an objective voice that was not directly involved in the controversy.

Finally, I provided social support for the athletes. I served as a nonbiased, objective source of support. I was someone from outside the ski community with whom they could discuss matters and, if needed, vent their frustrations without consequences. Interestingly, for instance, at the same time I met with the coaches regarding the Olympic selection controversy, I provided similar support for the athletes involved.

Who Was Involved?

I worked with a number of individuals in this consultation, including members of the aerial and acrobatic or ballet teams. The athletes I had the most contact with, however, were the mogul skiers. This was the direct result of the head coach's commitment to mental training. Specifically, I worked with

---

1. This consult was made possible through a U.S. Olympic Committee Sport Science and Technology Sport Psychology Network Grant.

14 World Cup mogul skiers during Phase 2. Hence, there are more skiers on the World Cup team (14) than end up going to the Olympics (7). Originally, five made the Olympic team, but due to the selection lawsuits and resulting arbitration, two mogul skiers were added.

Two coaches (a head and an assistant head coach) and a full-time athletic trainer/physical therapist were with the team the entire year and were involved in the program. Then, at the Olympic Games, a team leader (an administrator/organizer) was involved. During the regular year, this individual served as the program manager for the team, but seldom traveled to training and competitions. Finally, at the Olympic Games, the U.S Olympic Committee assigned a medical doctor and athletic trainer to be with the team. The team leader and USOC medical staff were not involved in the sport psychology consultation, although issues involving them had to be addressed at the Games themselves.

Understanding Mogul Skiing

Mogul skiing involves skiing by oneself down a hill of approximately 300 meters and racing against a clock. As competitors ski down the course, they are required to weave in and out of a number of small mounds called moguls or bumps. Skiers also execute two ramp jumps, labeled the top and bottom air. Going off the ramp, the skiers execute specific maneuvers with names such as a helicopter or double daffy. They must land their maneuver and then get back into their turning rhythm.

Skiers are scored by rating the quality of their turns (50% of their total). Turns must be smooth and rhythmical, with knees kept together. Jumps are also rated and count for 25% of the total score with judges looking for height, difficulty of the skills executed, control, and landing. Twenty-five percent of the total score is dependent on top to bottom speed. Thus, a panel of judges rates the skier in all these areas, scores are accumulated, and top finishers are identified.

It should also be noted that skiers take two runs: a semifinals and, if they finish in the top 16, the finals. Skiers who make finals ski in reverse order (e.g., 16, 15, 14), with the top finisher in the semifinals going last in the finals. Normally on World Cup circuit, the semifinals and finals are held all on the same day. However, in the Olympics, the competition is conducted differently, with the semifinals and finals taking place 2 days apart.

Finally, there are different lines or route options to ski on the course. The skier can come down one, two, and three different lines (paths), and skiers spend most of the week figuring out which line is the fastest for them. Thus, different skiers will use different lines.

I should also note that I did some work with the aerials discipline of freestyle skiing. I will not talk about that in this article. I had a fairly good relationship with some of the aerial skiers, and they had equal access to me, but the coach was not that interested in the services offered. He and I had a cordial relationship, but he just did not place the same priority on the mental training program as the head mogul coach, Jeff Good, did. Coach Good was the reason I was so involved with the mogul team.[2] He believes in sport psychology, and we interact very well. He was constantly on the phone scheduling me to come to certain camps and competitions to consult with the athletes. The aerial's coach, however, although not dismiss-

---

2. In accordance with Association for the Advancement of Applied Sport Psychology Ethical Guidelines, participant confidentiality is maintained throughout this report. In cases where names of athletes or coaches are used, permission was granted by the athlete or coach mentioned.

ing or opposing the program, never made any effort to initiate contact.

Olympic-year Mental Training Schedule

Table 1 contains the Olympic-year mental-training consulting schedule. Because of the team's Olympic performance potential, the mogul coach was able to secure a grant from the U.S. Olympic Committee to support the mental training program for the year. The consultation began with me attending the World Championships in Japan in January 1997. Coach Good did not expect me to, nor did I feel comfortable, actively approaching the athletes regarding sport psychology issues at this event because I had not interacted with them for over a year. However, because the event was being held on the same course as the Nagano Olympics, he wanted me to observe ("be a fly on the wall") and learn what I could because that would help the team in the Olympic year. Several athletes who had worked with me during Phase 1 sought my services (usually after the event), but this was the exception, so I did only a few consultations at the event.

Following the World Championships, I did not see the team until May, when I went to what I labeled the May start-up of kick-off camp. It was an off-snow training camp held at the Olympic Training Center in Colorado Springs, Colorado, and it represented the start of the new season. Specifically, the previous season finished in March, so the athletes had a month off before coming to the

Table 1. Nagano Olympic Campaign Sport Psychology Consultation Schedule

February 1–10, 1997	World Championships, Nagano, Japan (Moguls, Aerials, & Achrobatics)
May 8–10, 1997	Mogul Olympic Season Organizational Kick-off Camp, Olympic Training Center, Colorado Springs, Colorado
September 3–7, 1997	Mt. Hood, Oregon On-snow Mogul Camp
October 2–6, 1997	Winter Park, Colorado Preseason Mogul Camp
November 13–17, 1997	Mt. Hood, Oregon On-snow Mogul Camp
December 30–January 3, 1998	Gold Cup Olympic Trials, Lake Placid
January 30–February 1, 1998	Breckenridge, Colorado World Cup
February 1–15, 1998	1998 Winter Olympic Games, Nagano, Japan
March 27–30, 1998	U.S. National Championships, Snowbird, Maine

camp. At the camp, we focused on having the skiers focus on and discuss questions such as "What are my goals for the next year?" and "What do I want to accomplish?" In addition, in conjunction with the coaches, the athletes were asked to devise strategies and a plan for achieving the stated goals.

The next two training camps I attended were held at Mt. Hood, Oregon, in September and October. The team goes to Mount Hood because there is a glacier there, so they can ski during the North American summer and early fall, although the weather tends to be inconsistent because of rain and fog. I would spend 3 or 4 days with the team at these camps (which typically lasted 10 days). During the part of the season these camps were held, the skiers focused a great deal of their time working on skiing technique and form. Because of this, the bulk of the consulting work dealt with athlete frustration and athlete-coach communication as the skiers struggled through the process of honing their skills. Team relation concerns also arose because the team lived in very close quarters at these camps.

An on-snow camp was held in November and was significant because it immediately preceded the World Cup season, which began in December. Mental preparation was often discussed at this meeting.

In January of 1998, I attended the Olympic trials in Lake Placid, New York. The winner of this event automatically qualified for the Olympic team whereas the other slots on the team were decided based on World Cup finishes. In addition to observing the competition, I met individually with most of the skiers in an effort to discuss seasonal progress to date.

At the end of January, I attended the Breckenridge World Cup, after which the team immediately departed for the Olympic games in Japan. This was the event where the team-selection controversy occurred.

Finally, in March of 1998, I attended the final event of the ski season: the U.S. National Championships. We scheduled a consult at this event because there is a tendency for some Olympic athletes to "get down" after the Games—whether they were really successful and accomplished a lifelong dream or failed and had to deal with their disappointment. We also expected several athletes to consider retirement. Unfortunately, this did not turn out to be a good time to debrief the team. The athletes were so drained from the long season that most were too tired to even meet. However, the few athlete and coach consults that were held were very successful. Hence, even though the timing was poor, the head coach and I felt that holding a debriefing, career transition, and refocusing session was very important and should be scheduled in the future.

Intervention Strategies

The intervention strategies that we used throughout the program included group or team meetings, individual athlete consultation meetings, and coach briefing and debriefing sessions. The group meetings were formally structured as the head coach and I had set goals, outlines, and specific agendas for each session. These sessions, however, did not take place in formal classroom settings, as more often than not, we met in a living room of one of the condominiums where the athletes stayed, with some athletes lying on the floor and others crowded onto a couch. Although not planned (we did this because meeting rooms were not available) in many ways, this informal arrangement was advantageous as the skiers were a casual group who felt at home in such environments.

Although group meetings were held approximately four times per year, individual athlete consultations were held every time I had contact with the team for those skiers who desired to meet. So, typically, we would do something as a group, and then the athletes and I would schedule individual sessions. Again, because office space was typically not available, we met where we could, whether it was sitting out on a porch, driving up to the mountain in a car, or even waiting in a garage on one occasion. In these meetings, I generally asked the athletes how they were doing, how they were progressing relative to their yearly plans, if anything was bothering them, what was working right, and if there was anything I could help them with. Often, they raised questions or had specific issues they wanted to discuss. Out of the approximately 14 athletes who attended these camps, on average I would see from 7 to 10 athletes. So it is important to recognize that not everyone wanted to meet with me every time. In fact, some people never wanted to see me whereas others met with me every time.

The third intervention strategy involved holding coaching staff briefings. Typically, when I arrived at a camp (or talked on the phone to the head coach just before arriving) I received the coaches' and/or staff's perspective on the status of the team and individual athletes. They conveyed their impressions of the skiers relative to such things as performance improvements; injury status; distractions; and levels of motivation, stress, and frustration. On some occasions the coaches and staff members also indicated that I needed to see certain team members. Moreover, at the end of my visit, I always debriefed the coach as to the status of the team and individuals (e.g., "The team is really stressed right now" or "Athlete X could really use some extra attention and positive reinforcement"). Both the athletes and coaches knew that I did this and that I always protected the confidentiality of athlete concerns relative to issues that they did not want conveyed to the coaches. Finally, an added benefit of these coach-briefing sessions was that it allowed me to provide social support

to the coaches. Often, the coaches were under great stress, and they needed to vent their own frustrations. At other times, they used the occasion to bounce coaching style and communication ideas off me, because I was an objective source not involved in the politics of the team or their organization. In all, this was one of my most valuable roles on the team.

Phase 1 Group Meetings (1992–1994)

Phase 1 group meeting topics are listed in Table 2 (see Gould & Damarjian, 1998). Because the team had never had a mental training program before, we began with an introductory session on "What is sport psychology and mental skills training?" I defined what we do in the area and explained that we would not be talking about clinical psychological concerns—I was not a shrink, but a mental coach. So the goal was to provide a real understanding of what I was there for, my role with the team, and to motivate the athletes to take part in the program.

Further inspection of Table 2 shows that we discussed mental preparation and energy management. We also focused on visualization and imagery. As it grew closer to the Lillehammer Olympic Games, a group meeting on staying focused at the Games was held.

Phase 2 Group Meetings (1997–1998)

The Phase 2 group meetings (see Table 3) built on Phase 1 because most of the athletes in Phase 2 had taken part in Phase 1. A general session on goal setting and planning was held at the start-up camp in May. This was actually a review of goal-setting basics (Gould, 1998) with a heavy emphasis on explaining why setting goals and performance planning are important considerations for peak performance. Athletes also did self-assessments and completed individual

Table 2. U.S. Freestyle Ski Team Mental Skills Training Phase 1 Team Meeting Content
(From Gould & Damarjian, 1998)

Major Area	Specific Content Description
Introduction	* What Are Sport Psychology and Psychology Skills Training? * Psychological Skills Training Myths
Goal Setting	* Goal-setting Exercise (Long-term Dream Goal, Dream Goal This Year, Realistic Current Season Performance Goal, Monthly Goal, Next Practice Goal) Based on Orlick (1986) * Staircase Goals * Evaluating Goals By Using Goal-setting Principles * Factors to Consider and Areas in Which to Set Goals * Common Problems in Setting Goals * Individualized Seasonal Goals
Mental Preparation And Energy Management	* Optimal Zones of Functioning: The Relationship Between Emotional Arousal and Athletic Performance * Determining and Controlling Optimal Emotional Arousal Levels * Complete a More Extensive Skiing-Specific Competitive Reflections Form Based on Orlick's (1986) Original Form * Formulate a Race Mental Preparation Plan for Optimal Performance Formulate Emergency "Shrink" or "Stretch" Mental Preparation Plans for Use When Faced With Less or More Than Normal Time Available for Mental Preparation * Formulate Refocusing Plans for Coping With Unexpected Events and Distractions * Arousal Management: Psyching-Up or Chilling-Out Strategies * Nideffer's (1985) "Centering" Breathing Relaxation and Focusing Strategy * Thought-stopping Exercise (Bump, 1987) * U.S. Olympic Committee Sports Mental Training Relaxation and Energy Management for Athletes Brochure Distributed and Discussed
Imagery-Visualization	* Observe Orlick and Botterill Coaching Association of Canada "What You See Is What You Get" Video and Respond to Worksheet Questions Examining Uses of Imagery, Tips for Using Imagery, and Ways They Can Use Imagery * Summary of Key Points of Video * Sports Imagery Training Guidelines Based on Martens (1987)—What Is Imagery?, How Does Imagery Work?, Why Use Imagery?, Developing Imagery Skills, and Motor Imagery Guidelines
Staying Focused at The Olympics	* Understanding and Embracing the Olympic Challenge * Keys to Olympic Success (Staying Focused by Following Mental Preparation Plans, Challenge. Having Fun, Keeping Things in Perspective, Expecting and Preparing for the Unexpected, Staying Cool Under Pressure) Exercise Identifying Olympic Challenges (Positive and Negative Distractions) and Methods of Coping With Them

skiing goals that related to their long-term objectives.

A very well-received session was held on Olympic lessons learned by athletes and coaches. Content for this session was derived from the results of a research project conducted on all the U.S. Atlanta Olympic Games athletes and coaches (Gould et al., 1998). The project's purpose was to identify what went right and what went wrong relative to factors influencing Olympic performance. As part of the interview results from the project, Atlanta athletes and coaches identified lessons learned that they would recommend that future Olympians consider in their quest for Olympic excellence. For example, some of the lessons conveyed included

1. Successful teams and athletes have a "single-minded focus." This single-minded focus helps them make appropriate decisions relative to distractions that arise at the Games.
2. Peak performance results from a complex interplay of many factors—including many small details. Athletes must pay close attention to these small details. Detailed, focused, and consistent preparation is needed.
3. There is a fine line between training intensely to gain an edge over opponents and going too far and overtraining.
4. Team relations and cohesion are key factors for success.
5. Olympians must be ready to deal with distractions generated from a variety of sources at the Games. They must be care-

Table 3. 1997–1998 Olympic Year Campaign Mogul Sport Psychology Team Meetings

Date	Topic
May 9, 1997	Introduction to goal setting/Importance of planning (60 minutes) * athlete self-assessment * big-picture goals * individual goal sheets
September 5, 1997	Preparation for Nagano: Lessons learned from Atlanta Olympians (60 minutes)
October 4, 1997	Olympic season plan explanation (Jeff Good, Head Coach) (60 minutes) * set big goals and see self achieving them * see everything in a positive light * adopt attributes of role models * thrive on pressure, not stress
November 14, 1997	Coping with adversity * identify sources of adversity/stress * strategies for coping * centering

ful to draw energy from the Olympic excitement, while not getting too caught up in the distractions.

Approximately 50 of these lessons were included in a handout and discussed with the team. So these were little tidbits of knowledge and principles that might help an athlete's preparation for optimal Olympic performance. What made this session especially powerful were comments from some of the skiers who were previous Olympians. They made comments such as "Yeah, that's right" and "Watch out for that." Members of the team would then further discuss the principle or lesson involved and would learn from one another.

A third group meeting was held on the plan for the Olympic season. The head coach actually made this presentation because it concerned all aspects of the program (although the head coach and I discussed the presentation content). Specifically, this presentation focused on the team's proposed journey for reaching its goals and a rationale for why things were being done in the way they were. Emphasis was also placed on maintaining a positive perspective and on expecting and thriving on stress, not fearing it. This was an important presentation because it provided a backdrop to tie individual skier goals to a larger plan or picture.

Finally, in November, a group meeting was held on the topic of "coping with adversity." In this meeting, the skiers were asked to identify the specific kinds of adversity they might face during the season (e.g., poor performances, poor start to season, injury, inappropriate comments from teammates). Then, as a group, we discussed ways to deal with or prevent each adversity source. For instance, some of the women on the team reported that the men at times could be too crude and lewd in their behavior, and this caused stress on extended trips to Europe.

Everyone agreed that sometimes such teasing got out of hand and agreed on a signal to inform those saying such things to "stop" when things had gone too far. So, in essence, the group pooled their experience relative to possible sources of adversity and ways to possibly cope with them. I also reviewed Nideffer's (1985) concept of centered breathing with the athletes.

Individual-Athlete Meeting Topics

Table 4 summarizes the topics that were discussed in the sport psychology consulting sessions between myself and individual skiers summed over all skiers during the year leading up to the Olympics. These topics were compiled through an examination of all the consulting notes made during the individual meetings with the 14 mogul athletes. A rough classification of the topics discussed in these sessions resulted.

The topic most frequently discussed was seasonal plans and goals, which arose with 71% of the skiers. However, it should be noted that these were not formal discussions on the topic. Rather, much of the time, it was very informal and unplanned. For example, I would ask the skier how he or she was doing and the skier would respond by saying that he or she was very frustrated. Often, the specific source of frustration focused on a specific issue that was related to some big picture plan and goals. For example the skier might indicate that "I stink and will never get these new turns." However, after we discussed why the person made such a statement, it became apparent that the athlete was frustrated because it was the preseason and he or she was working on a great deal of detailed technical changes to the skiing and was not skiing well or perceiving any success. Reminding the skier of the bigger plan for the season and setting process goals lessened the skier's current frustration and

Table 4. Summary of Individual Consult Topics for All Mogul Athletes

Topic Description.............( ) Number and Percentage of Athletes Discussing Topic
Seasonal goals/Plans ....(10–71%)
Coach-athlete relationship-Communication...............................(7–50%)
Mental preparation routine...(5–36%)
Confidence ....(4–29%)
Stress management ....(4–29%)
Fun ....(3–21%)
Frustration with judges' placements/results/progress ....(3–21%)
Jet lag/Travel planning..(3–21%)
Thought stopping/Distractions..(3–21%)
Dealing with pressure to make team ....(2–14%)
Decision to attend opening ceremonies/ Olympic focus distractions..............(2–14%)
Fatigue-Burnout...(2–14%)
Focus on hill ....(2–14%)
Lack of coach time/attention ....(2–14%)
Mental preparation [singles vs. doubles] ....(2–14%)
Career transition ....(1–7%)
Dealing with camp setting/team issues ....(1–7%)
Expectations ....(1–7%)
Injury/Injury recovery...(1–7%)
Imagery ....(1–7%)
Motivation ....(1–7%)
Overanalysis of technique..(1–7%)
Perfectionism...(1–7%)
Personal issues off mountain ....(1–7%)
Refocusing...(1–7%)
Team issues..(1–7%)

allowed him or her to see it in the proper perspective (Hardy, Jones, & Gould, 1996).

Coach-athlete relationship and communication was another frequently discussed topic (by 50% of the skiers). For instance, a skier might say, "Coach never listens to me," or the coaches would come to me and say, "That athlete has an negative attitude. You need to talk to that athlete." In such situations, I might instruct the athlete on how to approach a coach in a nonthreatening manner. If the coach was concerned with the athlete's attitude, I tried to work that notion into my meeting with the athlete and then offer suggestions on why and how better communication could be fostered.

Mental preparation, competence concerns, and stress management were discussed with approximately 30% of the skiers. Even though these were world-class athletes, at times they lacked confidence and needed to manage considerable stress. Moreover, given the competitive nature of World Cup skiing, they had to develop mental preparation routines if they hoped to attain consistent success (Gould, 1998; Orlick & Partington, 1988).

Given the business like-nature of elite sport, many people would think that having fun is not relevant to these athletes. This is not the case, as some of the athletes have been skiing at this level for well over 10 years and get very tired of the circuit. Finding ways to help these athletes sustain the enjoyment of skiing is critical to success. Similarly, all the skiers indicated that they started the sport because of the "fun" of such things as going fast, hitting a big air (jump), or being outdoors. Yet as they moved up in the skiing world and it became more professionalized, they could become too serious and lose the fun element. Ironically, this often resulted in poor performance. It could be alleviated, however, by having the skier focus on having fun and remembering what was fun about the sport.

Jet lag and travel came up in meetings with 21% of the athletes. These were usually younger athletes who had never been to Europe. I made suggestions such as making sure they kept very well hydrated on flights to Europe, refrained from caffeine and alcohol intake, and set their watches to the destination time as soon as the plane took off. Similarly, I recommended that they bring some of their favorite packaged food in case they were not comfortable with the food at the destination. That way, they could have a precompetition meal that they liked.

Thought stopping was another technique that 21%, or three, of the skiers discussed.

This typically involved teaching the skier to replace a recurring negative thought (e.g., "I will get hurt again") with a more constructive one (e.g., "chest up").

Frustration in dealing with failure or other types of things were topics of focus with three skiers (21%). Often, they just needed to vent their feelings to a socially supportive other. On other occasions, I found it was effective to put this failure into perspective (e.g., it is preseason, and they are learning and will fail more) or have them focus away from outcome to more process or performance goals.

A wide variety of topics arose in my meetings with one to two skiers (7 to 14%), ranging from fatigue and burnout to career issues. Handling the pressure to make the team was a topic that seemed specific to the Olympic year. It was a special concern for the men because as a group, other than Moseley (the person who ended up winning Gold at the Games), few skiers had established themselves as clear favorites to make the team. At times, this resulted in a very tense and competitive atmosphere that the skiers had to cope with. In contrast, the women had a clear pecking order, and unless someone did not perform as expected, it was fairly clear who was going to end up on the Olympic team.

Singles versus dual format was a topic of concern for several skiers and related to a new format used for some World Cup events. Specifically, in contrast to the traditional "singles" format where one skier skied down the course against the clock, a second "duals" format was implemented where two skiers skied down the course in a side-by-side competition. Several skiers performed much better in one format than the other, and we discussed differences in their mental preparation and focusing techniques used in each format.

Lastly, the topics listed in this table are misleading if they are interpreted as always

Table 5. Summary of Individual Athlete Contacts and Topics Over Olympic Season

Event/Camp/Date	Skier A	Skier B	Skier C
1997 World Championships			
May Start-up Camp		* Fatigue * Frustration With Outcomes * Seasonal Goals	
September On-snow Camp	* Build Coach-Athlete Relationship * Jet Lag/Travel	* Concerns With Plan * Coach-Athlete Communication	
October On-snow Camp		* Dealing With Camp Setting * More Individual Training Time * Coach-Athlete Communication * Mental Preparation Routine	* Seasonal Goals * Personal Issues * Having Fun
November Dry-land Camp	* Coach-Athlete Communication * Pressure to Make Team		
Olympic Trials			
Breckenridge World Cup	* Opening Ceremonies/ Olympic Focus		
Olympic Games			
Total # of Sessions	3	3	1
Olympic Team Member	Yes	Yes	No
Gender	Male	Female	Female

(continued on page 61)

being discussed independently of one another. This was not the case. For example, focusing on long-terms plans and goals was often used as a method to deal with frustration whereas mental preparation routines, fun, and thought stopping were often techniques discussed at the same time as stress management.

Although Table 4 provides information as to the topics that most often arose in individual skier meetings that took place during the season, some information is lost because it does not identify what issues were discussed with specific skiers and when in the season these concerns arose. For this reason, Table 5 lists the topics discussed in each meeting

Table 5. (continued)

Event/Camp/Date	Skier D	Skier E	Skier F
1997 World Championships			
May Start-up Camp			
September On-snow Camp			* Seasonal Goals
October On-snow Camp		* Frustration Regarding New Technique * Seasonal Goals * Belief in Self * Thought Stopping	
November Dry-land Camp	* Dealing With Pressure * Focus On Hill	* Mental Preparation for Europe * Seasonal Goals	
Olympic Trials			
Breckenridge World Cup			
Olympic Games			
Total # of Sessions	1	2	1
Olympic Team Member	No	No	No
Gender	Male	Female	Male

(continued on pages 62–64)

held with the 14 skiers consulted during the Olympic year. Also included are when during the season the topic was discussed, the total number of consulting sessions held with the skier, the skier's gender, and whether the skier made the Olympic team. Not listed is the mandatory goal-setting session held with me, the coaches, and the physical therapist at the Colorado Springs kick-off camp in May.

Inspection of this table reveals that some athletes met only once with me (e.g., Skier C), whereas others met as many as seven or eight times (Skiers I and J). Individual differences are also notable. For instance, in the four meetings held with Skier G, coach communication and mental preparation were repeatedly discussed. In contrast, with Skier I, a wide range of topics was discussed ranging from perfectionism and fun to stress management and confidence. Studying these individual cases reflects both the consistency and variation involved in consulting with world-class athletes.

The Nagano Games: February 1–15

It is important to understand the schedule the athletes must keep when participating in an

Table 5. (continued)

Event/Camp/Date	Skier G	Skier H	Skier I
1997 World Championships			* Perfectionism * Fatigue/Burnout * Over Analysis of Technique
May Start-up Camp		* Seasonal Goals * Mental Prep. (Duals vs Singles)	* Seasonal Goals/Plans
September On-snow Camp	* Coach Communication * Coach Attention/Time * Travel	* Dealing With Frustration	* Coaching Attention/Time * Coach Communication * Mental Prep. For Semifinals
October On-snow Camp		* Mental Prep. Routine (Duals vs Singles) * Coach Communication	* Fun * Motivation * Coach-Athlete Communication * Mental Prep.
November Dry-land Camp	* Coach Communication * Mental Preparation In Gate	* Mental Preparation (Dual vs Singles)	* General Check In
Olympic Trials	* Mental Preparation In Gate * Dealing With Poor Results		* Confidence * Stress Management * Deal With Expectations (note: 2 Sessions)
Breckenridge World Cup			
Olympic Games	* Dealing With Poor Performance * Coaching Trust-Relationship * Seasonal Goals/Plan (note: 2 sessions)		
Total # of Sessions	5	4	7
Olympic Team Member	Yes	No	Yes
Gender	Male	Male	Female

Table 5. (continued)

Event/Camp/Date	Skier J	Skier K	Skier L
1997 World Championships	* Seasonal Goals/Plans		
May Start-up Camp	* Injury Recovery		* Mental Prep. (Duals vs Singles) * Disractions
September On-snow Camp	* Seasonal Goals * Injury Recovery * Mental Preparation * Imagery	* Seasonal Goals/Plans * Olympic Year Distractions * Team Issues * Coaching Attention/Time	
October On-snow Camp	* Mental Preparation Routine * Refocusing * Seasonal Plan	* Mental Prep. Routine * Olympic Year Distractions * Coach Communication	
November Dry-land Camp	* Fun	* Confidence * Stress Management	* Career Transition * Seasonal Goals
Olympic Trials	* Staying Focused	* Distractions * Mental Prep. Routine * Minimize Distractions * Focus	
Breckenridge World Cup			
Olympic Games	* Confidence	* Distractions * Mental Prep. * Lessons Learned * Coping With Stress (note: 2 sessions)	
Total # of Sessions	7	6	2
Olympic Team Member	Yes	Yes	No
Gender	Female	Male	Male

Table 5. (continued)

Event/Camp/Date	Skier M	Skier N	
1997 World Championships			
May Start-up Camp			
September On-snow Camp		* Confidence * Coach Communication	
October On-snow Camp	* Seasonal Goals/Plans		
November Dry-land Camp			
Olympic Trials			
Breckenridge World Cup			
Olympic Games			
Total # of Sessions	1	1	
Olympic Team Member	No	No	
Gender	Male	Male	

Olympic Games. Although each team's schedule will be unique, many teams would follow the same general pattern of the U.S. freestyle mogul team.

The Olympic schedule is built around the time the team competes in the Games. The mogul team competed early, so we actually arrived before the Games officially opened. The aerial team competed later in the Games, so they arrived a week later, after the Games were well underway.

The mogul team traveled from the United States to Osaka, Japan, as the first leg of their journey. It was not a relaxed trip, and by discussing the specifics of the schedule, some of the popular myths about the glamorous lives of elite athletes should be dismissed. The team left from Breckenridge, Colorado (the site of the last World Cup event before the Olympics), and awoke at 3:30 in the morning.

We loaded the bus with all the baggage, skis, and ski equipment at 4:00AM and left at 4:45. After a 2½-hour bus ride to Denver, we took our first flight to San Francisco and then caught a flight to Osaka, Japan. Almost 30 hours after our awakening in Colorado, we arrived at the U.S. processing hotel in Japan. Upon arriving in Osaka, checking into our rooms and taking a shower, we immediately went through U.S. team processing and accreditation. One issue that a sports psychology consultant needs to be familiar with is that all the female athletes are gender tested or must have their gender accreditation cards with them. (This is required because several decades ago there was considerable controversy surrounding alleged gender changes of athletes in efforts to gain competitive advantages in the Olympic women's weight events [e.g., shot putt]). So now all female athletes either have their gender identification card or must be tested. It is a simple test, but if a woman has not gone through it before, it can cause some stress (e.g., "What do you mean I've got to get tested? I mean, can't you tell I am a woman?"). There is some other medical documentation done at processing, as well as credentialing.

The most exciting part of processing for the athletes is uniforming. The athletes received all kinds of clothes—a parade uniform for Opening Ceremonies, medal-stand warm-ups, jackets, boots and shoes, uniforms, rings, watches. I think the U.S. package for the athletes and coaches included almost $4,000 worth of clothes. In fact, they left this part of processing with three huge duffel bags full of clothes. Tailors were even present to alter and fit the clothes.

Then there was a team briefing on the third day where the athletes are introduced to U.S. Olympic officials and given some basic information about the village, sports medicine, media, security, etc. After that, we flew to the Matsumoto airport, followed by a bus ride to Nagano. The team arrived in the village and their credentials were checked. Then they went to the American section of the village, checked into their rooms, and received a 30-minute briefing by U.S. Olympic staff relative to security and village rules.

The fourth day involved getting settled in the village. The team also participated in a press conference, then some training (mostly easy skiing to check out the course), and finally received some ski-team uniforming.

The fifth day involved a much-needed day of hard training (two 2-hour on-hill ski training sessions and one off-hill team stretch). The team also trained hard on the sixth day. Additionally, the team moved from the village to off-hill housing so that we would be away from the village distractions and only have a 10-minute (versus a one-hour) drive to the competition venue.

The course was closed on the seventh day because that was the day of Opening Ceremonies. Because semifinals were held the day after Opening Ceremonies and with the coaches' urgings and in accordance with a long-term Olympic plan, the team elected not to participate in the Ceremonies. This was a very difficult decision for our athletes because participating in the Opening Ceremonies is exhilarating and the memory of a lifetime, but it also involves being on one's feet for an extended period of the time (3 to 5 hours) in the cold. So it can have a very negative performance effect on those athletes who compete the next day.

The 8th day was the semifinals event. Practice runs took place in the morning and the competition at mid-day. Those who failed to make finals opted to move back to the village (a very good move), because it was awkward for them to be around those who made finals and for those who made finals to know what to say to them. The 9th and 10th days were training days, and the 11th day was the Olympic finals. Like the semifinals, the finals involved morning practice runs, a course check, and mid-day competitions.

On the 12th day, the team moved back to the village and focused on enjoying the rest of the Games. The 13th day involved a team photo and more fun and relaxation on one's own. We attended a General Motors sponsor reception and a hockey game on the 14th day, and then we traveled back to the United States on the 15th day.

Although participating in the Olympics is one of the most exciting events of one's life, it is still a very serious business trip for those athletes who want to perform well. There is not a great deal of free time, especially for the coaching staff who spend almost every waking hour trying to create a positive social emotional environment for the athletes while controlling numerous potential performance-disrupting distractions. The athletes have more time and try to maintain their normal mental and physical preparation routines in an environment that is very different from the World Cup circuit. It is critical that they draw excitement from the village and associated events without getting so caught up in them that they lose their high performance focus.

Participants Seen

I consulted with five of the seven mogul athletes during the Olympic Games. The five athletes I saw were the skiers I most often consulted with during the Olympic year, whereas the two I did not consult with were individuals I seldom saw during the year leading up to the Games. We (these two athletes and I) got on well socially, and when I consulted with them in the past, things seemed to go well, but they chose to do things by themselves in an independent fashion. Both of these individuals did not perform well at the Olympics, although one had a very good World Cup season. Hence, the athletes I spent more consulting time during the year I saw more at the Games.

The number of individual consultation sessions with the five skiers I saw at the Games ranged from two to four contacts. One performed very well and won the Gold medal, two performed well, one performed well all week, but made a small mistake at the end of a run that took her out of the medals, and one had a poor outing and failed to make finals.

Finally, I saw both mogul coaches. I roomed with the head coach, and we talked every day about how to create the best performance-enhancing environment for the skiers. The assistant coach and I talked on four or five occasions, especially in regard to one particular skier. The ski team's athletic trainer/physical therapist and I also met on several occasions, at times discussing particular athletes and, on other occasions, staff relations.

Topics Discussed

Table 6 lists the 1998 U.S. mogul team athletes, the number of consulting sessions I held with each at the Games, and the topics discussed. An inspection of this table reveals that much of what was done dealt with mental preparation, stress management, and performance-focus concerns—usually not mentally preparing the athletes, but reassuring them to stick with their normal routines, trust their training, be confident, and help them deal with potential distractions. I should also note that these Olympic consulting preperformance sessions, which lasted from 10 to 25 minutes, tended to be much shorter than the 45- to 90-minute sessions held in the Olympic year. Seldom did I suggest any new strategies. Rather, I focused on reassuring the athletes and reminding them to do what had worked for them the entire season.

Another issue I spent considerable time discussing with the skiers was performance debriefing. For those who failed, debriefing involved providing emotional social support and allowing them an opportunity to vent if they were frustrated or cry from the disappointment. Additionally, they needed to begin to refocus and set new short-term performance and process goals as the World Cup ski circuit began again shortly after the Games. For the athlete who won the Gold medal, we discussed how his life would change as the result of his success and how to maintain the performance focus that allowed him to be successful in the face of all new distractions (media appearances, business opportunities, and endorsements).

Other than debriefing sessions, in many ways, because the team had worked on mental preparation all season, my major focus at the Games was helping behind the scene—helping the coaches deal with distraction control and providing an environment conducive to a high-performance focus. I learned

Table 6. Olympic Games Consulting Athlete and Staff Contacts and Consultation Topics

Participant	Total Contacts	Meeting 1	Meeting 2	Meeting 3	Meeting 4
Skier I	4	Expectations/ Stress	Reassurance/ Fun	Perf. Assessment	Debrief
Skier G	3	Team Selection	Poor Perf./Future Goals	Poor Perf./Future Goals	
Skier K	3	Distraction Control/ Focus	Mental Prep./ Dealing with Family Distractions	Champion Stress/ Lessons Learned	
Skier A	2	Olympic Focus	Perf. Debrief		
Skier J	2	Reassurance/ Confidence	Perf. Debrief		
Skier F	0				
Skier B	0				

that with a team that was mentally trained, the vast majority of staff and consultant time is spent on trying to keep things from distracting the athletes, whether they be the media, family and friends, transportation problems, or security. The Olympic environment is a circus that can easily distract the athlete and coaches. At the same time, one does not want the athletes to overfocus and not draw excitement and positive performance energy from the Games environment. As the great U.S. speedskater and one of the most successful U.S. Olympians of all time, Bonnie Blair, told our team at processing, "Being an athlete at the Olympic Games is like being a kid in a candy store. The secret is to taste all the candy (enjoy the Olympic excitement and special events), but not get a stomach ache while doing so (get so caught up in the excitement that you become dis-tracted, deviate from your normal performance routine and perform poorly)."

Program Evaluation

Performance and Performance Results

One of the difficulties of conducting a sport psychology intervention program is that the consultant does not receive definitive feedback as to how he or she may or may not have contributed to athlete performance. This is a hard situation for a consultant. Typically, if the coaches and the athletes ask a consultant back, that indicates that the services were valued. Sometimes, however, the consultant is not asked back and no one says why. For example, my Phase 1 involvement was curtailed because of severe financial difficulties with the team (e.g., many staff members were let go and coaches fired), but no one ever came out and told me this. So a good deal of uncertainty is built in to the process.

Another way to evaluate effectiveness is to examine athlete performance (recognizing the consultant is only one performance influence among many). The mogul team's performance was solid. On the men's side, Jonny Moseley placed first and won the gold medal. We also had a person place 10th, and that is probably where this individual should have placed for his first Olympics. He did a good job. We had two men fail to make finals. What is interesting about this is that these two athletes made the team as a result of a selection-process lawsuit and arbitration. The NGB and coaches wanted to bring only athletes and coaches who they thought could make it on the podium, but this was not clearly specified in the selection criteria, so the two athletes won their arbitration.

Now in fairness to the two competitors who did not make finals, the lawsuit was difficult (e.g., you are not on the team and in a legal fight and then you're on it) and did not create a good performance environment in which to function. However, the results did seem to validate the coaches' original decisions.

On the women's side, we did not medal, which was disappointing because we had a good deal of depth on the team. Specifically, after semifinals, two of our athletes were seeded two and four. Both had won medals in previous Olympics—one was a gold medal winner, and the other, a silver medal winner. One skied very well, but the course iced up, and she fell to eighth. The other skied better then she had all year, had medal run going, made a minor bobble, and dropped to fourth.

So our women's results were very disappointing. In fact, I had trouble not crying because I knew how hard these women had worked. So, on one hand, you are happy because one person won the gold medal on the men's side (that was one of the primary team objectives—win at least one gold medal). On the other hand, you are totally dejected for the women because you know how hard they worked to do well at the Games and how much they deserved medals.

It is important to recognize that for me, however, I wanted to feel that way. I want to be objective in my work, but I also want to be part of the team. Hence, I identified with the athletes, and they were my friends, and I wanted to be with them through the highs and lows. So for me that is an important component to the consultation process.

Participant Interviews

After the competition, I had the opportunity to interview three individuals and learn about their evaluation of the sport psychology program and their Olympic performance efforts. These include two athletes, one was the gold medal winner and the second was a medal winner in Lillehammer who had a disappointing eighth-place finish in Nagano. The head coach was also interviewed.

Liz McIntyre. One athlete interviewed was a three-time Olympian who had won a silver medal in a previous Games. She is one of the mentally toughest athletes I have ever worked with. Unfortunately, the Nagano competition did not fare well for her. Liz felt that mentally she did the best job she could, but the course turned unexpectedly icy and changed on her. Hence, although she skied the best she could under the conditions, an eighth-place finish resulted. Immediately after finishing, she skied over to me to see if I had a radio to let the coaches know that the course iced up, so I think her evaluation was correct.

Liz's experience really taught me an important lesson. She was ready to perform, and she had done everything right, but she just ran into some bad luck. What I learned from Liz's experience is that to win an Olympic medal, you must avoid bad luck. You must do all the prerequisite mental and physical training and preparation, and you must avoid bad luck and sometimes have some good luck. I always knew this, but never realized it emotionally before observing Liz at the Olympics. What elite athletes are doing is dealing with probabilities. With training, they increase the probability that they can have a peak performance, but sometimes factors outside their control (e.g., the course conditions change) prevent them from having a good outcome, no matter how hard they work.

It is also important to note that I wanted to interview Liz for several reasons. First, she was very experienced, having participated in three Olympics. Second, she was extremely involved in the mental training in both Phases 1 and 2. Third, she is very intelligent, and, I felt, would have a good feel for what program elements would and would not work for her. Finally, we had developed a very good relationship and I was confident that she would give specific feedback about my consulting style. Typically, athletes and coaches are not specific relative to their feedback about mental training—just saying everything was fine or good.

Relative to me and my consulting, Liz indicated that a major strength was that I gave very specific feedback and concrete suggestions of techniques she could employ or practice. A weakness was the fact that I was not with the team enough during the year to be totally integrated into it (like the athletes and coaches), and hence, I did not always know everyone's day-to-day idiosyncrasies. Moreover, at the start of the Games, in informal conversations, I asked Liz some questions about how Nagano compared to the Lillehammer Games. She indicated that it was best not to talk about previous Olympics (as she liked the Lillehammer rural village set-up better than the urban Nagano venue), because she was in Nagano and she did not want to think about which was better. In

essence, Liz was in Nagano and, like it or not, was going to make it work for her. Finally, she felt that my role at the Games was appropriate, as it is best to sit back and wait for athlete requests for contact and not initiate such support on one's own.

In terms of the mental training, Liz was very pleased with the sport psychology services provided. After working with me, she felt she was better able to maintain focus and better able to cope with daily hassles and distractions. A case in point was her work with thought stopping and thought control. The year prior to the Games, this was identified as an area she wanted to improve. Hence, she practiced keeping her focus and controlling her thoughts by practicing thought stopping and control as she did sprints in her backyard and later during training runs. Liz indicated that what she learned helped her a great deal at the Games because there was an unexpected change in the normal start signal (from the announcer saying "1, 2, 3 Go" to "1, 2, 3" and recorded voices of children yelling "Nagano" instead of "Go"). She found this change distracting, but was able to use her focus and thought-control skills to keep it from interfering with her performance. In addition, when Liz found the course to be unexpectedly icy during her final run, she reported using all her thought-control skills to stay task focused.

When asked about her impressions of moving out of the village and up on the hill, Liz indicated that it was very positive for her. Not being a city person, she liked being in the scenic mountains. She also appreciated not having to take the hour bus ride each way, and she liked being away from the media.

Liz was also asked what mental training advice she would give to future Olympians. This included appreciating and realizing the importance of the mental aspects of performance. In addition, she felt that, at the Olympics, one needs to learn to go with the flow, as everything will not be as one desires and if one tries to fight all the changes, one's energy will be drained. Finally, she emphasized that it is the athlete's choice as to whether or not he or she gets rattled by unexpected events or the behavior of others. An individual cannot necessarily control the occurrence of such events and circumstances, but he or she can control reactions to them.

Lastly, Liz was asked her opinion of why some members of the team do not use at all, or infrequently use, the sport psychology services provided. She indicated that everyone on the team feels performing well in competition is more mental than physical. However, some do not work on mental skills development because they are afraid others will see it as a sign of weakness or that it is not within their comfort zone. Finally, many just do not know how to develop such skills.

Jonny Moseley. Jonny Moseley was a first-time Olympian who performed extremely well in Nagano. Sitting first after the semifinals and being America's first hope for a medal at the Games, he handled the pressure well and won the gold medal. Jonny's interview was very interesting as he revealed that, although talented, he was pretty "scattered" in his thoughts until the Olympic year and that mental training helped him quite a bit. The interview focused on what aspects of the mental training he felt worked and did not work for him. What was really interesting about this interview was that I was unaware of the influence of some of the things that he mentioned worked for him.

Jonny is a bright individual but indicated that in the past he was "sort of scattered" in his approach to his skiing. Both he and his coaches felt that prior to this season, they never knew what he was going to do from week to week relative to his mental preparation and performance.

The first important point that arose from the interview was that the year before the Games, Jonny made a conscious effort to improve his mental game. He met regularly with me and the assistant coach in an attempt to develop a more consistent mental-preparation routine. We also talked a great deal about how to handle the pressure of the Olympic year.

The biggest change reported by Jonny was his more organized approach to mental preparation. He worked on developing a consistent routine (although it was not highly mechanized). Moreover, in previous years, he had reported that he would try to get "psyched up" before big events, but this season discovered that finding his rhythm and relaxing were more effective and led to more consistent performances.

Relative to the Nagano Olympics themselves, Jonny indicated that he set aside time each day to relax, whether that involved watching a favorite video, going for a walk, or day dreaming. Moreover, because of the extra distractions accompanying the Olympics, he took his time between practice runs and focused on "making each one count."

Not surprisingly (being the favorite going into the finals), Jonny indicated that thoughts of "what if I win" and how that would change his life kept running through his head. Moreover, he said it was "difficult to be yourself when these thoughts are constantly playing in your head." He dealt with this in three ways. First, he constantly asked himself, "Is this me?" to make sure he did not fall into the trap of trying to act like what others expected and, in so doing, unknowingly lose his focus. Second, he set aside time each day to dream, so dreaming did not interfere with task-relevant thoughts on the hill. Finally, he (and the rest of the team) moved out of the village and stayed in a more isolated location near the venue several days before and during the competition itself. This allowed him to avoid both village and media distractions.

Two mental training techniques that Jonny used and reported worked well for him were centered breathing (Nideffer, 1985) and making a list of things to focus on. Specifically, he used centering (a technique all skiers were taught as part of their mental training) in both practices and competition ("2 to 5 times in the gate") and indicated that he thought it was effective because "when you center, you feel athletic." Moreover, "people don't bother you," and it is "easier to focus your thoughts." Relative to making a list of things to focus on, Jonny wrote out a list of what he called "tangibles and intangibles" to concentrate on. This list included items like technical cues (e.g., "chest up") and reminded him to keep things in "perspective." He read over the list every morning before training runs. He perceived this as critically important because it organized his thoughts. Finally, Jonny noted "that it really surprised me that I'd do something like that" (write out the list), but it proved to be quite effective for him.

Jeff Good. As the head coach of the U.S. Mogul team and three-time Olympic coach, Jeff Good was committed to sport psychology and mental training. When asked the reason he wanted me with the team at the Games, his response was to give the athletes a "focus point" or another person to speak with and get advice from someone other than the coaches. He felt that I provided a consistent, objective voice, and I was an individual who knew the athletes and coaches, as well as their and the program's objectives. Finally, Coach Good indicated he wanted me available at the Games in case any emergencies arose—as sort of an "insurance policy." He felt little need for me to "psych up" athletes because the skiers (with the help of the coaches and myself) were mentally prepared for the Games.

When asked what made me more or less effective, Coach Good indicated that positive characteristics included my professional attitude and approach to working with the team, the trust that existed among the coaches, athletes, and me, consistent contact with the team in the year prior to the Olympics, and his (the head coach's) priority placed on the mental training program. He also felt it was important that I knew my role on the team and "was a key ingredient," but did not try to be the "whole cake." A weakness was the fact that I had not traveled to Europe with the team prior to the Games and, therefore, did not know the day-to-day mannerisms of the athletes.

Coach Good felt that he and I had developed a good working relationship due to several factors. First, although maintaining confidentiality, I debriefed the coaches on major issues occurring with the team. In addition, when arriving at a camp, the coaches also briefed me as to the psychological climate of the team and individual athletes. Second, Coach Good felt it was very useful for me to meet individually with the coaches and talk to them not only about the team, but also about the stress and pressure placed on them as coaches.

Coach Good spoke extensively about the importance of "trust" for a sport psychology consultant. Specifically, he indicated that a consultant must be able to have candid and honest conversations with athletes and coaches. He or she must also be perceived as part of the team, live like the athletes ("in the trenches"), and be totally integrated into the program.

When asked about the role of mental factors at the Olympic Games, Coach Good indicated that the Games are different and impose structural changes (e.g., housing, opening ceremonies) that do not mesh with an athlete's normal preparation routine for a World Cup ski event. The athletes and coaches must be flexible enough to "go with the flow" without letting things disrupt their game plan.

Relative to dealing with distractions at the

Games (a major concern for Coach Good), Good felt it is important that the staff and coaches create a physical and social environment for the athletes with as few distractions as possible. Critical to this is to make the athletes aware of plans and possible distractions (e.g., roommates, training dates, dates moving in and out of the village) well ahead of time. At the same time, however, athletes do not need to know all the details (prevent information overload), just what directly impacts them.

Finally, when asked what psychological characteristics discriminated the three Olympic medalists he had coached from the other skiers, Coach Good indicated that it was their confidence to make use of everything available to them (e.g., sport psychology, nutrition, strength, and conditioning). They were not afraid to try new things, but at the same time, would take the good parts and filter out or not use less useful aspects of these programs. He also said that these three athletes were very motivated to work hard on their own.

Recommendations and Consulting Lessons Learned

A number of recommendations for improvement and consulting lessons learned were identified by myself and those interviewed. One mentioned by Coach Good and Liz McIntyre was to travel with the team to Europe, although this was not economically feasible during this consult. As McIntyre indicated, traveling with the team would allow me to know the athletes on a daily basis and learn their mannerisms and idiosyncrasies. They felt this was important because one of the difficult things about a 2-week Olympic campaign is reading the mood states of the skiers (e.g., determining if they are normally grumpy in the morning or whether this is a signal that something is wrong and the athlete needs help). Spending 8 to 10 days with

them during the World Cup season would help alleviate this situation. Additionally, it would further integrate me in as a part of the team.

Other lessons that I learned from the coaches and athletes that hopefully will help me to be more effective as a consultant follow.

Understand the Difficulty of Winning Medals.

First, it is very difficult to medal at the Games. As previously discussed, preparation is necessary but alone not sufficient for winning medals. Athletes need to avoid bad luck and hopefully get some good luck. I do not mean to imply that that those who win medals are merely lucky, but it is important to recognize that an athlete can do everything right, and sometimes it does not work out as it is supposed to. So, as consultants, we had better go into the Games with our eyes open regarding this issue.

Try Not to Do Too Much or Be Too Helpful When Working at the Games.

Volunteers, particularly sports psychology consultants, must not try to do too much or be too helpful at the Games. Even if you feel guilty at times, the most appropriate intervention may be doing nothing. Doing nothing is much harder than it sounds. You may not think that, but when the sport sends you all the way to the Games and you see an opportunity to help, you want to go over and help. However, certain athletes may not be receptive to assistance, or you can unknowingly "hover" over the competitors and not give them enough space. Many times, it is important to back off or realize that the team needs some space and wait for them to request your services. That was probably one of the biggest things I learned from my experience in Nagano, which was validated by head coach Jeff Good in his interview.

Make Efforts to Fit in With the Team.

Coach Good felt that one of my major strengths as a consultant was that I integrated well with the team and adapted to them and their lifestyle, as opposed to attempting to make them adapt to my needs. For example, at training camps, if the coaches were sleeping on the floor, I slept on the floor. I did not complain. I did what everyone else did. I did not try to make the team adapt to me. I adapted to them. So that was a pretty effective method of fitting in with the team, even though I did not know I was doing so at the time.

Create a Positive Social Emotional Climate at the Games.

It is critical that a positive social emotional climate be engineered for the athletes during the Olympic Games. This certainly involves focusing on positive reinforcement and encouraging remarks. Reassurance is also needed.

In addition, as the competition approaches, do not overload the athletes with information. What was really interesting at Nagano was observing all the distractions that are present and that can potentially interfere with athletes' mental preparation and performance. For example, the U.S. Olympic Committee processing is absolutely necessary, but somewhat distracting. Athletes receive such information as a book on protocol, two drug-control books, city transportation maps, and information on "flag etiquette" (this is important because in our country our flag is revered and an athlete improperly using a flag can create a major controversy), and a poster of every U.S. Olympic Committee person at the Games and what their job is (so you know from whom to obtain assistance and what they look like). Then, once at the Games, there are newsletters coming out every day and media briefings. Although this information is useful, it can cause "informa-

tion overload" for many of the athletes because they are asked to process much more information than they are used to. At the end of the day, we are trying to create a positive social emotional environment that gets simpler and simpler for the athletes.

The mogul staff created a positive social emotional climate by securing housing outside the village near the venue for 5 days surrounding the actual Olympic competition. This allowed the coaches to limit the information athletes had to process. At the same time, they were careful not to create an environment that was so isolated and focused that the athletes thought too much about the Games and their performance. For instance, provisions were made so that the athletes could watch their favorite movie videos, go for hikes in the woods, cross-country ski, attend other events, and work out. So they were active, but they were not being overloaded or distracted in a negative way. This took a great deal of staff effort, especially from the coaches.

In fact, relative to creating a positive social emotional environment, the coaches are the unsung heroes. They spend almost every hour of the day thinking about one thing: how to create a positive social/emotional climate and avoid the distractions. Behind the scenes, however, they are going crazy. For instance, a sponsor was scheduled to provide food services at our out-of-village housing, but the day we moved to it, the coaches learned that the sponsor would not be there for 3 days. This was a major obstacle that had to be overcome. This took a tremendous effort on the part of the coaches and team leader. The obstacle was overcome, and interestingly, the athletes never knew about the problem.

Minimize Questioning in Front of the Athletes.

One way the coaches limited information overload was by requesting that the mogul staff not ask questions in front of the athletes. For instance, questions such as "What is the bus schedule?" and "What are we doing tomorrow?" are important. However, Coach Good felt that when staff asks questions in front of the athletes, it makes the athletes nervous and creates uncertainty. What is really interesting is that, based on his Olympic experience, the athletes do not hear the answer—only the question. Hence, he recommended that although we certainly needed to pose these questions, they should not be posed in front of the athletes.

Be Aware That Athletes and Staff Are Very Sensitive at the Games.

Athletes and staff are very sensitive and can be influenced by little things and events that would not normally affect them. For example, our team leader and assistant coach had a minor argument one day (like a brother and sister would) over a mix up in leaving the training bibs at the village. What struck me about this minor disagreement was that it was tension induced, and soon after it started, the two parties realized that they were wasting time arguing, apologized, and took care of the problem in their usual professional manner. It is important to recognize that Olympic tension will influence the staff as well as the athletes.

Remember That Minor Remarks Can Unknowingly Influence Athletes.

Consultants can influence athletes and coaches by unknowingly making certain minor remarks. For example, I have a habit of greeting people by saying, "How ya doin'" instead of saying, "Hi." However, innocently uttering this phrase at the Olympic games the day before someone's finals, especially if the athlete does not know you very well, might be interpreted as "Does he think I've got a problem? Is something wrong?" So it was really important for me to

recognize that that kind of innocent mannerism might be misinterpreted by athletes, and thanks to Coach Good, I was able to do so.

Help Athletes Avoid Energy-reducing Distractions.

Helping athletes avoid energy-reducing distractions and maintain a performance focus is critical to Olympic success. Major distractions are addressed below.

Opening ceremonies. As previously stated, deciding whether to attend Opening Ceremonies is a difficult decision for athletes who must perform a day or two later. Usually, the organizing committees do an efficient job of transporting the participants in and out of the ceremony, but athletes can be on their feet 5 to 7 hours, and in the winter Games, the weather can often be very cold. At the same time, these ceremonies tend to be very motivational for a team or individual athlete. Although no definitive solution can be offered relative to whether one should or should not attend Opening Ceremonies, it is most important that coaches and competitors consider the tradeoffs of doing so.

Media distractions. The Olympic Games often have more media personnel in attendance than athletes and coaches. Olympic athletes and coaches, then, may often need to deal with more media coverage than at any time in their careers. Ways of helping athletes cope with these potential media distractions include having them take part in media training prior to the Games (the U.S. Olympic Committee does this for all teams), hiring sport-governing-body media coordinators who understand the demands of high-performance sport and protect athletes and coaches from overcommitted media schedules while promoting them and their sport, and, establishing clear rules about when it is and is not appropriate to deal with the media (e.g., no interviews on competition day until after the event).

Family distractions. An athlete's family

and friends can be a major source of support or a very negative distraction at the Olympic Games. The key is for the families and friends to understand the demands of high-performance sport and realize that their athlete may not be able to socialize with them at certain times (e.g., see them the morning of the competition or go out to dinner the night before). Like the sport psychology consultant, family members and friends must be aware of how the athlete could misperceive their innocent comments. The best policy, then, is, prior to the Games, to educate and discuss the optimal role families and friends can play in the Olympic experience. That way, strategies and procedures can be derived that are in the best interest of the athletes.

Staff interference. An important lesson I learned at the Olympic Games was that the sport-governing-body staff can be become a distraction unless on-site performance-related roles or tasks (which do not interfere with performance) are clearly specified. For example, the U.S. Mogul team athletes are used to having their assistant coach and maybe the trainer at the bottom of the hill when they finish a practice run. However, in Nagano, I was present as well as the team leader, a U.S. Olympic team trainer, a U.S. Olympic team doctor, the ski team trainer, and a media person. There were just too many people present trying to be helpful, and the coaches and athletes were being crowded. Based on his previous Olympic experience, the head coach assigned everyone specific roles and/or had them move to more unobtrusive positions. For example, I often videotaped practice and competition runs while, during the semifinals, our team leader helped escort the athletes through the media after competing their runs. So the head coach had a job for everybody. Assigning such roles was critical in eliminating performance-interfering distractions and should be considered in Olympic planning.

Provide Social and Psychological Support for Coaches.

With so much focus on the athletes at the Games, it is often forgotten that the coaches are under much stress and that there may also be the need to assist them in their Olympic quest. For me, the coaches are the unsung heroes of the Games because of the tremendous pressure placed on them to help their athletes produce results; moreover, because of the size and politics of the Games, coaches do not have as much control as usual over the practice and performance environment. Recognizing this state of affairs, the U.S. Olympic Committee has developed a high-performance "coaches' house." In Nagano this was a small apartment in the village. In addition to serving as a high-technology video-feedback center, it provided an important haven of social support for the coaches. The coaches could go to the house after a long day and relieve some of the pressure placed on them. They were able to relax, have some refreshments, and get away from everything for a while. Moreover, everything said was kept confidential as only coaches and sport science and coaching staff were allowed in, so they could vent their frustrations if needed. In essence, this was an important psychological support center for the coaches.

In addition to consulting directly with athletes, Coach Good identified both consulting with coaches and providing general psychological support as important services I provided the mogul coaching staff. Sport psychology consultants, then, should view coach consultations and support as important aspects of the mental-training consultation process.

Be Aware of the Need for Absolute Trust.

The athletes and coaches must absolutely trust the sport psychology consultant. This point came out in interview with Coach Good and emphasizes the importance of establishing long-term working relationships between athletes, coaches and consultants.

Remember That Coach Support Is Critical.

Coach support is critical. The only reason I was able to do the work I did with the mogul team was because of the tremendous support of Coach Good. We had developed a great working relationship, and our styles and personalities meshed well.

Conclusions

No two Olympic Games or teams participating in the Games will be alike, so in interpreting this case study, it is important to recognize that the topics discussed and effectiveness of particular strategies will always need to be customized to the individuals and situations involved. However, based on my Olympic journey as an educational sport psychology consultant and mental coach, a number of general guidelines and principles have been identified as starting points for other consultants to guide their practice. Moreover, being better aware of the unique nature of the Olympic Games environment can help us better assist athletes and coaches in their quests of Olympic excellence. It is hoped that this article helps consultants better assist athletes in achieving their Olympic goals.

References

Bump. L. A. (1989). *Sport psychology study guide*. Champaign, IL: Human Kinetics.

Gould, D. (1998). Goal setting for peak performance. In J. Williams (Ed.), *Applied sport psychology: Personal growth to peak performance* (3rd ed.; pp. 182–196). Palo Alto, CA: Mayfield Publishing Company.

Gould, D., & Damarjian, N. (1998). Mental skills training in sport. In B. C. Elliot (Ed.), *Training in sport: Applied sport science* (pp. 69–116). Chichester, England: John Wiley & Sons, Inc.

Gould, D., Guinan, D., Greenleaf, C., Medbery, R., Lauer, L., Strickland, M., Chung, Y., & Peterson, K. (1998). *Positive and negative factors influencing U.S. Olympic athletes and coaches: Atlanta Games assessment* [U.S. Olympic Committee Sport Science and Technology Grant Final Report]. Colorado Springs, CO: US Olympic Committee.

Hardy, L., Jones, G., & Gould, D. (1996). *Understanding psychological preparation for sport: Theory and practice of elite performers*. Chichester, England: John Wiley & Sons.

Martens, R. (1987). *Coaches guide to sport psychology*. Champaign, IL: Human Kinetics.

Nideffer, R. (1985). *Athletes' guide to mental training*. Champaign, IL: Human Kinetics.

Orlick, T. (1985). *Psyching for sport: Mental training for athletes*. Champaign, IL: Human Kinetics.

Orlick, T., & Partington, J. (1988). Mental links to excellence. *The Sport Psychologist, 2*, 105–130.

Lessons From Sport Psychology Consulting

Keith P. Henschen

As I walked through the dressing room of the NBA team with which I had been working for the last 3 years, I sensed that the atmosphere this morning was a little different than usual. Rather than jovial, it was very tense; in fact, you could probably cut it with a knife. Today, all NBA teams had to reduce their rosters to 12 players. The problem was that we had 14 players, and all but our first-round draft choice (who had signed a guaranteed 3-year contract) were veterans. The harsh reality was that 2 veteran players would have to be released after practice today.

As luck would have it, during practice on this very day, one of the players received a serious injury that would keep him out at least three-fourths of the season. Immediately, he was placed on the injured-reserve list; now only one player would have to be released. As the 2-hour practice came to a close, all eyes were on the coach. Finally, the coach called one of the players over for a private conversation. This player had been in the NBA for over 10 years and had been selected for at least one All Star competition. I watched the coach explain his reasoning, and then he and the player moved away from each other. As the players started to go back to the dressing room, I noticed that the released player left the gym at the opposite end of the floor. This was strange, because he was still in his workout gear. A couple of minutes passed, and then I followed him outside and found him sitting on a bench. I sat down with him but said nothing. After a few minutes of silence, this giant of a man (around 7 feet tall) began to tremble and sob. In a few seconds, I found myself crying right along with him. Here were two grown men, sitting on a bench in the middle of a college campus, sobbing their eyes out. After what seemed like an eternity but was closer to a half hour, the player looked at me and said, What do I do now?

Such is the life of an applied sport psychology professional. What a powerful experience. As I look back on the situation, I feel comfortable that I handled it to the best of my ability, but only time will tell. My philosophy in working with performers at any age has always sprung from a holistic perspective. Their joy is my joy, and their pain is my pain. If I am going to be part of their successes, I must also be available during less successful times.

Regarding the released athlete, I had known him for the past 3 years and considered him to be a friend as well as a professional basketball player or client. We had dined together, had played golf together, and had exchanged ideas and philosophies. He was a human being in my life—as was I, in his.

When the emotional release was fairly well finished, both of us returned to the locker room, fully expecting it to be empty of players. It was not. Eight of the players had showered, but had waited for us to return. One by one, they shook the released player's hand and assured him of their continuing friendship. I waited for the player to shower and to collect his gear; then I went with him to his apartment. Only later in the afternoon did I feel comfortable enough to leave him by himself. For the next 2 days, we spent a lot of time together as he prepared to leave town and return to his place of permanent residence. Since he was near the end of his career (in basketball), I asked if he would like to counsel with someone in his home area concerning career transition. He said he would appreciate that, so I immediately arranged a referral for him.

This may seem like a sad scenario, but it is one that occurs all the time in professional sports. I still receive telephone calls periodically from this former player and delight in the fact that he has readjusted to a normal lifestyle and is once again enjoying life outside of athletics.

Holistic Approach

As I stated before, my philosophy and my modus operandi have always been based on a holistic perspective. When I work with a performer, I view him or her as a total person. I frequently come to know not only a player's performing life, but also his or her spiritual, social, and intellectual pursuits. They are not just performers to me; rather, they are unique people. Athletes in particular are not special people, as society is prone to believe; they are merely people with special physical talents. I treat these talented athletes no differently than I do anyone else. I marvel at their physical deeds just as I do the work of an artist, an actor, or a poet; but I admire their accomplishments—not necessarily the people who perform them. My holistic approach means that I am involved in the following aspects (with their consent) of my clients' lives:

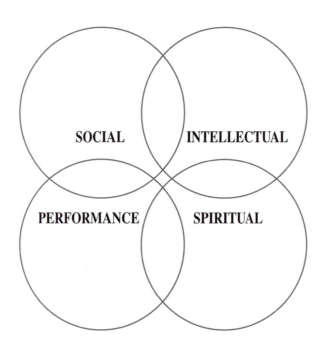

Of course, with younger performers I am very careful not to intrude into some of these aspects of their lives (i.e., social, spiritual) unless they or their parents specifically request it. I do not purposefully display my value system to the athlete unless it is deemed important to all the parties involved. Young performers are particularly vulnerable and impressionable, so it is essential that I show the most ethical behavior at all times.

Cultural Implications

Since I employ a holistic approach, it has been crucial for me to broaden my understanding of the cultures from which many of the athletes with whom I work have their roots. The following vignette emphasizes some of the issues I have faced.

One of my first trips as an international sport psychology consultant was with the Senior United States Track Team, to Great Britain (87 athletes—both male and female) for a quadrangular meet against Russia, East Germany, and Great Britain. The head coach called for a team meeting in New York just before we left; at this meeting, I was introduced as the sport psychology consultant for the trip. I only knew, personally, about 10 of the athletes. As the trip began (on the plane), I noticed that very few of the Caucasians interacted with the African Americans. It didn't appear to be a big problem, but it was evident. The coaching staff, on the other hand, had a mixture of ethnic backgrounds and seemed to interact very well. Once we arrived in Great Britain, this pattern of segregation continued and seemed to be the norm rather than the exception. After 2 days on the trip, I had counseled with 12 athletes (11 White and 1 Black). I realized at that point that the Black athletes were hesi-

tant to use my services. Was it me? Was it because I am White? Was it a cultural bias, or was it that they were not familiar with sport psychology?

Not wishing to make an issue of this, I decided to see if I could make some inroads into the African American group of athletes. During each meal, I struck up a conversation with one of the Black athletes and then sat with that athlete and his or her friends. On the fourth day of the trip, two Black athletes finally asked some questions concerning sport psychology and requested some time with me. This seemed to break the ice, as more Black athletes began to request help. On the 7-hour flight back to New York, I sat with one of the Black athletes. He asked about my background and, eventually, about my experiences with African Americans. I thought the latter question was strange, but I answered it. What this athlete said next has stuck with me. He said, "As you know, you are rare. Very few of you sport psychologists can work with the Black athlete. Most sport psychologists don't understand our culture!"

This interaction left me to ponder the validity of the words spoken: This athlete was right on target. The United States has very few African American sport psychologists, yet the majority of athletes at the highest levels in some sports are Black.

If Whites are to work effectively with athletes who come from different cultural backgrounds, then we must understand these cultures thoroughly—an awesome challenge! Many sport psychologists assume that their knowledge of performance in particular and people in general is the most important factor in working successfully with performers. This simple assumption is erroneous. To establish rapport and to eventually become effective in consulting, it is imperative that the sport psychologist understand the athletes' value systems, patterns of behavior, reinforcement preferences, cultural pressures and expectations, and general philosophies of life. Any observant individual realizes that all cultures are different. Traveling in different countries and adjusting to cultural differences is analogous to the challenges faced by the sport psychologist who works with athletes of varied cultural backgrounds. People may look the same the world over, but the determinates of their behaviors differ greatly.

Speak the Language of the Athlete

If there is one element that has helped me communicate with athletes, it is my ability to speak their language. I have made it a point through the years to stay abreast of current slang and frequently-used terms from the cultures I deal with. Does this mean that I always talk like them? No, but I do listen carefully and use some of the phrases or terms judiciously. The novice consultant must use care in this area. It is really apparent to the athletes when someone is trying too hard to speak the language, and that is a turn-off to them.

Speaking the language of athletes involves using words and examples with which they can readily identify. They will be impressed with your ability if you can deal with their problems at *their level*. If you use the language of a particular sport, athletes then realize that you know enough about the sport to discuss it intelligently; this also helps when interacting with coaches or management.

I must admit that speaking the language of the athlete can have a negative side. When presenting at clinics, I will sometimes throw in a few cusswords (i.e., *damn, hell, bullshit*), but never the really offensive ones or the "magic" words. This may offend a few people, but most of the athletes laugh because they understand the humor. It definitely is an attention grabber, but it can also have some negative effects. At one clinic in particular, after a lecture of about 45 minutes in which I used about four cusswords, a coach asked if my cursing ever interfered with my ability to work with highly religious athletes. Initially, I thought this was a strange question, but then I realized that I should use my colorful language less often. Actually, I have had great success with religious athletes because they quickly realize (one-on-one) that I admire and respect their devotion to their values. I guess I speak too often the locker room language of the athlete—one of my faults.

Gender Issues

One evening at dinner, my wife posed a very candid question. She asked, "Are you ever attracted to any of the beautiful athletes whom you counsel?"

Now, how would you answer this question? You could attempt to change the subject, provide a nebulous response, or pull a "President Clinton" and flat out deny the truth.

I was in an interesting situation, but true to my personality, I immediately answered, "Of course I find them attractive." Then I asked, "Why would you ask that question?"

She said that she had recently read an article stating that the highest percentage of psychologists' misconduct or unethical behavior is centered around sexual relationships. My next comment probably saved my bacon. I told my wife that even though I am at the end (the very end) of what could be considered middle age, my eyes still appreciate beauty wherever it occurs. Next, I said that finding someone attractive and allowing yourself to be attracted to someone are completely different scenarios.

In fact, this is a very real problem in our field, as it is in all the helping professions. When I first entered the field of applied sport psychology I was counseled by a leader in our field that the very first issue to get out of the way in any counseling situation is the sexual issue. Due to the nature of the consulting relationship, transference and counter transference can become problems if they are not recognized and dealt with appropriately. It is the consultant's responsibility to monitor his or her feelings and to make sure that he or she stays within appropriate boundaries. If a consultant feels his or her control slipping away in this area, then the consultation should be terminated immediately and a referral made.

Another gender issue that can confront male consultants, as they get older is that their clients can come to view them as father figures if they are not careful. I do not believe that this attachment is as dangerous as sexual attraction, but it can escalate into an awkward situation. Naturally, if your approach to counseling is holistic, you will deal with various aspects of an athlete's life; if your counsel is good, respect and admiration will be natural consequences. Handling this respect and or admiration is your challenge. A technique I have utilized successfully when counseling women is to talk frequently about my wife and daughter. When the opportunity arises, I make sure to introduce my wife and daughter to those athletes with whom I am working. Also, when I work with high school- or college-age females in my private practice, I generally do the consulting at my home. My wife and my children, when they were younger, are always in close proximity. This minimizes opportunities for an undesirable consequence and sends a message that my family life is solid. All of us are human, so it is important that we structure situations so that there are virtually no opportunities for transgression.

As a male sport psychology consultant who works frequently with female performers, I operate on one basic principle—*Leave your ego at home.* I do not need to soothe my male ego at the expense of my values. All males, as we progress in age, like to perceive ourselves as still being attractive to the opposite sex. We can fulfill these desires by remaining ethical and by relishing the appreciation our clients extend to us for our help, rather than by allowing relationships to evolve into problematic areas.

General Reflections

As I write this chapter I wish to share the general principles that I have learned during my career in applied sport psychology. In the previous section, I revealed one of those principles—leaving your ego out of the picture. Now I would like to share some other important lessons.

Limitations. If there is one thing that I do know, it is what I don't know. I once heard that a wise man knows that he doesn't know it! None of us, as sport psychology consultants, is perfect, and we all have limitations. We must recognize our personal limitations and, of course, try to improve on them. We will find it difficult—and sometimes impossible—to work effectively with certain individuals, because of our limitations. Our personalities are naturally more pleasing to some people than to others. This is not a weakness, just a fact of life. Just as teachers in a classroom, we can stimulate some students, while others will fail to appreciate our style. The following example illustrates the point:

*During my opening remarks to a college women's tennis team, I noticed that one athlete was inattentive and, apparently, bored—either by me or by the subject matter (group dynamics). As was my practice, I asked each of the athletes to complete a few (3) psychometric assessments and return them to me in a few days. I would then **assess** them and provide individual feedback* *during our weekly sessions. All of the young ladies returned the tests fairly quickly, except one. This player (the bored one) had to be reminded three times to turn in the tests, and it took her 4 weeks. I asked the coach if this was her pattern of behavior (being late) and the coach said, "No, she is normally just the opposite." In the meantime, I had already had two or three individual sessions with each of the other players on the team, and they were busy improving their mental skills.*

Finally, the tests from this particular athlete were turned in, and I scheduled an individual session with her. The session was a disaster. The player was noncommunicative and quite defensive. Finally, at the end of the session, I asked her, point-blank, "Why the attitude?"

She said, "What attitude?" So I responded, "Hey, it is obvious you don't want to be here. Is it what we're doing, or is it me?

She looked startled but then showed great candor. She said, "I think it might be you. It's not that I don't like you, but you are so dominant, and I try not to be dominated."

I think my response really floored her. I said, "I appreciate your feelings and I am glad you voiced your concerns." Then I asked her if she was still interested in developing some mental performance skills, and she said she was. I suggested that maybe she would feel more comfortable working with Jamie (one of my doctoral students). She said she would be willing to give it a try.

The final report on this situation was that my graduate student established a great rapport with this athlete and worked with her for 2 years, until the tennis player graduated. Jamie (the graduate student) told me a few years later that the player had a problem with a dominant male in her life and that my behavior reminded her of that male. The athlete appreciated the fact that I didn't take her uneasiness personally.

Again, my philosophy in counseling is the same as my philosophy in teaching: If my limitations are such that I can't help a person, somebody else probably can. So I leave my ego out and recognize that I have limitations; at the same time, I attempt to help the person find a counseling environment that is comfortable for him or her.

Competencies

My advice to any sport psychology practitioner is to stick to your competencies. It should also go without saying that your training dictates the general areas in which you should have expertise but that training does not always result in actual expertise. Experience *and* training are the normal ingredients of expertise. I fail to understand the unmitigated gall of clinical psychologists who, without experiences in the field, market themselves as sport psychologists. My area of competence is performance enhancement, and I believe it would be highly unethical for me to promote myself in any other area of sport psychology. It takes a lot of experience in a variety of areas to become effective in applied sport psychology, and knowledge in the clinical area is only the beginning. For those individuals who have psychological course work, it is imperative that they supplement this knowledge with supervised applied internships. Psychology is the foundation; application is the process. It is not enough to have the scientific psychological knowledge; you must also master the art of application.

Art of Application

I realize my statements in this section will not endear me to many colleagues, but I believe these things must be said. There is an *art* to applied sport psychology. Great people in any endeavor are actually artists. Not all great sport psychologists adhere to the same processes, but they attain all the same results. Their approaches to application are uniquely individual, yet they are based on the same principles. When I contemplate the names of the premier sport psychology practitioners of the world, a number of great people readily come to my mind, but no two of these individuals utilize identical procedures or processes. What they do have in common, as the artists of applied sport psychology, is their adherence to the following principles:

A. *Be yourself.* You must know yourself and be yourself to be effective. Knowing your limitations and which techniques to employ are essential. My success, however limited it may be, has resulted because I am who I am. I have never tried to emulate someone else's style. Yes, I have learned from others and have incorporated their methods into my repertoire— but in my own way. When I think of artists, I always think of Frank Sinatra and his song "My Way." If you are not yourself, the athletes you are counseling will recognize it immediately, and your charade will lessen your effectiveness. There is only one Michael Jordan, one Vince Lombardi, and one you. There are no techniques in our field that are secret, but the ways in which different counselors employ these methods are definitely unique.

B. *Please yourself.* The first priority of any human behavior is to please oneself. You must enjoy what you are doing, or you will cease doing it emotionally. It pleases me to help others attain their potential.

Helping others to master their challenges and to overcome their struggles gives me great inner joy.

As I sat in the audience in the Special Events Center at the University of Utah and witnessed the NCAA Women's Gymnastics Championship, I became very emotional. I watched as the young ladies I had been counseling and teaching for the last year performed almost flawlessly in routine after routine. Here was a collection of collegiate gymnasts, ranked fourth in the nation, who were on the verge of winning another national championship in front of 15,000 cheering fans. As a team, they came together and—in event after event—put the mental skills we had been practicing into performance. As I sat there and wept openly, my wife looked at me and asked, "Why are you crying?" I explained that these were tears of joy (in fact, as I write this section, I am weeping again). This was not the first national championship team I had worked with (this particular team had won eight previous championships while I was their sport psychology consultant), but it was the most pleasing to me. Because I knew the adversities these athletes had endured— injuries, eating disorders, family problems, and excessive challenges—it pleased me greatly to see them performing so well. I was really happy!

When I say that you must please yourself, I realize that it may sound hedonistic and selfish, but I firmly believe that you must receive great pleasure from the process and not merely from the results. Every artist enjoys wholeheartedly his or her creative expression.

C. *Use your intuition.* Intuition seems to be one of the most mysterious cognitive abilities of humans; each of us is blessed with varying degrees of this phenomenon. I attribute many of my successes to the use of intuition. Long ago, I learned to listen to my soft inner voices or to my feelings to direct some of my decisions. Again, I think intuition is probably a combination of knowledge and experience that is stored somewhere in the recesses of our memory. This information becomes available to each of us in a variety of situations, but we frequently fail to heed the prompting of this powerful, natural human ability. Instead of utilizing this gift, we do exactly what we try to teach our clients not to do—we employ our analytical thought processes. In other words, we try to think our way to success rather than relying on intuition. My greatest accomplishments in terms of counseling have resulted not because I knew exactly what to do, but because I was willing to listen to my inner guidance.

D. *Cultivate confidence and a positive self-concept.* Confidence, in my experience, is not a global concept; rather, it has very specific manifestations. Great performers and great applied sport psychology consultants are not necessarily confident people overall, but they are very confident within their realms of performance. Also, high-level performers frequently are not the highest scorers in the area of self-concept. My statements probably will not be well received by researchers in sport psychology, but I believe they are valid. Most of us have high self-concept and high self-confidence in some situations but not in others. Here is a case in point: One of the players with whom I work is a perennial NBA all-star and is recognized as one of the best players ever to play in his po-

sition. I would offer that he has an above-average (but not excessive) general self-concept. He believes in himself, but only in certain situations. His confidence in social situations is very low, but put him on the basketball court and his confidence soars. The old adage that confidence and self-concept are synonymous with success is only partially correct.

E. *Learn to use the tools in the toolbox.* Each athlete is unique; therefore, a particular athlete will respond to one technique better than to another. The best applied sport psychology consultants are those who have a variety of tools in their toolboxes and know when to utilize each of them. If you advocate or become proficient in the delivery of only one method, you are doomed or limited to success with only a few performers. Not only must you have a variety of techniques at your disposal, you must also master the application of a variety of procedures within a given technique (e.g., breathing, progressive relaxation, and/or autogenic training).

The greatest abuse I see in this area involves the general concept of goal setting. Goal setting seems to benefit some individuals, but it also evidences frequent negative effects with other individuals. The bottom line is that the modification of human behavior and/or emotions requires the availability of a plethora of tools. The challenge is to practice these techniques until you are proficient not only in their delivery but also in your sense of which of them to use at a particular time. If you want to be an effective force in applied sport psychology, your toolbox should be packed with tools.

F. *Be passionate.* Unless you are passionate about what you do, you will eventually find yourself merely going through the motions. Having worked in this field for around 30 years, I still find myself excited about going to work every day and working with performers. I remain committed to the discipline of sport psychology and hope to continue to contribute my voice to the field. I am convinced that what sport psychologists do in the applied area makes a difference in the performance of the majority of individuals with whom they come into contact. When my passion subsides, I will retire.

G. *Be compassionate.* From a number of the experiences I have related in this article, it should be clear that I genuinely care about other human beings. My holistic philosophy requires that I get to know many individuals at a very personal level and learn to care sincerely for them. I love to watch people learn new skills and overcome challenges and adversity. In the process, I feel the hurt, the pain, and—sometimes—the agony they are enduring. Compassion is a necessity in the helping professions.

H. *Have a method to your madness.* Every applied sport psychology consultant should work from a theoretical framework to guide his/her actions. Consultants need a plan or strategy so that they are not just shooting in the dark. For each group or person with whom I work, I develop a plan of action, with checkpoints along the way to evaluate progress.

I. *Use your counseling skills.* The final principle that all great applied sport psychology consultants follow is the employment of counseling skills. All of my doctoral students are required to complete a general counseling allied area as a portion of their doctoral studies. Why? Because in applied sport psychology, your effectiveness is grounded in your counseling skills. Interviewing effectively, listening skillfully, communicating well, using noninvasive methods of probing, and monitoring nonverbal messages—all are essential in applied sport psychology. If your counseling skills are weak or limited, your chances of achieving success in applied sport psychology are very remote.

Other Considerations

I was right on time for the appointment, and as I entered the boardroom of X Corporation, I was impressed by who was in attendance. A week previous, the general manager of an NBA team had called me and asked if I would be interested in joining their staff as a sport psychology consultant. I said, "Yes, I would be interested." The general manager then asked me to attend a meeting where sport psychology services would be discussed and I would be interviewed for the position. In my excitement, I neglected to ask who would be at the meeting, so I was a little surprised to walk into the room and find the entire coaching staff (4 men), the trainers (2), the team doctor, the general manager, the president, the director of player personnel, and the team owner in attendance. So much for a small, intimate meeting. After the customary formal introductions, the general manager facilitated the meeting and the questions began. The president immediately asked me what I could bring from sport psychology that would make the team better. In response, I explained that individual mental-skills training, group dynamics for the team, input into the drafting process, and consultation with the coaching staff were all areas in which I might contribute. My response seemed to sit well with most of the people in

*the room, but I still sensed some reluc-
tance. The head coach then asked a
very pointed question: "We tried this
before and it didn't work out. Why do
you think you can be successful where
someone else wasn't? Also, three
fourths of our team is Black, and the
previous consultant was also Black,
but the players wouldn't accept him.
You are White, which probably makes
it more difficult—again, why do you
think it will work for you?"*

*My answer was very candid. I replied,
"I am familiar with the previous person you hired, and he wasn't really in
the field of sport psychology. His expertise was in social work. Our training and approaches will probably be
totally different. As I understand it, he
tried to be 'one of the guys.' Look at
me—I am in my late forties, gray-
haired, and have no desire to 'be one
of the guys.' I do want to be accepted
by them, but not as a peer—rather, as a
resource. I know your previous consultant was Black, but I don't think my
skin color will be a detriment once the
players get to know me and what I do.
My work in track and field at the
Olympic level involves many African
Americans. I think you already know
something about my reputation, or you
wouldn't have called me."*

*The head coach continued. He said, "I
don't know about all this stuff. I sure
didn't have it when I played in the
NBA."*

*I chuckled. "Hey, a lot of things have
changed since you played in the NBA."
Everyone laughed, but then I continued,
"And the players are different, society's
expectations are different, the money is
different, and the lifestyles of the players have changed dramatically. I realize*

*you are a little hesitant to include this
area in your sports medicine team, because of previous experiences, but I pre-
dict that either you do it now as a pre-
ventative measure or you will have to
include it later to deal with crises."*

*The next question was a beauty. The
owner asked what I would do the first
year. My answer floored him! I said,
"Very little. I would spend most of the
year being present at practices, at
shoot-arounds, and in the locker
room." I stated that before I could be
effective with either the players or the
coaches, they would have to feel comfortable with me as a person and with
the field I represent. I also told him that
I would not want to travel with the team
unless there was a particular need. In
addition to being around the team
when they were home, I said, I would
take every player (individually) to
lunch to get to know each of them personally and to allow them to become
acquainted with me. Other than that, I
would do very little the first year.*

During this meeting, I did not promise the
world or try to sell an unrealistic product. I
was merely myself, and I attempted to convey the importance of the psychological side
of performance. A disbelieving head coach
is a common problem but not one that cannot
be overcome. In fact, I probably worked
more with the coaching staff the first year
than I did with the players. Once the coaching staff is in your corner, you have won half
your battle of acceptance.

When working with professional athletes,
there are a couple of other imperatives. First,
stay in the background. You are in this situation as a resource, just the same as any other
member of the sports medicine team. Do not
try to be part of the action; rather, stay out of
the limelight. The athletes will quickly take

note if you are always there when reporters or television cameras are in the vicinity. The athletes are the show, and what we do for them in terms of sport psychology contributes only slightly to their success. In other words, do not overvalue your contributions, and always give the credit to the athlete.

Second, be a pro, not a fan. At the professional level, you will be working with the greatest athletes in the world. This is exciting as well as challenging. Remember, though— these are not special people; they are merely people with special physical talents. If you get caught up in being a fan rather than being a professional, you will compromise your credibility. Athletes need reality from you, not adulation. This is true at all levels of competition. Never, never chase athletes around to get their autographs. If you do, you become just another groupie.

Summary

In this article I have shared some of my reflections and experiences as an applied sport psychology professional. I, of course, have very few answers as to what a sport psychology professional should always be or do; I can only share what has been successful for me. Simply, my limited success has come about because I have been able to detect the issues behind the issues. Obvious issues are seldom the ones that really demand work.

The only other piece of advice I can give, which has been effective for me, is to read avidly. I enjoy digesting information from almost all fields and then applying these materials creatively to my work in sport psychology. These creative applications have nourished my enthusiasm and replenished my zest for change. When I discover a concept in physics or chemistry that is applicable to sport psychology, I am elated. After all, isn't the application of information the essence of understanding?

Experiences With Application of Action-Theory-Based Approach in Working With Elite Athletes

Dieter Hackfort

Introduction

Within a few minutes of our first meeting, coaches and athletes are quick to emphasize what an important, predominant role psychology plays in their sports, and how psychological factors are of the utmost importance, critical for success in competition. When athletes or coaches (together or alone) request my assistance and we commence our working relationship, they usually understand that I am familiar with various sports, that I have worked with Olympic athletes and professionals, and that I have a great deal of experience in mental coaching. Nonetheless, I ask them to tell me about their special situations, including the main aspects of their sports training and competition—the purpose of this being to expand my knowledge base in their particular sports or disciplines.

Sometimes athletes or coaches recount personal problems that confront them; however, most of the time they refer to their sports or disciplines in more general terms. They explain what is special about their sports and what a sport psychologist should know when confronted with athletes in these sports. They also may refer to problems that arise from their psychosocial environment, such as marital, coaching, or educational problems. In the case of an athlete who has

not experienced success for a long period, one single problem or cause generally does not account for his or her lack of success. More often, the problem is a combination of elements, consisting of personal factors, factors related to the task (sport at hand), and environmental factors. In my work, a first step is to learn the subjective definition of the situation and to determine the methods the athlete or coach has implemented to deal with the problem up to that point.

In this chapter, I use some examples that are, in some respect, typical of my work and that might have a fundamental meaning in applied sport psychology. Applied work should be theoretically based. Here it is based on an action-theory perspective in psychology. This perspective was originally termed *Handlungspsychologie*, which might be better-labeled *Handlungs psychology* or *action psychology,* though the latter is not a precise representation of the words. This conceptual frame is elaborated with special reference to acting in sports, and it is a prevalent perspective in German academic and applied sport psychology (Hackfort, Munzert, & Seiler, 2000). I present here limited information to clarify the perspective for a sufficient understanding of the practice described. I do not provide a "case report" approach but refer instead to selected examples of concrete problems, representing fundamental aspects and central issues that confront me in my applied sport psychology work.

Issues Concerning Action Situations

A fundamental assumption of the action theory is the constellation built up by the person, the environment, and the task. The individual interprets this constellation. The situation definition depends strongly on the action the person must organize and realize. Both objective and subjective factors influence the way a person handles a downhill situation, and the concept of the person's competencies influences his or her decisions, action plan, and means of realizing that action plan. The execution of the action influences the person-environment-task constellation and the following definition of the (next) action execution. A person becomes aware about the person-environment-task constellation as soon as he or she defines a goal. Actions as goal-directed behavior are intentionally guided and purposive activities of a human being. (Animals are only able to organize behavior at a lower level; that is, without reflections and rationality.)

On the background of his or her individual definition of the situation, the athlete is using strategies from personal experience that are representations of his or her understanding and orientation. These strategies are "naive," as they are not systematically developed, applied/realized, and evaluated. This, however, does not mean that they are unintelligent methods. They are expressions of the naive psychological concept of the athlete or the coach. For the professional sport psychologist, it is very important to learn about such concepts and strategies as the psychologist should comprehend the athlete's actions and the reasons and attributions for these actions, as these can be con-

sidered as a starting point. It is also necessary to be informed about such concepts, beliefs, and convictions to prevent resistance or inability to change.

When an alpine ski racer came to see me after a very serious accident in a World Cup race, he asked me what he could do to repress and forget this experience. First, I asked him for the reason he believed that it would be better to forget this accident. He explained that, in his opinion, an "extinction" would be a precondition to face racing situations again, which for him meant to "touch the limit." If he could not repress the incident, he thought there would be an inhibition and this would hinder his efforts to be successful again. He expected help to overcome the cognitions and pictures about the accident in his mind. I convinced him that repression did not mean that such thoughts would never appear again and that he should have been learning something from that situation. Learning from that situation might have served as the best protection for such an accident never to happen again (which might be unrealistic in this sport) and might have increased the probability of appropriate coping with such a situation. Thus, repression was not the correct strategy, but rather coping with the experience and coming up with a better alternative. He accepted this advice, and we started to analyze the situation.

After a short time, it turned out that it was not the first accident this ski racer had had. Previous accidents had not have such serious (physical) effects and (psychological) consequences, but he (step by step) could remember (in a semihypnotic state) seven accidents. He was astonished about his recollection of seven accidents, which made it very clear for both of us that he had been quite successful in repressing memories of accidents up to that point. This did not mean that these experiences had not been of any influence on subsequent actions and that this strategy was not appropriate for his health and performance.

Further analyses of the accidents revealed that frequently "signs of trouble" had started as early as the evening before the race. After practice, when he knew his time and ranking, he had reflections about the strategies he planned to use to be successful, and these pushed him towards his limit (task-oriented analysis). He was occupied with worries and cognitions (imaginations) about his public reputation. Fear of failure, an extremely high level of aspiration, and unpleasant feelings came to his mind. He became aware of his negative feelings when he was resting on the couch for a massage by the physiotherapist. The massage was aimed to enhance his relaxation, but the cognitions about his strategies were strong, and he experienced alarming signals, which indicated to him that he was in a less than optimal condition. He slept for only a few hours. The next day, in the lift that took him to the race, he had extremely unpleasant feelings. He vomited and responded to his colleagues' questions by referring to his bad stomach as a physical, not a psychic problem. In addition to the athlete himself, two other people could have or should have become aware of the psychic nature of the problem in this situation, but nobody had talked with the coach, and a sport psychologist was not included in the team at that time. All this refers to an environment-oriented analysis. In the prestart situation, the athlete tried (with some degree of success) to suppress his worries and to ignore his negative feelings (person-oriented analysis).

To take his feelings as signals, and especially fear as a signal for danger, was my next message for the athlete. I explained to him that feelings, and especially negative feelings, stem from something real. They have a meaning and occur as more than just something to impede optimal performance. These feelings have reasons, make sense, and they are of functional meaning with regard to action regulation. To ignore such signals makes it impossible to harness them and react to them in an effective manner. To be sensitive for such feelings makes it possible to initiate safety strategies in time and to protect against threatening circumstances.

To handle his body sensations and to become focused, I taught him a relaxation-activation technique and a strategy for concentration. For relaxation, deep breathing was used, combined with differential muscle activation and relaxation (legs and arms). For the prestart situation, the athlete learned to turn his attention from disassociative cues to inner associative cues (relaxation-activation of the leg and arm muscles). Next, he turned his attention outward to the periphery of the course and then to the center of the course (attention narrowing) to reduce the width of attention. This strategy was practiced first in training sessions, and then in competition in Eurocup races; then, finally, it was successfully realized in World Cup races. His colleagues were very surprised that he was back in the circus in such a short time after his accident, and they commented that he was demonstrating a new style with regard to his character.

At the beginning, I was not very sure if the accident and the psychological rehabilitation were the major problems. I reflected also on psychotherapy and considered the alternative of placing the responsibility in the hands of a psychotherapist. I discussed this with a colleague and with the medical doctor of the athlete who had served the national ski racing team for many years. Both encouraged me (as a sport psychologist) to work with this athlete. Once I recognized his emotional and mental coping strategies, I decided to begin working with this skier.

Issues Concerning Action Regulation

Actions are subdivided into various phases (anticipation phase, realization phase, and interpretation phase) that are characterized by particular regulation processes. In the anticipation phase, planning and calculation processes are of utmost importance. *Planning* refers to the hierarchy of goals, to the way or course of execution, and means of performing an action. *Calculation* refers to costs and benefits, necessary input (e.g., exertion) and possible output (gain), and it is closely connected with motivational processes (e.g., aspiration level). In the phase of realization, especially, tuning and processing are of major importance. Whereas *tuning* refers to the psychophysiological activation (psyching up, psyching down, etc.), processing refers to the psychomotor execution (e.g., mental training, visualization, etc. are techniques aimed to improve or enhance preconditions in this area). In the phase of interpretation, especially, controlling and evaluation processes are important. *Controlling* refers to whether the set goals have been achieved. *Evaluation* refers to "judgments" about the degree and significance of discrepancies and attributions following successful or unsuccessful performance or outcome.

Some fundamental aspects in the analysis of action regulation can be illustrated by a brief report on work with an athlete from the Nordic combination skiing sport who had problems with the ski jumping discipline. The focus here is on the process of calculation, definition of the aspiration level, and decreases/increases of self-confidence.

The athlete was performing on the senior level for one year, and during this time, he was unable to repeat his performance from previous years when he belonged to the junior-athlete category. The level of performance in the group of senior athletes was higher than in the group of junior athletes, according to his coach, but this should not have caused a major difference. The coach argued that he could not understand why the athlete was unable to jump as far as he had done in the past.

Instead of an improvement, as was expected by both the athlete and the coach, there was a decrement in performance, and the athlete could have been eliminated from the team if he had not demonstrated a significant improvement in performance during the upcoming competitions.

When I asked both athlete and coach about the result in the last competition, they expressed great disappointment. When I asked them why it was disappointing, they explained that the athlete had been very good in training, but in competition he was not able to jump as far as he had done in training. After that, I asked them to tell me his best jump in competition and in training. He had jumped 69 meters in the competition and 78 (best jump) meters in training. Next, I asked them what they had expected for the competition, and they answered 78 meters. If he had been able to jump 78 meters, he would have made a good placing and would have had no problems staying on the team, but now he might be eliminated from the team. When I asked if it would be realistic to expect the longest jump in competition, they were astonished. From comments of the athlete it emerged, he felt that only his best result from training would be accepted as a good performance in competition. In addition, he was not very aware about the differences between the best jump and good ones; he had clear causal attributions only for bad jumps. We discussed these issues (calculation, expectancy and aspiration level, and awareness about factors contributing to success) and came to some conclusions:

It would be reasonable to estimate a mean distance of jumps during the last week of training and to expect certain deviations. We operationalized, on the basis of experience and with respect to statistics, that the mean ± 1SD should define the zone of a realistic performance level and only jumps below this zone should be defined as failure. The task for the next training session was to shift up this zone (and not only trying to raise the mark for the longest jump). This should have heightened the probability of success without the risk of inducing further stress associated with improving the longest jump.

Both the athlete and the coach should pay more attention to successful jumps in order to identify significant elements associated with success (and not predominantly discuss bad jumps).

Elements (factors, determinants of success) should be combined in a brief "action plan for success." In this way, I tried to modify the expectations and establish a more realistic level of aspiration in an attempt to reduce the level of pressure experienced by the athlete. Because the athlete was not sufficiently aware of the elements associated with success, the hint to focus on successful jumps and to reflect on successful experiences should have heightened his self-awareness and positively have influenced his self-efficacy to ski jump.

The idea for such an intervention strategy is that pure practice (only doing, repetition of trials) is not sufficient for learning or development. Evaluation of practice is a precondition of consciously experiencing one's competencies as a special aspect of self-experience and self-concept. This is a cognitive representation and a basis for reflections closely connected with self-awareness (including self-efficacy). Self-efficacy in combination with a realistic level of aspiration is advantageous for experiencing success (including an internal attribution). Internal attributions of success are preconditions for the development of self-confidence. Trait self-confidence, combined with a realistic definition of the level of aspiration and an experience-based self-efficacy, leads to (actual, actualized) state self-confidence in a given situation, and this (self-confidence) corresponds with the situation-specific optimal (and not situation-unspecific maximum or ideal) performance.

Further aspects with regard to action regulation are concentration and decision-making. These were serious problem for a female archer. When she asked me for help, she had just been dropped from the national A-team. She told me that she had experienced poor results in the past national and international competitions because she was very nervous. To explain her competitive stress, she argued that it "cost" her too much time for the shots. Archers allow 150 seconds for three shots. After 120 seconds, a warning signal (yellow light) indicates that 30 seconds are left for completing the remaining shots. Very often, the athlete had released only one shot up to this signal and then became nervous because the two remaining shots had to be executed in 30 seconds. I asked her the reasons for taking such a long time for the first shot. She answered that the first shot was very important: If the first shot was poor, a final good result was almost improbable, as the level of performance was extremely high and very tied for the top archers.

After talking about the situation in more detail, it turned out that she often aborted the first shot, sometimes two times, because she was not sure she was aiming the arrow into the center of the target. After lifting the bow, and while aiming, she tried to focus on the center of the target; then, she noticed that she was shaky in that position and tried to refine it. However, when it was getting shakier and shakier, she lowered the bow. After about 105 seconds, she noticed that competitors on her left and right side had already completed their shots (world-class athletes only need around 105 seconds on average for the three shots). This observation initiated further doubts about her success and further increased nervousness. As a consequence, the last two shots were usually completed under stress, with insufficient concentration.

It was my belief that her problems occurred because she did not appear to have an appropriate strategy for concentration (attentional narrowing), aiming, and decision-making (shot release). We discussed possibilities to overcome these problems and developed the following strategy (some minor aspects and supporting measures have been omitted in this description): The target consists of circles of various colors. The outermost ring is white. The target is then made up of black, red, and light yellow rings. The centermost ring is dark yellow. After lifting the bow and correctly positioning herself for aiming, the athlete looked to the edge of the target and pointed with the tip of the arrow to the middle of the white ring. Following this, she proceeded to point from one ring to the next, moving her focus from the edge of the ring to the middle. As her aim reached the middle of each ring, she repeated to herself the color of the ring. When she reached the middle of the center ring, she said to herself, "Shoot" and released the arrow. This strategy assisted the athlete in organizing her concentration and aiming into a process that led to the decision. The decision was no longer connected with thoughts such as "Shall I?", "Is it good enough?", "Is it better now?", "No, should be better now, no. . . ." The point at the middle of each ring acted as checkpoints for the athlete's aim. The movement from one checkpoint to the next alleviated the impression of shaky hands, which was a sign of nervousness for her. During the following training sessions through practicing the strategy in sets of three shots, the athlete successfully developed a rhythm for the strategy. This enabled her to complete all three shots in a 108-second timeframe. A few weeks later, the athlete won a national competition and requalified for the national A-team. The following world championships were very successful for the team.

Some time later, a coach of the national rifle-shooting team informed me that one of his female athletes had a problem with her shooting during the final stage of a competition. It appeared to the coach as if "she wanted to do it too good." She did not appear to be as determined in her routine in the final stages of competition as in the first part of competition. I informed the coach about my previous experiences with the archer. This interested him greatly. An appointment was made with the athlete in to discuss the problem and possible methods of overcoming it. She was interested to start working on it immediately. The concentration and aiming strategy used with the archer was adapted to satisfy the shooting situation. Additional elements, such as breathing and self-talk, were incorporated into the process. Again, this strategy proved successful, and both athlete and coach were satisfied. The athlete is still one of the best shooters in Germany. The basic structure of the strategy described here appears to be of fundamental importance. Further explanation of this idea is included in the following section.

Issues Concerning Orientation Regulation

The development of an action plan requires exploration of two issues: first, the intentions and aspired goals and, second, opportunities. The action situation is analyzed to identify an intentional orientation (goals, subgoals) as well as an instrumental orientation (ways and means to realize interventions). These are related to the processes in the anticipation phase of an action, previously described and characterized as orientation regulation. In sports, where the task is to hit a target, such as golf or shooting, the environment is not ever changing, and other competitors do not try to obstruct performance. However, in sports such as soccer or basketball, the first step of the requested action should be to check the environmental circumstances (e.g., light, weather, noise, and ground) and to consider the relevant cues in the environment (external action space) with regard to the action. The orientation for this process is external. The concept of the environment then has to be related to the person's actual self-concept. The athlete's self-concept should include appraisals of actual abilities and emotional state (internal action space). The actual self-concept can be considered internal in orientation. When these two concepts are related to each other, the relationship between environment and athlete becomes a function of the concept of the task, which is adjusted for this connection. The process of bringing together the self-concept with the concept of the environment in order to define what has to be done (concept of the task) is considered an internal-external orientation.

The requested action to complete the task is an external realization of an internal concept. This conceptualization is fundamental for understanding the functional meaning of mental training (mental rehearsal, mental practice). Based on this conceptualization the psychologist determines what has to be done (concept of the task) and the conditions under which it needs to be done (external and internal conditions: concept of environment and self-concept). An understanding of how it can be done (action concept) is developed. This concept is the basis for action regulation in the realization phase of an action. Thus, it is of significant orientation. The concept as a set of answers to the question "How do I have to complete the task at hand?" consists of a number of aspects, such as instrumental instructions and imaginations. However, the concept also refers to emotional aspects, such as mood, feelings, and especially a feeling for the movement, which has to be executed. These aspects are often neglected. In particular, this feeling for

the movement is very important for the orientation immediately before and during the execution of the movement.

The orientation for an effective action has to take into consideration cognitive and emotional aspects. Actions consist of cognitions, emotions, and motions. In order to carry out the most suitable action, it is necessary to work on the integration of cognitive, emotional, and motor processes. This is one of the main reasons for the necessity to consider psychological competence in all efforts to improve actions, not only in the sporting domain, but also in other contexts, such as industry. In the sporting context, it is important to consider not only competition, but also and especially training. As psychological competence is based on special qualifications and sport is a special setting, specialists are necessary. Hence, sport psychologists as the relevant specialists, should not only be consulted when there is a problem (e.g., emotional problems, stress, nervousness) and/or before a competition, but should also be integrated into the training process and the team of consultants working with the coach and the athlete continuously.

In summary, the outlined orientation regulation follows an external–internal-external perspective. First, the external action space (external orientation) is evaluated and defined. Second, the internal action space (internal orientation) is evaluated and defined. A relation is established by defining the concept of the task. An action concept is developed, including cognitions and feelings. Through mental practice, the feeling for the requested movement is amplified, and thus, the feeling can serve as an orientation in the action-regulation process when executing the movement. Third, the anticipated action (outside orientation) is realized, and the process of execution and the results are evaluated. After explaining this concept to the athlete, it is important for his or her orientation regulation to keep in mind the process "from external to internal to external."

Individual orientation regulation is sometimes influenced by the orientation of others—not only in team sports. I further explain this by using an example from working with the German national weight-lifting team. Before the Olympics in Seoul, a national (final) competition took place for the selection of the eight Olympic team members. Soon after this competition, I noticed that in the team of eight athletes there were two groups. One group comprised those who had already reached their goal by being selected as members of the team. This group was very relaxed, and their concentration in training was significantly reduced. The other group consisted of athletes who were medal contenders. For the athletes in this group, stress was significantly increasing, and engagement in training was heightened. In the first group were two athletes who had a close friendship with two athletes in the second group. This caused some concerns in interpersonal relations between the athletes and conflicts during training sessions. I talked about it with the national coaches and explained to them that the interests of each group were very different. As a result, we decided to develop two training groups with special considerations for training, such as times and locations. In addition, sharing of rooms was changed. Following this intervention, there were no further troubles, as the orientations in the training groups were now similar. Three athletes of the team from the second training group won medals (one silver and two bronze medals), which was an unexpected success for the team.

An essential mental basis for being able to organize and realize movement actions under various external and internal conditions is the availability of an action concept. For example, when something occurs that was not expected and the athletes are under stress, some athletes lose control (control about the situation, self-control, control about the movement actions) because they do not have an elaborated action concept. This refers to the cognitive concept of which the athlete is aware. The elaboration of such a concept is described in the following section.

Elaboration of an Action Concept

A professional golfer had a problem of being too unreliable to improve results and obtain a higher ranking. In one tournament, he played well, but in the next tournament, he was unable to make the cut (the cut divides the players after two rounds and the top 65 ranked players and ties go on to play the third and fourth round). After a very good round, he often played a very poor round or vice versa. When the "drives" and "long shots" were good, the "short shots," and especially his "putting," were poor or vice versa. These experiences led to manifestations in his attitude toward playing golf and his self-concept as a professional golfer. He believed that his mental skills were lacking and asked me to help him to overcome his limitations. After a further interview and some tests, I decided to work with him and to focus on the elaboration of an action concept.

The procedure I followed to develop the action concept was established frame by frame. To achieve this, I considered special modules of the environment (situations, problems, actions, etc.) that are considered (by the athlete and by myself) important aspects of the desired action concept. As already mentioned, it is important to learn from the athlete his or her beliefs, strategies, thinking, reflections, and self-concept and to understand where the athlete is coming from. Usually athletes have an inconsistent self-concept in which some elements are well represented cognitively, and others are neglected and not developed at all. Sometimes the athlete is not aware of beliefs, strategies, and other aspects that determine his or her actions, in which case the behaviors are guided by implicit concepts. In talking with the athlete, he or she may become aware of their self-concept, which is a good starting point from which to work. Often, missing links or elements insufficiently developed can be identified, and the inconsistencies, highlighted. The elaboration of an action concept strongly depends on good cooperation with the athlete and, in most cases, with the coach.

To refer to standard situations, elementary tasks and fundamental actions make it possible to develop the frame and get hints for basic elements. Such standard situations in golf are the first stroke from the tee with the driver, long distance shots on the fairway, chipping situations (ball in the rough or in the bunker), and putting on the green. For such situations, the golfer chooses a special club and follows a special routine, which can be regarded as an action concept closely connected with the chosen club. Choosing a club is the consequence of the definition of the situation, and it is connected with an action concept for solving the task. This special action concept can also be regarded as a module for the action concept for the round (18 holes, one day in the tournament). The action concept for the day consists of, for example, a module for precompetition exercises including warming up, a module for the various situations with the single clubs, a module for strategies between the holes, and a postcompetition module with special regard to recovery and cooling down.

In the case of this professional golfer, the actual routine did not protect against large deviations in performance of specific shots. The golfer was not sufficiently aware of the functional meaning of the movement feeling, and he did not consciously refer to his inner state when taking his starting position

for the drive. He was not sure about linking the test stroke and the drive. We elaborated the following action concept: When it was his turn to play a shot, he went about two meters behind the ball, which was teed, and figured out the target area for the drive. Next, he took his position for the drive, made a step backward, fixed the ball with his eyes, breathed out to a point where he felt neither tension nor relaxation, visualized the movement of the stroke, and recalled the movement feeling. Next, he executed the test shot, rested at the end of the stroke, imagined the flight of the ball, and "sucked in the feeling of that shot like a dry sponge" (such metaphors may be helpful in communicating with the athlete and providing orientation especially with regard to the feeling). After taking the position for the drive, while breathing out as mentioned, he visualized the movement of the shot and executed the drive like "painting the image of the shot" guided by the movement feeling.

In general, new modules are integrated into the frame and combined with already elaborated modules of the superior action concept, which is written like a script. The single modules are written on small slips of paper/stickers (Post-it notes) that can be easily supplemented and that are arranged on a sheet of paper in the format of a letter. The athlete works with this script, marking the most important aspects of the action concept. I ask athletes to mark the three most significant aspects of the action concept, important aspects (red marker), cognitive aspects (with a blue marker), and emotional aspects (with a green marker). When we notice that an aspect in training is forgotten, the module (sticker) is placed higher on the script. By working with the script, the athlete becomes increasingly aware about the significance of some aspects and keeps these in mind in training and competition. If the athlete has good experiences completing the

ACTION CONCEPT (GOLF)

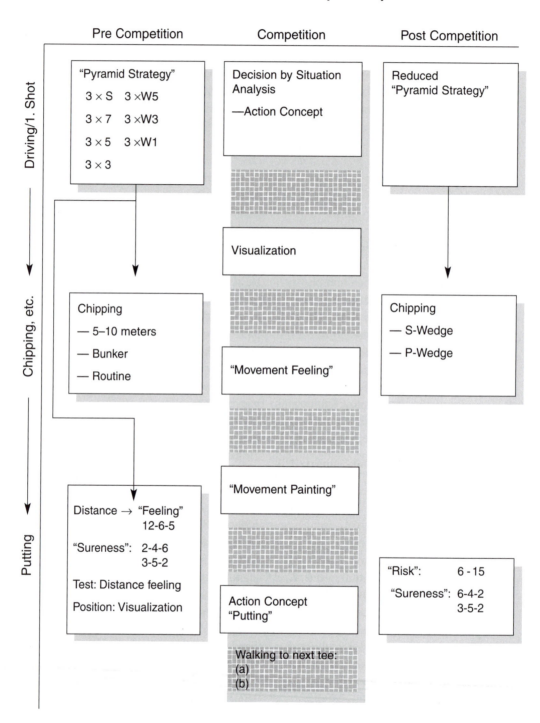

	Pre Competition	Competition	Post Competition
Driving/1. Shot	"Pyramid Strategy" 3 × S 3 ×W5 3 × 7 3 ×W3 3 × 5 3 ×W1 3 × 3	Decision by Situation Analysis —Action Concept	Reduced "Pyramid Strategy"
		Visualization	
Chipping, etc.	Chipping — 5–10 meters — Bunker — Routine	"Movement Feeling"	Chipping — S-Wedge — P-Wedge
		"Movement Painting"	

Putting	Distance → "Feeling"
	       12-6-5
	"Sureness": 2-4-6
	           3-5-2
	Test: Distance feeling
	Position: Visualization
		Action Concept "Putting"
		
		Walking to next tee:
		(a)
		(b)
			"Risk": 6 - 15
			"Sureness": 6-4-2
			            3-5-2

Figure 1.
Action Concept of a golfer.

action concept in training, he or she is able to execute it successfully in competitions. The athlete becomes increasingly convinced about the meaning and value of that action concept and develops growing self-confidence.

The sport psychologist can play an important role in developing the script with the athlete. The sport psychologist not only is in the role of a mental coach, instructor, advisor, or counselor, but is also in the role of a moderator, who is moderating the elaboration of the written script representing the action concept of the athlete. The elaboration of such an action concept refers to physical, mental, and emotional aspects. In Germany, we talk about a psychodidactic approach. Figure 1 provides an impression of an action concept (personal information is removed) that is an example of a result of this approach.

The action concept also serves to transfer a performance intention to an action intention by action-goal setting. Performance goals are often idealistic and not realistic, as specific circumstances and actual conditions are not sufficiently considered. Performance goals, in addition, are often influenced by others (in elite sports, the mass media also play an important role with regard to this issue), inducing pressure and stress. Action intentions direct the attention from a performance intention induced by focus on the result to the process of the performance. Concentration on the process and visualization are helpful in executing the action concept.

Final Remarks: Psychological Training

Coaches and athletes often regard psychological training with respect to psychophysiological tuning, emotional and motivational processes, and only sometimes with respect to cognitive processes (except mental training). It is my view that psychological training has two broad domains. The first is related to specific psychological functions, which includes cognitive processes (e.g., attention, imagery, decision making), emotional aspects (e.g., anger- or anxiety-control, frustration tolerance), and motivational tendencies (e.g., control of the aspirational level, persistence). The second domain is related to the organization of training, which includes developing training situations in which action concepts can be mastered with the intention of being successful in competition. Like training in general, psychological training is also a systematic (with respect to the objectives, the plan for the process of training, and the evaluation of the results) process of optimization. Psychological training refers to psychic functions and psychological means.

When asked about the significance of psychological training in a TV interview, I answered: "If skill training, endurance and power training, and tactical training cover 99% of the performance potential, and psychological training can contribute only 1% to the best possible performance, those who are engaged in skill training, endurance and power training, and in tactical training 100%, must be foolish because they risk that an opponent may be successful by a difference of 1% of training engagement. If psychological training only has a 1% potential, it may be the decisive 1%."

Reference
Hackfort, D., Munzert, J., & Seiler, R (Editors, 2000). *Handeln im Sport als Handlungspsycholgisches Model (Acting in Sport from an action-psychology model)*. Heidelberg, Germany: Asanger.

High-Performance Sports and the Experience of Human Development

Sidónio Serpa

João Rodrigues

Introduction

The decision to write this article was made during the Olympic Games in Atlanta. We were in Savannah, where the sailing competitions had been held, the day after their conclusion. Sidonio Serpa was having lunch with João Rodrigues, who had finished the competition in seventh place. We talked about how the Olympic tournament had gone, about his assessment of himself and the outcome of his efforts, about what he was feeling at that moment and what he had felt during the competition, about the sailing team and the atmosphere within it. We talked about many things during the meal and afterwards, when we visited a large bookshop. It was there that I bought the fantastic autobiography of Greg Louganis, *Breaking the Surface* (1996), and, by a stroke of incredible coincidence, I came across, for the second time in my life, Victor Frankl's work, *Man's Search for Meaning* (1984), which I had mentioned to João over lunch. These two books, although not dealing with sport psychology, are perhaps among those that have provided the most important food for thought for my work with athletes. Frankl and Louganis were for João and me, respectively, travelling companions on the return flight to Lisbon.

Before the Games, João had been number 3 in the world ranking and the European windsurfing champion in the Mistral class. Furthermore, he had been World Champion in the previous season. When the Portuguese Olympic sailing team set out for the United States, he was their bright hope for a medal, the *gold* medal, which many people on the team thought he could bring back to Portugal. In fact, through the first third of the competition, João Rodrigues was the great *star* of the team. In the end, everyone's attention had turned to the crew of the 470 class, Hugo Rocha and Nuno Barreto, who also had an important international record and conquered a bronze medal.

I asked myself whether João would be disillusioned; if he would look at all he had been through over the past 4 years as a wasted investment, so clearly directed towards the Olympic Games.

Anyone who has ever been on the inside of the Games understands very well that a seventh place is only possible for athletes who belong to a world-class elite. In fact, in this competition there were former world champions who finished below that position. It is for that reason that, besides the medals given to the first three finishers, diplomas are given out down to the eighth place. However, that is not how the public regards the Games, as they play the role of consumers of the creation of gods and idols, sold by the powerful media. Only the winners appear to deserve respect. Isn't the man in second place the first of the last-place finishers?

How would João feel in the face of this apparent failure and the fact that being the star at the outset, he was quickly relegated to a secondary position, hidden by the medal won by his companions in the 470 class? He was, in truth, a potential candidate for a gold medal and that was the way he was seen by those who follow closely the evolution of sailing in Portugal.

It is true that I had never heard him say that the winning of a gold medal was the object of his participation in the most important sports competition in the world. It is also true that when journalists asked him questions about his objectives in the Games, he would answer "to be in harmony," in harmony with the elements that interact in the regattas—the board, the sail, the sea, the wind—but above all, in harmony with himself. I knew that he meant that the athlete and the person he was should be complementary facets of an integrated and harmonious whole.

I remember very well what he had said in Lisbon during a meeting with the whole Olympic team, as part of the program of psychological preparation for Atlanta. We were a few weeks from departure. As they discussed each athlete's perception of his or her participation in the Games and his or her personal objectives, João gave an original reply. He said he looked forward to the event as a "very beautiful party" in which he would take part with all his might and that he would desire to enjoy it the best he could. Like at a wedding of very close friends, he would take his best clothes and enjoy the party with the most positive spirit of involvement in the collective commemoration; he

did not say that he would consider his Olympic participation as just another competition, not giving it more importance so that he would not be placing himself under pressure that might disturb him. Nor did he take the opposing position that this was the objective of 4 years of work, and, competing among the best in the world, he would try to win a medal. He gave neither one nor the other of the most common answers. The Games to him were a very beautiful party that he would attend with his best suit and his best disposition!

It is true that these were the concepts that he transmitted, but now that the Olympic Games were over, would he feel satisfied, successful, and in harmony, or would João-the person be disillusioned with Rodrigues-the athlete because the latter had spoiled the party for the former?

I asked him that very question during that lunch. He said no, that the objective of experiencing that event intensely, of seeking to meet each challenge of the competition efficiently, had been reached. He had totally dedicated himself seriously and professionally. The results depended on the interaction of the quality of his performance with that of the others, and six others had been better. Nothing weighed on his conscience. He felt he was within the limits of the harmony he had sought for before the Games. His lack of anxiety over the medal as a fundamental objective of his participation in the Games had not been a bluff. Essentially, he was concerned that the managers and technical staff of the Portuguese Sailing Federation who had given him so much help and treated him so well over the last 4 years would be sad. Fortunately, according to him, the duo of Hugo Rocha/Nuno Barreto had succeeded in winning a medal, which rewarded the Federation for its work. I didn't insist further. Months later, I came back to the point. During one of our periodic sessions, I said to him:

In Savannah, after the Olympic competition, I asked you if you were disillusioned with your results. You told me you weren't. I let it rest there because I didn't want to open any wounds there might have been. But now, after these months have gone by, how do you feel about it?

He looked at me with a deep and serious expression, thought for a few seconds, then answered:

Sidónio, when I'm worried and something is weighing on my conscience, I think about it at night, in bed, and I have trouble sleeping. I can guarantee that I haven't lost a minute's sleep over my final standings in the Olympic Games!

Going back to our conversation at lunch, he commented how his adversaries were generally unhappy with windsurfing and competitions once the Olympic races were over. The last year, especially, they had lived like nomads, going from regatta to regatta, from country to country, occasionally getting to make a brief visit home, which they almost stopped feeling was theirs. They had competitions and more competitions. Many of them were under the additional pressure of fighting to conquer the right to be selected to represent their country in the Olympics. João noticed this fact, but he didn't share this collective feeling of having had enough and wanting to put the surfboard away for a few months. In fact, he confided to me that he was trying to contact his university in Lisbon to sign up for the World University Championships, which were to be held 2 months later. Since he had finished his licentiate degree in mechanical engineering at the most prestigious Portuguese school a few months before the Games, he was eligible to participate in that competition. He was ready and willing to get back on his surfboard and do more racing.

He also talked to me about those who came in ahead of him in the Olympic competition. "They were better than me. They deserve my respect," he told me. "That's why I was at the awards ceremony when the medals were given in order to congratulate them."

This was the longest, most profound conversation about what was involved in his participation in the Games since the races had begun. Up until then, and already in Savannah, we had talked at length during the relatively long period in which we were there before the beginning of the competitions. The last *psychological conversation* had been on the eve of the first day. He called me on my cell phone and said he would like to speak with me. We met in the Olympic dormitory. It was a sort of final self-assessment, a review of the internal state of affairs. At the end, he said to me, "Well, that's it., Now it's up to me! I'm the one who has to resolve the problems on my own." We never did reflect together again on the questions about his psychological adaptation to sports competition.

My work with the Olympic Sailing Team had begun about 2 years before Atlanta. The athletes and the coaches had been very favorable in their acceptance of the inclusion of a psychologist on the technical staff, which for the first time in Portuguese sports was present at the Olympic Games. However, the extent of the psychological intervention depended in large part on what the athletes themselves asked for. Some perceived the psychological work as a fundamental element in enhancing their performance. Naturally, because they were different persons, the approaches were also different, but, in general, the desire for personal discovery and perfecting through sports was common. It is interesting to note that those who made the most systematic use of the psychological accompaniment were among those in the international scene who were placed in the highest levels of sports achievement. This may suggest that there is a precise moment in the maturation of an athlete when he or she recognizes the psychological element that is integrated in the overall process of improvement in sports. This maturation itself is perhaps determined by such factors as the psychological and social framework in which the young athlete is trained and the methodology of that training.

My work with João Rodrigues over the 2-year period in which I followed the process of his Olympic participation concentrated on deepening his self-knowledge based on reflections on his experiences in sports. Naturally, the fundamental questions that stood out had to do with the meaning attached to sports activities in the context of personal development. Sports and life became associated with each other in a common set of problems. The whole work, which was aimed at perfecting his sports performance, gained meaning in the process of evolution of the *athlete-person*. In reality, we can conclude from what many high-performance athletes say, that the sports project takes on meaning when it is integrated in an overall project of life, and João was very clear on that.

It was a matter of organizing cognitions and feelings that would provide the most appropriate answers to the situations of athletic competition and, therefore, those of life. Personal experiences were gradually and progressively perceived within a single, unifying logic. Sports became a means for the promotion of self-awareness and self-knowledge on a path of adaptation needed for the harmonious interaction between the person and his or her surroundings. A real consistency between personal goals, motivational guidelines, and instrumental processes was being cemented. An intellectual structure that consciously integrated thoughts, feelings, and behavior appeared. The result of this was a more efficient management and

regulation of the psychological processes, which, in turn, brought about the rise of homogeneity in the top athletic performances.

In this context of integration, the participation in a process of training-competition in high-performance sports, the problems surrounding the social role of the athlete arose. He or she is, at once, a victim of pressures and constraints, a model in society, and a generator of progress in the society in which he or she participates. The top-level athlete must be aware of this. It was in this sense that many times in our conversations, João Rodrigues manifested his desire to share with others the discoveries that his evolution in the sport had given him. Now that he had completed a cycle of maturation with the Atlanta Olympic Games, it appeared to me that it would be a challenge for both of us to prepare a joint text. In it, we would transmit to others interested in the subject our joint experience of joint evolution, in a framework of humanistic references we both believe in. This was the proposal I made during that lunch in Savannah, the headquarters of the Olympic sailing competitions.

The text that came out of this was the result of about 20 hours of taped conversations we had over the following months, and of its preparation in the light of psychology. In addition, it is organized according to the *Integrated Model of Psychological Training* (Serpa & Araújo, 1996), which has been under development in the Sports Psychology Laboratory to provide a basis for psychological research and intervention in athletic training.

The Integrated Model of Psychological Training

In this model developed by Serpa & Araújo (1996), psychological training is viewed as an integrating element in the process of athletic training. The psychological factors evolve with the maturation of the athlete throughout the course of his or her career. Furthermore, there is a constant interaction with the other dimensions of the athlete's life. On the other hand, during a certain phase of the athlete's career, the most important questions that arise are the result of the level of involvement in the sport and the specific demands of that participation at a given moment of the process. The type of work carried out and the psychological intervention are also distinct, according to the various phases and occasions.

The intention is that the process will develop specific skills that facilitate adaptation to sports situations. Simultaneously, there is an appeal for the athlete, from the initial stages, to participate actively in the analysis of his or her reactions and in the reflection on goals and objectives. This contributes to an intellectual structure in which attitudes and concepts are organized to support any adaptive reaction of the individuals to internal and external demands.

None of the psychological work can be

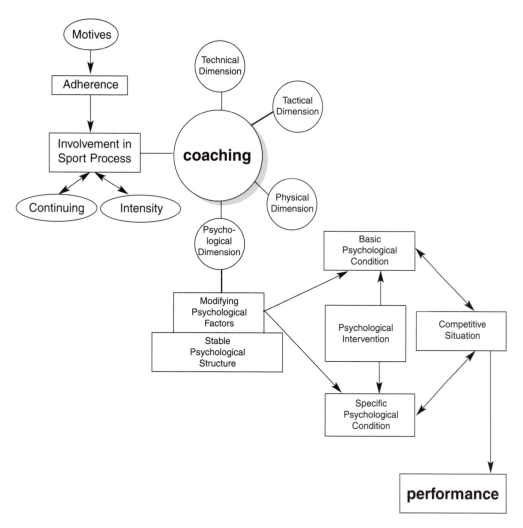

Figure 1.
Integrated Model of Psychological Training

separated from the other training components, which include the technical, tactical, and physical aspects. It is the sports problem-situation that will promote the overall development of the athlete.

The *Integrated Model for Psychological Training* (Figure 1) proposes that adherence to the sports process is a result of a set of motives or reasons that the young person seeks to satisfy in the activity he or she has chosen. In participating in the sport, the athlete may find the desired response. Sometimes, the knowledge gained from the experience will lead to an evolution of other interests in the athlete's life. In any case, the athlete will tend to remain active in the sport, dedicating himself or herself to it with varying intensity. The way in which the coach understands the reasons for the young person's participation, respects them, and finally, causes them to evolve through the management of tasks, is perhaps the first moment of the psychological preparation of the athlete, who will be led to continue his or her participation with a progressive involvement or to give it up. The truth is that the motivational valences are not stable. Rather, they evolve in a search for meaning that links the activity to the goals of the essential motivations of human beings. The attitude of the coach in the different phases seems to follow a deterministic pattern in the formation of characteristics that facilitate success.

Research has concluded that one of the variables that conditions the behavior and emotions of the athlete in the training-competition process, which reflects on his or her performances, is the cognitive character of his or her sports orientation. This can range between two extremes: concern about the *athletic result,* on one hand, and concern about the *task* they perform, on the other. Formed through the processes of interaction with others and with the world, the type of interaction between the coach and the athlete

should be an element controlled by the former so that it is correctly managed.

Studies on the career of an athlete find that it is made up of various phases with differing characteristics, which are related to the levels and types of participation, equally distinct in nature. For example, based on the work of Bloom (1985), Salmela (1994) refers to the *initiation stage*, which essentially consists of playing, the fundamental features being the fun and joy of participation. Those who have reached a level of excellence tell about the pleasure they feel at improving themselves, free from the pressures of being forced to produce athletic results. Their choice is entirely free, and many times is informal.

The next stage, *development,* begins when young participants who are gifted with differentiated qualities take note of the fact and become involved in a more demanding and formal training process different from the "playing around" they were formerly involved in. Their perception of their status changes. They are no longer *kids with a knack for sports*; they are now thought of as *athletes.* Performance now becomes the fundamental concept, and *the game* gives way to *the work.* In this, however, they still find pleasure in the constant striving for perfection. In this phase, they assume a set of rules of behavior and restrictions in their lifestyle, especially those that relate to their free time, special diets, or their social life. They commonly develop a permanent attitude of self-analysis.

The *specialization stage* corresponds to the period in which sports becomes the center of the individual's life project and in which the individual reaches the highest level of performance. Involvement in sports is total, not only from the point of view of carrying out the tasks of training and competition, but also in the time spent thinking about, studying, and dreaming about the elements that condition an athlete's results and evolution. The high goals that the athletes pursue and that justify their living are made part of their inner being and come to have a relevant social role in a context more or less broad, depending in part on the impact their sport has on society.

From the above, it can be concluded that the psychological approach to training has different forms. The initiation phase essentially consists of the type of pedagogical guidance given by the coach in order to develop the intrinsic motivation and promote a positive motivation for the task and the fulfillment of personal objectives in a pleasant atmosphere of fun. This is a key period in the acquiring of attitudes and concepts.

Beginning with the specialization phase, training principles are followed and specific techniques and strategies are used. When there is, then, a relatively stable psychological structure, the focus is on psychological factors—emotional, cognitive, and behavioral—that are used for adaptation to the demands of practice and competition.

Thus, we are within the nature of intervention that fits in the psychological training concept proposed by Serpa & Araújo (1996):

> a planned, systematic, multidimensional process for the stimulation of the modifiable psychological characteristics, as well as the management of the nonmodifiable ones, by means of a consistent set of strategies and techniques which develop the capacity to adapt, directed at the sports development of the athlete. (p. 2)

Just as in the physical training, by respecting biological and methodological principles, foundational qualities will be developed, upon which later progress is accomplished to meet the individual potential.

The development of the *basic psychological condition* must be taken into account, including emotional, cognitive, and behavioral factors of a general nature. These are indispensable for the subsequent work on the *specific psychological condition.* The former includes factors such as the capacity for emotional control and activation, the adaptation of the processes of concentration, the resistance to stress, the volitional qualities of dedication and combativeness in which self-motivation assumes a special importance, the attitudes and behavior of autonomy, the capacity to analyze situations and oneself, as well as the social adaptation. As for the development of the specific psychological condition, the following aspects should be taken into account: aspects related to the athlete's adaptation to the particularities of the results in the respective sport, such as the development of his or her capacity to deal with the specific demands for concentration and activation, the psychomotor control, or the adaptation to the decision-making demands of the sport.

The intention is that, in accordance with the training principles, the athlete be provided with situations that stimulate the acquisition and development of the components of those two types of psychological conditions. This occurs as a result of the interaction between the individual's characteristics and those of the competitive situation and the task associated with the particular sport, in the context of a general involvement (Figure 2).

It should be stressed, however, that the individual develops fundamental elements as a result of interaction with his or her involvement in general and with the social environment in particular. These situations involve the significant adults, such as parents and coaches, who are part of his or her stable social-psychological environment. These are the wider reaching conceptual and attitudinal aspects, which are related to a clear perspective of the sports project that is integrated

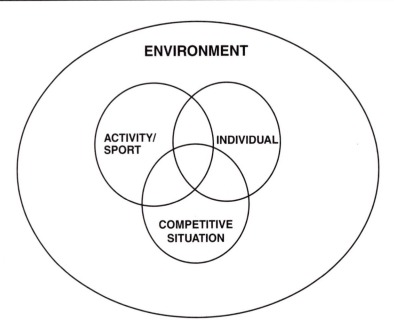

Figure 2

into one's own life project and which determine the use of sports as a source of personal development. The consistency and orientation of these factors determine the character of the athlete's cognitive-emotional reactions that later affect his or her performance and outcome.

Published work is essentially concerned with the techniques and strategies that develop and optimize the psychological factors of the performance, through the capacity to manage the cognitive and emotional components. Besides the vast amount of material published in the scientific journals of sport psychology, some books have dealt with the theme in a developed manner. Examples of this are the chapters by Burton (1993), Suinn (1993), Zaichkowsky and Takenaka (1993), Rotella and Lerner (1993), Nideffer (1993), and Crews (1993), which make up the section "Psychological Techniques for Individual Performance" of the *Handbook of Re-*

search on Sport Psychology, edited by Singer, Murphey, and Tennant (1993). Likewise, Hardy, Jones, and Gould (1996) and Buceta (1998) deal with this theme. The article by Le Scanff (1998), published in an important French psychology journal, *Bulletin de Psychologie,* develops an interesting approach inherent to psychological preparation to be included in the normal sports training.

The approach in this article is more phenomenological. We believe that preceding the process of adaptation to a sports situation, there must be a psychological training that promotes a consistent attitude that fits the sports project into the overall project for life. The athlete must learn to project the sports activity in a process of personal development that will thus give meaning to the sports experience. In this way, we looked at this work from the perspective of the formation of a psychological structure within which all the trainable factors of performance ought to be taken into consideration: the personality, the significant relationship between the instrumental means provided by sports and the goals inherent in human motivation, as well as the existential aspects inherent in the relationship between the individual and his sport. To this end, we take the experience of an athlete in a high-performance competition who agreed with us to reflect upon the course of his life during an Olympic season.

An Experience of Personal Development

This section takes up the reflection on the experience of work with João Rodrigues in his preparation for the Olympic Games in Atlanta. We present the process of personal development of a high-performance athlete, based on his relationship with the situations inherent in the sports training and competition, or in a broader sense, with the world. Surely, the high level of international performance is not foreign to the process of maturation that took place in the 4-year period leading up to the Games. We try to understand the development of the relatively stable psychological components that are the basis for the performance factors. These factors are trainable and allow for more technical and segmented intervention.

It is, therefore, on the specialization stage of João's career that we focus our attention. In fact, the elaboration that he came to perform on his experience in the sense of seeking fulfillment through the sport of sailing is probably explained by the *need for self-fulfillment,* which is the highest level of Maslow's pyramid of the *hierarchy of needs.* The relational theory of personality (Abreu, 1998; Nuttin, 1965) associates this process with axiological needs. The concepts, personal orientation, and reflections that characterize this period in the career of an athlete require a certain level of personal maturity, which not all athletes

achieve in a similar way, possibly because the closest and most deterministic social involvement does not allow it.

With respect to social involvement, it is important to note that the case being studied had all the characteristics reported by Bloom's research (1985). From the very beginning, the stable home environment provided affective support, which was instrumental and fundamental. In a climate marked by a very positive attitude towards the sport, the father, as well as the brothers, was a passionate practitioner of windsurfing. On the one hand, the incentive and support that facilitated involvement in the sport were always present. On the other hand, there was a complete absence of pressure regarding any obligation to achieve competitive results. The coach who guided him from a certain point onwards and became his friend followed the same type of values and helped him to organize his activity.

Up until the Olympic Games in Barcelona, the first in which he participated, he took windsurfing somewhat lightly, driven mainly by the great pleasure he felt in the enjoyment of the freedom to navigate in the open, limitless spaces and in the joy of perfecting qualities that were making him progressively more efficient in the task. The fact that he lived on an island, Madeira, provided him with the natural surroundings that were a strong attraction for him "to jump" into the sea, which he had always learned to live with and with which this sport allowed him to have a constant interaction, with the aid of the winds that provided the required mechanical energy:

I have a tremendous passion for the sea. That is what led me to this type of sport. Madeira is an island, and it is impossible not to look to the sea. Windsurfing was the only sport I found in which I can always go further, where

I can define the obstacles and succeed in overcoming them, for example, try out a new maneuver which appears almost impossible to do, explore better the characteristics of the board-sail set. There are other sports in which the obstacles are unsurpassable for me, so I lose my motivation and interest (Rodrigues, personal communications, February.19.1997).

His participation in competitions came about in a natural way, and the good results soon began to appear, first in Madeira, then at the national level in confrontation with participants from the whole country. At 16, he was champion of Portugal for the first time and ended up becoming the habitual winner of the national competitions.

There were international events also, but he did not achieve the good results he had had in Portugal. Although circumstantial reasons led him to go 2 years without participating in competitions, he never stopped training. He found the energy to continue dedicating himself to training sessions, searching to improve his technique, and one day in speaking with a director of the Sailing Portuguese Federation who asked him if he liked to sail. The answer was obviously affirmative, and the director told him, "Then don't give up now, because one day your chance will come!"

That comment had an important impact:

When I didn't really feel like training, I thought about his words, saying that my day would come, and I would go out to sea. I never thought that it would be a medal, a title. I think it was a test of my patience because there were a great many competitions held for boys my age, Portuguese and from other countries that I knew about. That made me regret not being there with them. But there was always the hope

that one day I would be there, too! (Rodrigues, personal communications, February.19.1997).

It is evident that from an early stage, the essential motivation resided in the intrinsic aspects inherent in the pleasure of overcoming challenges. Possibly, there were also motives of a social nature, of the affiliate type. The desire to be with the others could, in some way, be related to being part of an elite group, and in that context, participation in events was perceived as prestigious. Here, too, resided the challenge. The immediate satisfaction that many times characterizes young people gave way to a long-term goal. Many other excellent athletes refer to this aspect, such as Greg Louganis (1996), for example, in his autobiography.

Then came the opportunity to participate in his first Olympic Games, in Barcelona, 1992. The fact that he had been the habitual winner of the events in Portugal was associated with the culture that the surrounding society transmitted to him. This led him to establish result-oriented sport goals. Although he had the notion that he was not prepared for "places of honor," he felt that the 20th position was the worst he would allow himself to finish. For months, he trained with that perspective. He decided to put off his university studies at the faculty of engineering and interrupted his academic activities for a year.

It was precisely this participation in the Olympic Games of Barcelona that became a critical life event in the João Rodrigues's sports career, a generator of ulterior personal development, as reported by Danish, Petitpas, and Hale (1995). For these authors, these critical events are points of change in the course of an individual's life when opportunities for evolution and growth appear. The personal response depends on the individual's resources in hand before the event and his or her preparation to cope with it, as well as on the individual's personal history. In reality, there is a continuity in the process of a person's life, during which a system of logic is being constructed, which underlies the responses of adaptation to the critical life events. Next we introduce the essential elements of the interviews with Joao Rodrigues. Some theoretical comments are also included.

The Opening Ceremony of the Barcelona Games was the key moment in which I realized that a sports project was something more than the simple search for results. I knew I wasn't prepared to achieve a result of international importance, no matter how much I wanted to. I remember it as if it were today: I was adoring the fantastic spectacle of the Opening Ceremony. I suddenly looked to one side and saw someone crying. It was a foreigner in his 30s who couldn't control his emotions. That confused me greatly because I couldn't understand what was going on with him. I shouldn't have been feeling the same thing, although it gave me goose bumps, and was very moving, but that was more because of the show, which made me feel somewhat apart from what was really happening. Perhaps I had not explored myself enough. . . . I then saw the importance that the Games could have. They were, after all, more than a mere sporting event which justified my spending a year away from my studies, but which deserved more and better training than I had done. That was when I really understood that I should try again and that that moment was nothing more than a stage in my career.

What do you mean, "try again"? Do you mean try harder to achieve a good standing?

No, I didn't think I would go to Atlanta and win anything. At that moment, I looked back and understood that things were being done wrong. It was not just the athletic preparation, which may have been faulty, but most of all the wrong way in which sports, competitions, and the Olympic Games, were viewed. That person right there beside me who was so moved meant something that I was not able to understand. I became aware that sports should grant a higher pleasure, one I was not able to feel. In fact, there I was, under an incredible stress because I knew I had no chance to do anything special at the Olympic competition. The week before, I had had a stomachache and insomnia. And what was more, I had bad memories of Barcelona, since the year before I had come in close to last place in a meet I had participated in. The final result in the Games was what was normal for my level at the time, although previous international competitions had given me expectations of finishing at least 20th, and I ended up in 23rd. That was very hard for me to take, because everyone around me thought I would be in the top 20, and I ended up taking that to heart and making it my goal.

Then when did you decide to change your "attitude" towards the sport?

On the trip home from Barcelona, when I was about to reach the Portuguese border. I told myself that I had to change something. But I would have to think a lot about what I would change. Possibly I should change my way of thinking, the way I viewed the sport. I had to try and understand what windsurfing meant to me! But it was not just about the sport that I had to reflect. It was everything having to do with school and sports. I didn't like it at all that I had gone a year without studying. I felt that it had been a waste of time. I felt perfectly useless, that I had lost a part of my life for nothing. I had given up my academic activities, but neither did I have anything to show for it in sports.

Do you think that period was a total waste of time?

I thought so at the time, but I now realize

that in the end I gained by it. Because sometimes it's important to go down, to fall, so that you can see that it is possible to climb even higher. And from that moment on, I really did change a lot! Not only in relation to my training, but also in relation to my school life. I clearly established two fundamental goals for myself that I really wanted, as well as the way to achieve them. They were within my realms of sports and studies. I knew that I could evolve a great deal and that I was not using my abilities. It was as if I were using a large truck that was nearly empty, which was an enormous waste of energy!

Was your "new way of being" immediately clear to you?

No. But one thing I really wanted was to put aside the fear of failure, the fear of not being able to succeed. I felt that many times. Even about the "new attitude." When I set these goals for myself, to improve in windsurfing, to finish my university degree and go to the Games again with a good level of performance, many times, I had the sensation I couldn't do it.

Did you ever think about giving up?

The possibility of stopping and taking the easy route again did occur to me. But I had already tried that route once, and it didn't fulfill me at all. I didn't like it. I hadn't grown as a person. I stayed at the same level. I decided then that I had to abandon those pessimistic thoughts and try things in a positive way. No matter what happened, I would never give up. I would always try to reach a plane that was a little higher. And that's what I did from that point on, involving the two projects and passions that were most important to me, sports and the university. That implied a change in the plan for my life.

How did your life change?

Mainly in the way I organized my life and the way I began to put my efforts into what I

did. The social part of my life was drastically reduced because there wasn't time for everything. Everything that I did from that moment on was centered on those two vectors and neither of them was more important than the other. Neither of them could be excluded because I knew that if I excluded one, the other would stop working. That's exactly what had happened before Barcelona.

Wasn't it difficult to put your social life on a secondary plane?

No. I'm involved in an individual sport, and the sea is very large, where at times it is difficult to find someone. In a certain way, I was already used to it. On the other hand, I had such a passion to do windsurfing that when I went out with friends in the afternoon, I was always looking at my watch thinking that it was a waste, not being out at sea. I've always had good friends who have known how to understand my options, keeping up the great bond between us, even though we have little time to be in contact.

Your decision to put your sports activities and your school activities on the same level went somewhat against what is usual. Many people have the idea that it is almost impossible to be successful at university and in high-performance sports at the same time.

That's true. But that was an even greater challenge and, therefore, interesting! I wanted to harmonize the two things, all the more because they had told me that it would be impossible! It's just that when I entered the university, in one of the very first classes, the professor told us that when one enters the faculty of engineering, the rest of one's life has to be forgotten because the course is very difficult. And he specifically said that high-performance sports were incompatible! That, as a matter of fact, was right in line with what the greater part of the persons around me said. It was more or less in this perspective that I lived until Barcelona. It was for that reason that I interrupted my studies for a year. After all, it was only one year, and one doesn't go to the Olympics every day! It was a dream of mine. And there I went. . . .

The truth is that you reached that goal of participating in the Olympic Games. What was missing after all?

It's that I chose the easiest solution. Giving up my studies was, in a certain way, running from the difficulties at the same time I did something that gave me a lot of pleasure. In the end, I had a strange, empty feeling . . . an inner void. Something was missing there. . . . It wasn't just going to practice more times, dedicating myself more to sports in a quantitative point of view. I think it was necessary to use that situation for growth, growth as a person. And to raise my sights, because they were set too low.

What do you mean by raising your sights?

When I say raise my sights, I don't mean my goals as an athlete because up until Barcelona, I don't think I had ever set my sights on any goal, in the sense of being an outstanding windsurfer, of winning a certain international competition. Seeing I wasn't a top windsurfer, any time I went to sea, it was to obtain the best possible showing, which was so vague it was like not having a goal at all. Raising my sights means developing the capacity to use all my resources. To synchronize them all.

To do that, you had to be aware of the way you functioned in the two areas—know yourself better.

Exactly. And I finally understood that both of them could be integrated in one and the same logic. I tried to find a way for them to help each other. It's that I had told myself that I had to finish the 3 remaining years of my course (of a total of 5) without failing any subject and making up the ones I was be-

hind in. And I would also continue to ride my surfboard and improve my skills. So I had to change both the way I studied as well as the way I trained.

How did you do it?

The first thing to do was to be 100% in each of these activities. When I trained, I really trained, and when I studied, I really studied! I would have to use my head when I was riding my board in order to understand the logic of my adaptation to the problems brought about by each situation in windsurfing, but I also had to feel physically fit to perform in my studies. Besides that, the pleasure I got from doing sports was a factor which greatly helped me recuperate and be efficient in my studies.

You found elements that could be transferred from one activity to the other.

That's true. Later, our conversations allowed me to understand that I was using the same logic to resolve windsurfing problems and engineering problems, as well as viewing the competitions and the exams as motivating challenges to find appropriate solutions. Little by little, I was developing a way to study, a bit unconsciously, through which I was learning the essential foundations for each subject, which allowed me to build a "pyramid" in which things were being fit in without limits. For that reason, the most interesting part of university was the exams, where I put to the test my skill at solving difficulties until I reached the final answer. It gave me an enormous pleasure. If we could measure the speed of thought at those times, things were passing through my head so rapidly that I was already foreseeing the following steps, and things fell into place, leading me to the answers. It was like in the races!

Were you completely involved in the task?

Yes, completely involved. However, when I went for an exam, I never went thinking about it. I didn't take a watch because I knew that if I looked at the watch and there was little time left, I would get nervous and lose the involvement which would let me flow through the task of resolving the problem. Each question was solved step by step. I was aware that what I was doing was well done.

Was this a game to you?

I never thought of it as a game. I rather thought of it as a challenge.

And did you always achieve this involvement and this flow in the resolution of the exam?

No. When there were factors that worried me and I felt that I wasn't controlling them, things didn't go well. For example, when I thought that I had only that one chance, when I was forced to have a good result, the effort was much greater.

With weaker results?

Exactly. Like in windsurfing. The same thing happened. I had to stop worrying about the result of my behavior. I concerned myself with finding and understanding the bases for my adaptation to situations, with improving my skills, bettering the quality of my reactions to the demands of the world of the regattas and to those my adversaries created for me. To do that, I had to know myself better all the time and the elements with which I worked, as well as concentrating on what I was doing, "unattaching myself" from the results it would produce.

If I understand what you're saying to me, just like in your studies, you concerned yourself with understanding the process upon which you were acting so that the result, in this case, athletic, would appear as a natural consequence. The understanding of the process of windsurfing consisted in being aware of the way to ride the board and function in harmony with its components, the water, the wind, the opponents, etc. The consciousness you were developing about your-

self also played a determining role in this.

That's the way it was, in fact. Sports and studies were two complementary and fundamental pieces in my personal development, which fit together perfectly within a unifying logic.

Was it after Barcelona that you evolved in this way, seeing that before that you would have been more concerned about the results of your participation in the races? Did you see things more from the outside, ignoring the essential linked to the process?

To a certain extent. In the competitions, I was concerned about the result, but in the practices, I didn't know very well what I was doing there. If I was supposed to sail for 3 hours there, I went to sea with no concrete goals to achieve in that task. It was only afterwards that I began to reflect permanently on the way to increase efficiency at each moment and with each maneuver. I went from being a "car driver" whose only concern was to operate the instruments so that the vehicle would get under way, to the situation of being an "engineer" who wants to know his machine better and better so as to get the maximum out of its potential. And there I was the machine and the engineer!

What special care did you start to give the "machine"?

I had to understand the way the "machine" worked in order to get the maximum performance possible out of it. And it's so thrilling to work with machines, knowing that we can always increase their performance, changing something here, tightening a nut there, altering a parameter in its operation. . . .

It's the professional perspective of the engineer that's speaking.

Point taken. But it was exactly the same thing riding the surfboard. My performance was low, and so it had to be improved, which meant studying the elements of that system made up of the board and myself. I concerned myself more with the mechanics of the board. I gave more attention to the "fuel running the machine," which was me, changing my diet. I reviewed the "system of maintenance," being more careful, especially with the physical preparation. The "system of storage" was also improved with more efficient rest and a better organized and more reinvigorating sleep. All in all, I perceived that in order to achieve ever-higher goals of personal improvement, I had to work all the elements within an integrated system for which I was responsible.

In this perspective, how did the academic life at the faculty of engineering influence your efforts to perfect the "machine"?

My studies helped me perfect the "hardware" essential to the development of the "software," which determined the behavior of the machine because, if the information were not efficiently processed, the mechanical part was not sufficient. And the intellectual demands that windsurfing put upon me helped my performance at the school, just as it gave me the physical conditions which were indispensable to the great demands of the studies. As a matter of fact, the intellectual training, which the university offered me, helped me understand and construct with great ease the logic underlying the accomplishments in the regattas. Although it was evolving in a progressive and unconscious process, my life began to be made up of a set of physical and intellectual elements, complementary and integrated.

Didn't the exhaustion from training make studying difficult?

On the contrary. For example, following a weekend during which I had had a very hard practice session, I could study everywhere. Even on the Lisbon city buses! I had achieved total concentration. As a matter of fact, before Barcelona, I had tried two alter-

natives: giving prevalence to studies and giving prevalence to sports, and neither of them worked. I got to the point where I would study until early hours of the morning, sleep a little, then get up very early to study some more. Doing it this way, I didn't pass some of my subjects, and I had low marks the first 2 years. After Barcelona, studying and training with total passion and dedication in both activities, I entered the third year of university with four subjects to make up—which I did—and I never failed another exam, and I began to have higher marks. In sports, on the other hand, I improved my performance immensely, obtaining results I had never had before.

▲▼▲▼

The dialogues transcribed here reveal the nature of the evolution that took place in João's attitude after the Barcelona Games. Participation in Olympic Games always marks the personal history of an athlete. I believe, however, that not all of them experience that event with a level of maturity combined with a sensitive moment that allows them to reflect so profoundly on their experience so as to decide to change course in their relationship with the world and themselves.

Danish et al. (1995), in their proposal for a life-development model, mention that the qualitative leaps that generate development are associated with critical events in the life of the individual. From these events, the professional who is providing psychological support to the athlete will use an efficient process for the establishing and managing of personal goals as an instrumental means of promoting development. I believe that the impact that generates changes in goals will be greater as these goals are intrinsically assumed. Their optimal influence will take place when the goals arise from the individual's becoming aware of the need for certain aims with existential meaning. Besides, the phenomenological approach of Frankl (1984, 1987) accentuates magisterially the importance of the meaning an individual attributes to his or her experiences as a factor that produces adaptation and growth.

This is what happened to João after his first Olympic Games. Besides, this effect was maximized by other contemporaneous events, among which stands out the fact that he was a student at one of the most prestigious Portuguese universities and he had not achieved the desired results. His participation in the Games equally involved two important events: observing the emotion of the participant who cried during the Opening Ceremony and being disillusioned for finishing below his expectations. All of this set off a process of existential reflection in which the sport, as being the central element, gained meaning as integrated in the vaster plane of a life project.

His perception of training and competition in sports thus underwent a restructuring that decisively influenced emotions and behavior in a deterministic holistic approach to an effort to harmonize all the elements.

From the motivational point of view, intrinsic motivation increased, but the pleasure of doing the sport lost its superficial character. In fact, it gained a meaning inherent to the stimulation of self-knowledge and the overcoming of personal limitations as a form of human improvement and development. Within this psychological dynamic, the motivational orientation was centered on the tasks and on the process, which is viewed as a continuum made up of diverse stages of evolution, like landings in a staircase. The search for the solutions to the problems posed by the activity became the principal focus of attention. The athletic results were relegated to a secondary plane, and their meaning was then to be found in the symbolic reference inherent in the quality of the path traveled. The aims he sought to achieve became clear, as did his operational reference goals and the processes by which these would be possible.

The anxiety and anguish that come from the concern for obtaining certain athletic results and the inherent doubt about the inadequacy of the personal resources have disappeared, replaced by the conviction that it will always be possible to find the road that will lead to successive qualitative conquests. This was the challenge that nourished the constant motivation along the line mentioned by Frankl (1987), when he affirmed, "today's man himself should create the tension which will make it possible to find the meaning to his life. He does it, making demands. He demands that he himself be the producer and he provides tasks of abnegation" (p. 2). Likewise, sports, in Frankl's (1987) view, has in this context an essential role, fulfilling the existential void that many times has originated in the lifestyle of Western society where possession and abundance of the means to live do not find correspondence in the "reason for living." Through sports he seeks "the knowledge about the absolute limits of Man. The individual expands with each step he takes in the direction of the horizon, and as the external horizons open up, the internal ones undergo a similar opening" (p. 2).

In the case we're dealing with, underlying self-fulfillment was a permanent test of the personal potential, through challenges related to participation in a competitive sport, with the evolution in his studies and the conjugation of these two areas, but always having in mind the search for the understanding of the logic underlying the processes, which allowed for the discovery and creation of adequate resources. The phenomenological, psychological, and biological aspects gained equal relevance along with the instrumental knowledge necessary for the resolution of the problem situations.

The new methodology that was appearing implied a systematic assessment of the dynamics inherent in the sport in particular and life, in general; the determination of areas of personal fulfillment to explore and develop; the optimization of the central points of individual competence; and the planning for life in terms of the options taken.

We found through this witness that sports and studies are not activities opposed to each other and in conflict. Contrary to the usual social perception, they are not mutually exclusive alternatives. Sports and studies appear here as being complementary and obeying the same logic on the phenomenological plane.

According to the social stereotypes and the values that emerge in the Western world where HAVING takes precedence over BEING, sports and the academic life have to be in conflict because they are disputing over prevalence in the realm of the same logic. In fact, the purposes that society finds for the two activities correspond to acquisitions apart from the fulfillment of the individual potential and inherent in the affirmation of the individual before others. They symbolize the power in the social context; that is the meaning that, in sports, is attributed to the medals or the sports titles that promote social prestige or material benefits. The grades in the schools and the diplomas that are obtained follow the same logic; furthermore, they are supposed to make new acquisitions and social positions possible through a professional distinction that favors them.

In this perspective, when these two vie for the honors of the prestigious social valorization on the same ground, the one that is closest to the reigning social values will gain predominance. Thus, it happens that, in a culture still marked by the Cartesian dualism, the acquisitions of a "physical" nature will be passed over for those of an "intellectual" nature. The academic domain will always beat the sports domain—unless through sports there are significant material gains. Just like men, societies have their price. They may condescend to accept a citizen who is culturally impoverished, intellectually wanting, and professionally inept, if that individual's bank account puts him or her at the top in relation to fellow citizens.

However, the sports-school conflict will not exist if the conception of the referenced citizen is placed within the perspective of the development of the BEING and not that of the growth of the HAVING (Abreu, 1998). Such activities will then be complementary because they both will contribute to the permanent development of the "person-athlete-student" through the instrumental means in which they are constituted. As they form a meaningful whole for the one who there finds a permanent challenge to the fulfillment of his or her potential, they contribute to the satisfaction of the social, cognitive, and axiological needs that are indispensable for human fulfillment and, therefore, for the happiness of the athlete-student and the consequent social harmony. In the line of thinking defended by Abreu (1998), study and sports should be organized activities that take on meaning for the individual so that both activities are included in a personal project for life. They would thus lead to the learning of an individual strategic plan associated with the development of self-knowledge. Contributing to this would be the development of the capacity to clarify and formulate goals, to carry out an articulated management of the useful information coming from the environment, to reflect on personal experiences, to interpret and understand one's own behavior, to discover personal resources, and to organize a structure of means-ends.

It is precisely this that João Rodrigues teaches us with the story of his experience: that it is possible to make sports and academic activities complementary, in using what is acquired from each one of the domains to better adapt to the other and, therefore, to life because both are meaningful in a perspective of personal development and not simply making acquisitions devoid of existential content possible.

In working with athletes, one of the functions of the psychologist or the coach should be to help them find their true inner goals and make a contribution to enable them to build a structure within a logic of overall improvement of the person. The techniques used many times in the establishment of operational objectives must be seen as mere instrumental means. On the other hand, it is essential to understand the level of psychological maturation of the athlete because that will determine his or her sensitivity and susceptibility to the more phenomenological type of process of reflection. In many cases, the more objective techniques will be the ones that will prove to be the most suited until the critical moment arrives when another type of approach is called for.

The Motivational Aspects

The integrated model of psychological training suggests that the adherence of individuals to participation in a sport is determined by a set of reasons, termed motives, that constitute forces that attract the individual to that sport. Participation in the sport can satisfy these reasons, leading the player to remain active, increasing the intensity of his or her behavior. Sometimes these reasons are transformed as a function of new interactions that have been established. What is important, both in the development of the subject and in the consequence regarding the athlete's persistence in the sport through the progressive challenges that present themselves, is the meaning that exists in the relationship between the sport and the final goals of the fundamental motivations of the person.

In this section, we will elaborate on Rodrigues's motivational process and its profound implications on investment in the sport of sailing/windsurfing.

The goals to be fulfilled that you have mentioned to me as being those that motivated you are in contradiction to those normally we expect to hear from a high-performance athlete. After all, you established for yourself the pleasure of doing the sport and personal improvement, even in competition, and you avoided putting importance on the standings, titles, medals. Isn't this really important when you participate in a meet of the level of a world championship or the Olympic Games?

In my perspective of sports, that is not the objective. It should be a vehicle for growth and development where pleasure has to be present. This is what constitutes the fun of competition. But I view the sport in a serious and professional way. I don't make life easy for my opponents! I seek to be perfect when I race in the regattas. If that is enough to win the races, so much the better, for me, for the Federation, for the sponsors.

And if it isn't?

I'll learn from the errors I made so that in the following competitions I can be on a higher plateau. But I will have a tranquil conscience because I will be certain that what I did corresponded to the maximum of my skills in that situation.

What meaning does a medal, or a place on the podium at a competition, have for you? You say you go to enjoy yourself, in search of your harmony, your development, but then, if you leave there with a gold medal, what does that mean?

Good question . . . Some time back I received a very beautiful trophy at a European championship. When I got home and was taking it out of the suitcase, it fell on the floor and broke. It was the most beautiful trophy I've received so far. I remember looking at it and thinking, "Well, I have to win another one." I wasn't very upset because the important thing wasn't the trophy itself, but the fact it was a symbol that I had tried to exceed my limits. And that is an indestructible personal credit! It's that I had, in fact, had a good performance, which, by chance, corresponded to a good result. In that competition in particular, I had finally conquered the taboo that I couldn't move with a weak wind. The trophy was only a symbol of that conquest of mine. That's something that isn't necessarily associated with a prize, nor does it disappear if the trophy's destroyed.

Isn't that perspective somewhat egocentric?

I don't believe so because my evolution contributed to the evolution of the class in which I compete, which in this case is the "Mistral." It's that if I evolve, the others will have to evolve, too. In order to catch up with me, they will have to try much harder, and they will have to go through things I went through. On the other hand, in a circular way, their evolution will put new problems before me, which will bring about new improvements. This permanent interaction is one of the central, generating elements of the sport, which also has a social outreach in making others enthusiastic about doing it, thus gaining new windsurfers.

It is true that, in making life difficult for your opponents, you take on the fundamental ethical element of sports, which is to contribute so that they too exceed themselves, but don't you think that, on the other hand, the sports titles can play a social role and for that reason become important?

I believe they can be socially motivating through the impact they have in the press. People like winners. I understand these reactions because I know what the idealized standards for sports are. But I can't allow myself

to drift with this current and assume that I have the obligation to win. My convictions, my ideals, my goals have to be so solid that these things pass me by. As a matter of fact, victories not only can be the source of anxiety, but the glory they bring are completely ephemeral. When I won the World Championship in South Africa in 1995, an Argentine, my opponent and friend, came to me and was very emotional. He hugged me and said, "The world is round, and now you are on the top of it!" That left me thinking. Then, when I arrived in Madeira, where I live, I was received with glory. There were a lot of people at the airport and public tributes, which I will proudly show my grandchildren. It all happened so fast that I really started to float. I stayed on the moon, and I paid dearly. I didn't land in time for the next World Championship, 3 months later in Israel, and I finished in 18th place! I went to the opposite side of the world, and, this time, the only ones waiting for me at the airport were my parents.

Did you suffer because of this?

More than anything, I learned from it. . . . As I said in an interview to a Madeirean newspaper (Freitas, 1996), it was the best thing that could have happened to me! I realized that, far more than titles or medals, one could gain experience that will serve us in life. It was the way I got my feet on the ground and began to understand why things were going wrong. I knew that I had to rethink my life and go back a ways in order to climb up. I had let myself slide into the valorization of the athletic results.

You wanted to win. . . .

That's true. Since I had won the previous World competition, I said to myself, "Well, there I'll have to win this!" I liked it so much that I wanted to repeat the experience. It turned out that it went very badly for me, and one of the main reasons was precisely that I wanted to win. I stopped thinking rationally. The starts, which are fundamental for the final position, were all wrong for me; I couldn't make the right decisions. In the only race in which I managed to go out in front, I fell and finished in 10th place. I had completely lost my concentration! Rather, I was totally concentrated on the final result I wanted to achieve. I was not concerned about myself. I was concerned about winning. It was the worst championship since Barcelona. As a matter of fact, I realized later that every time I want to win, I end up losing.

Did it happen again?

Yes, on other occasions. I think I finally understood. A curious thing happened to me in China. I accepted an invitation to participate in the Asia-Pacific Championship. I confess that the principal attraction for going there was to see China. I viewed the event with no great sense of responsibility, and things went well for me the first 2 days. At some point, I realized that this was a competition, which counted a lot towards the world ranking. Then my goal changed, and I began to think, "if I win this, I'll be no. 2 in the ranking." There, I lost! The most beautiful thing that happened to me was that I lost the championship in the last of the 12 races and in the last leg. When I finished, I didn't know whether to laugh or cry. I had made such a point of winning that . . . to rank no. 2 in the world had no impact in the press, but I thought it was a good idea and would please me. It's amazing how I had fallen into the same error 4 or 5 months after Israel. How badly that last race went for me! I made completely stupid mistakes, from falling to not seeing the buoy. My concentration was on another goal. My intuition, the instantaneous and correct response to situations, stopped working. The competition was practically narrowed down to me and a windsurfer from Fiji since the others were weaker and falling behind. I only concerned myself with beating

him. At the finish line, he beat me by a half a meter. That's hard to believe, isn't it? It was a good thing that happened to me!!

From what you describe here, we can conclude that contrary to what happened in these competitions where you had bad results, you don't think about a victory in the ones you end up winning.

It's normally that way. For example, in the World Championship in South Africa, it never crossed my mind that I would win. It was the first competition for which I had intentionally developed the following thought: "I trained the best I could; I am in the best possible shape; my goal is to sail the best I can, resolving each problem as it appears." What is certain is that I had no fear whatsoever of taking a chance. I trusted myself as I had never done before. This was particularly noticeable on the starts. Since I had trained a lot, both psychologically and technically, I was so confident that I always got off to a good start, like I had never done in any previous competition. No matter what the situation, I was always among the first to arrive at the buoys, which was half the battle for the final result. However, I was so involved in the task that, at times, I only realized I had won when I would look back at the end after crossing the finish line.

When you speak about the different levels of importance you place on the competitions, it's implicit that you will have key competitions for which you prepare yourself more carefully and where you place a more special meaning on your performance.

That's true. Normally the European and World Championships are the ones where I try to be prepared in the best possible way. I use the other regattas to learn and try to put in practice what I learned during the summer.

What's the difference between these regattas and the training sessions that also serve to learn and test yourself?

It's that in the regattas I have the intense opposition of the competitors who create problems for me. If I have worked well, I will know how to get around them. If I come in first, I conclude my work, and the path I'm taking is right. If I come in last, that means that there is something that I should change, and I have to find out what it is.

I see. But what leads you to attach a different meaning to certain events, such as the European and the World championships, selecting them as key competitions?

In principle, everyone will be at the height of his or her skills in those competitions. The challenge is greater, therefore, and I want to meet it.

In truth, it appears to me that the competitions are an instrument for assessment for you. By comparing yourself with the others, you get a measure of your state of evolution. In the competitions where the competitors are better prepared, the measure is more dependable, and you have a more accurate indication of your capabilities.

Yes, that's exactly the situation at the Olympic Games. There, too, just like the others, I want to do my best. Curiously, I find here a similarity with the exams at the university. What I wanted to know was whether I was going to succeed in resolving the problems, and the harder it was to obtain a good result, the greater the personal satisfaction it gave me. The competitions are, in fact, the "test bench" where I test the level of improvement I am at.

That is to say that you keep establishing successively higher landings. Aren't you frightened by the possibility of failing in your attempt to reach them?

Not at all. If it weren't so, records would never be broken. I have the idea that we can always go further, that there are thousands of things that can be perfected.

Your analysis of the psychological and motivational orientation you have in competitions points to two fundamental types, the consequences of which you have become aware of in your performances: the result and the task. Was there a moment in which that difference became clear to you?

There was. I remember a conversation with an Austrian windsurfer and friend during which he confessed that he no longer felt a motivation to win. For someone who had been champion of the world, any finish below first place would seem to have no meaning, but, on the other hand, winning at any cost was not what I wanted. There was something missing! This friend of mine told me then that what he most appreciated in me was the way in which I trained, the method I used. He further said that it was important to try to reach perfection, always seeking to do better, even knowing that it is impossible to be perfect. It was at that time that I became aware of what was wrong: I was forgetting the process of evolution and concentrating myself on the desire to win.

Did you "test" this change of attitude?

I can say that I did. In this phase of the crisis following the two world championships, there was one of the most important competitions on the international circuit in Hyères (France). I intentionally directed my concentration on the elements of performance. In one of the regattas, especially, I succeeded in concentrating completely. I didn't look at anyone else, I didn't concern myself with the others, only with myself. "By coincidence." I won! At that time, I said to myself that it was still possible. I had finally found what I was missing.

Can you explain?

I had come to understand that establishing goals centered on the athletic result didn't motivate me in actual practice, nor did it help me in the competitions. I was able to recover the goals inherent in the task I carry out during the regattas and which is part of an overall process of improvement.

In actual practice, how do you establish those goals?

I try to feel everything as much as possible—my body, each muscle, the water hitting against the board, the wind passing across the sail, past my body. I try each moment to put everything into harmony and reach perfection because in windsurfing, the board, the sail, and the windsurfer should be one. The most sublime moment happens when everything else ceases to exist and becomes "that"!

How do you reach this moment?

More than anything else, it's necessary to want to achieve it, which is quite different from wanting to attain a certain position or some type of material or social benefit.

Don't you have references by which you guide your behavior?

In training, for example, I sometimes establish task goals to perfect details related to change of tack or to what is necessary to improve the speed moving straight ahead. On the other hand, I also have goals, which refer to the optimization of my own bodily functioning since, even in competition, it is important to feel exactly the type and intensity of the effort I am putting out. One of my aims is to succeed in reaching "optimum performance" in which the greatest efficiency is achieved with the least effort, and each time, I have a better notion of how to get there, feeling the actions of my body, the position, the way the muscles work. When I concentrate on this process inherent in the system which I'm part of with the board, the sail, and the physical involvement, I am much more relaxed, I tire less, I move better. Everything is much more harmonious.

But on the other hand, the athletic results you have obtained have brought you another

order of benefits, of a financial nature, prestige and social recognition, etc.

Although that is true and sometimes pleasant, the only thing, which motivates me to windsurf and compete, is the enormous love I have for that. In no way is it to get my name in the papers, nor to earn money. I'll give you an example of the immense pleasure I have in riding the surfboard. When the Atlanta Games were over, I immediately thought how 4 more years of training would really appeal to me. I had not windsurfed during the month of August, and one day in September, as I left work at lunchtime, I looked at the bay of Funchal and saw it full of wind. It was a beautiful day, very windy. I was completely hysterical! I ate lunch quickly and ran to take my board out into the water. Of course, having eaten so quickly, along with the physical effort, I ended up feeling ill. I almost got indigestion. It was an almost infantile precipitation. But it had been so long since I had had that sense of liberty.

▲▼▲▼

The motivational process described by Rodrigues can be understood from the perspective of the relational theory of interests and personality (Abreu, 1998; Nutttin, 1965). In this constructivist perspective, the motives that are deterministic on the behavior of individuals result from the history of the interaction of the person and the world. Thus, the development of the personality is processed on the basis of the fulfillment of four groups of motives, which are considered primary because they are shown to be indispensable for the development and survival of human beings, seeing they are inscribed on the biological structure of the species. The biological, cognitive, social, and axiological needs are mentioned, as they relate to the metabolic transactions between the individual and his or her surroundings, to the organization of the information that the subject is gathering, to the aspects inherent in the interpersonal relationships, and to the reflection that organizes values, ideals and the meaning of life.

However, the instrumental means for the satisfaction of the mentioned needs or motives are not innately determined. In a very flexible way, they result from the life history of the individual, namely through the lessons being learned in his or her relationship with the world. In this way, the individual's interests are formed. The dynamizing force of these interests comes from the meaning that the individual attributes to them as a means of achieving the purposes inherent in the fundamental motives, which takes place in a process of subjective organization of a system of means-ends. Quoting Abreu (1998),

> the dynamic factors of behavior (motives or needs), as relational forces pointing towards an end, require a set of processes, activities and intermediate or mediating acquisitions, which are important or valuable for achieving the required relationship: it is here that the interests are located. (p. 67)

Thus goes the notion that the individual projects into the future a profound reason for his or her behavior, organizing himself or herself for it in function of a project for life that many times is being restructured in successive projects and in a genuine strategic plan. In this context, the motives are a permanently motivating tension for which the interests become the means of fulfillment.

> The state of satisfaction which accompanies the concrete satisfaction of a motive or the conclusion of a task in which we have invested time and effort is always transitory, because, having concluded that task, we again formulate new goals, throwing ourselves into new challenges. (Abreu, 1998, p. 76)

It is in the perspective set forth that we believe that sport has gained an existential meaning for the individual, in that it is an interest-activity through which the subject tends to satisfy his or her fundamental motivations. On the opposite side, when the connection sports-purpose does not find a meaningful relationship in the perception of the participant, a lack of motivation sets in, which is expressed in the lack of dedication and then abandonment.

The case we have been studying illustrates perfectly this motivational process. In fact, the involvement in the sport of windsurfing finds meaning in the relationship that João establishes between the sport and the fundamental motivations. As a matter of fact, the biological motives find a response in the activation of the organic systems, promoting physical development, health, and well-being. On the other hand, the existence of the athlete as a social being (social motives) is developed in the meaningful personal interactions that take place in the sports context, as well as in the perception and respect the athlete has in regard to his stature as a social model inherent in his being a notable athlete. The cognitive motives are equally satisfied in the permanent attitude of reflection and interpretation of the information that comes from his relationship with sailing, with a view to perfecting his adaptation to the world. Finally, his axiological needs find an answer in the clarification of the meaning of life and the values underlying the person-world relationship, which originate in the questions raised by this sports activity that thus assumes a profound personal meaning.

The motivational strategies, then, appear naturally. Windsurfing, as an essential element in his project for life, is prolonged indefinitely in time. The moments in training and each competition gain meaning as steps to be taken with a view to fulfilling the essential motives. The strategic planning occurs in this logic, containing the formulation of intrinsically assumed goals. Self-knowledge becomes a constant attitude on the way to the optimization of the dynamic relationship with the involvement. The competitions are moments for assessing the route, generating critical reflection, interpretation, and meta-cognition.

The development of autonomy is conscientiously sought after. It is revealed, namely, in the way he establishes his goals for each training session, according to the needs he feels as a result of a constant self-analysis. The phase of his career he is in now, as well as his level of personal and athletic maturity, gives him a certain independence from the coach.

The essence of João Rodrigues's motivational process is projected in his personal development. For this reason, extrinsic rewards do not have a mobilizing effect, and there was a certain existential void after he won the world title in South Africa. This goal, the moment it was achieved, eliminated tension coming from an extrinsic source, but it was not inserted into a course in which the intrinsic tension should persist in the direction of the aims that derive from the fundamental needs. The motivation only returned when the athletic results began to be viewed for their symbolic value projected in the information about the correction of the process, on the way to personal perfection. At that moment, he also became aware of the relativity of the athletic performance, of its limits and results. In fact, the personal limit is only momentary, in function of the individual conditions at the time. On the other hand, the success in obtaining the personal limit may translate into a lower result than that of his opponent, who at that moment may be in a more advanced stage. Nevertheless, the perception of success may prevail, associated with the conviction that he has achieved his potential under the circumstances, although he was inferior to his opponent.

The psychological preparation in sports, or the psychology of sports training, appears to be centered on the promotion of the maturity of the athlete so as to facilitate the perception of the meaningful relationship between sports and the motivational purposes. It would be like working at the level of "hardware," as opposed to what happens many times when the approach is centered on the imposition of a "software" made up of techniques that seek to artificially create a motivational energy that tends to run out in the short or medium term.

The athlete we have been dealing with developed a global and an inner perception of the sports performance. The process of training-competition is guided by a constant search for solutions by means of the identification of the problems, the blockading factors, and the factors of progression. The goal to be reached is the full harmony of the system of surfer-board-sail-surroundings, resulting from a perspective that integrates all the elements, associated with a profound involvement in the task. Volitional factors emerge as deterministic, and they are reinforced by the feeling of the emotional appropriation of the elements of evolution, which likewise nourish the intrinsic motivation. Curiously, this psychological approach to sports has many points of contact with the perspectives of Asian culture, as we find it very well described in the classic work by Herrigel, *The Zen in the Art of Archery* ("Zen in der kunst des bogenschiessens"; Portuguese edition, 1997). Western sports psychology, namely the Anglo-Saxon, which tends to break the preparation of the athletes into segments, will find great advantages in looking closely at the globalizing and unifying perspective with which the oriental philosophers understood the human being.

Epilogue: The Assessment of a Journey

The purpose of the preceding sections was to transmit and analyze the path taken by João Rodrigues over the period of one Olympiad. We dealt with the motives and the attitudes that made up the psychological foundations on which he has based his behavior. We examined the motivational process that gave rise to choices and strategic planning. We tried to understand his evolution as a result of the history of his relationship with the world and, especially, as influenced by processes of restructuring from critical events, due to the personal meaning in which they were clothed. With the help of this windsurfer's experience, which he agreed to share with any who would read this work, we sought, above all, to transmit the concept that sport can be an instrument that facilitates the fulfillment of essential motivations of human beings. In this way, sports will be a generator of personal development for those who participate. The psychological training of the athlete should go far beyond the teaching and training of a set of techniques and strategies aimed at optimizing psychological skills. It should be based on a process that stimulates personal maturity and a consistent means-ends relationship, in which the means consist of a participation in sports that is thought through and subjected to self-criticism whereas the ends are those inherent in the fundamental biological, cognitive, social, and axiological needs.

The psychologist, and the coach as well, should know how to use participation in sports as a vehicle for the development of athletes. To do this, they have to understand the athlete's level of maturity so as to stimulate his or her development in accordance with the distinct period in which the individual is found.

Because we have been following the course taken by João Rodrigues and the process of his reflection and psychological maturation, it would be interesting to "hear him" again on his assessment of this existential journey from Barcelona to Atlanta.

Having come to the end of this 4-year journey, what are your thoughts about it?

They were 4 wonderful years! The difficulty that was associated with them many times had nothing to do with sacrifice. They were 4 years of deep growth.

Can we say that it was what you imagined at the Portuguese border on the way back from Barcelona, when you decided to change your attitude towards sports and studies?

Ah, no! It was much better! When I crossed that border, if I had known it was going to be so good, I would probably have jumped up and down with joy for having made the decision. But those 4 years were much better than I ever could have imagined, in all respects.

What do you mean by "in all respects"?

In sport, in school, in my personal life in finding fulfillment as a person, in growth, in seeing the world in a different way, in . . . ah . . . everything. I think I evolved more in this last 4 years than in all the previous 20.

What do you project for the future?

I don't like to think about goals, which are too concrete, but it has never crossed my mind to abandon sports. Once again, I'm going to let things happen. As a matter of fact, I don't want to think about whether the next 4 years may or may not be as good as the previous 4. I hope that I continue to grow in the same way as I have up to now. Principally, I want to continue developing myself as a person, because I believe there are no limits for that. The more we learn, the more we become aware that there are many more things to be learned, many more things to be discovered. The path I discovered in these past 4 years was much more direct—from the inside out. Before, I was much more turned to the exterior without realizing how the inner life is as important and deterministic as what we do and what we feel.

Would you like to explain more about what you mean by "inner life"?

It's difficult to put into words. I remember that after the Barcelona Games, in spite of everything, I was very arrogant because I felt that the fact I had gone to the Games made be better than the others. Later, I was really upset when one of my brothers was riding the board better than I. Deep down, the inner activity implied remodeling all those things, concluding that one is always learning and developing. But we have to be the ones to discover that and have the humility required to accept it. When I really saw that there was something to be changed, I had to turn back inward and try to understand how I functioned at that level.

That's a complex process that needs time.

Sure. We need to be very relaxed in order to be aware of the signs that come from within, to understand what we really are, and the influence that society has over us. We need to understand whether what we do corresponds to what we really want or whether we are simply limiting ourselves to reacting uncritically to social influences. As I read once, we are made up of three "I"s: the one others think we are, the one we think we are, and the one we really are. I believe we only attain peace and harmony when those three are one and the same. What concerns me most is that the "I am" and the "I think that I am" coincide completely. What others think about me does not bother me so much. I can't open up their heads and put things in them.

From that perspective, the obsessive search for results may keep us at the level of "what we appear to be" to others and to ourselves, perhaps to hide what we don't know about "what we are" and what we are probably

afraid to discover. I think that a fundamental role of sport is to utilize the sport process to promote self-knowledge and, through that, to organize ourselves creatively so that we fulfil our potential. In that way we can find in sports participation an inexhaustible fountain, without any inhibitions from the objective level of performance. The best examples are given us by the "Masters" of martial arts who, notwithstanding the diminution of their physical resources, continue to practice their skills up until very old age, always seeking new subjective landings on the staircase of evolution.

I agree. It is in the difficulty of this process that I find the great fascination of sports as a way of establishing harmony between what I am and what I think I am!

Do you mean to say, then, that the fact that you were not an Olympic champion when you were one of the strongest candidates was not very important?

I don't know what would have been the sensation if I had won the gold medal in Atlanta. The sensation I have now is one of fulfillment. I feel fulfilled even though I placed seventh because my goal from the beginning was not the medal, but to finish with the notion that my performance had corresponded to the maximum of my potential in the competition. And I have a clear conscience. I like to think that if I had been the champion, I would have the same attitude to desire to learn, grow, and develop more; to think that I can always set my sights higher to perfect my resources and personal qualities. It took me 4 years to modify my internal structure, which had taken me to Barcelona with a clear goal regarding my standing, which I did not achieve, but which made me suffer and feel empty.

Before you began your Olympic competition in Atlanta, you told me that you would like for me to know that it wasn't the medal you were after. I believed you. but now, I would like for you to reflect on whether that corresponded to what your real "I" thought, or if it was your "wishful I" speaking.

I'll answer this way: After the Games were over, I never lay down sad. Normally, it's when I lie down that all the worries, all the nuisances come to mind, and I don't remember losing any sleep over not having won a medal in Atlanta. But I do remember spending many sleepless hours over the fact I didn't finish in the top 20 in Barcelona!

After Atlanta, didn't you go through a certain existential crisis commonly associated with the phase following the achievement of a very important goal, such as participating in the Olympic Games?

But for me the Atlanta Games were not a goal. They were merely a step in an evolving process, not a goal.

Then you have another step ahead.

I do. It's the Games in Sydney—not for the Games in themselves, which I have never thought of as an end, but rather as one more point to assess what windsurfing is going to help me do in the next 4 years. I even told myself that if I go to Sydney, I would not commit the same errors I didn't know how to avoid up until Atlanta. If I succeed in that, I will have learned from that experience.

It has been some time since João and I had the conversations that prompted this text. Other critical life moments have since been experienced by him, bringing about new restructuring and with it, new developments regarding his relationship with the world and with himself. His participation in the Atlanta Games and his licentiate degree in engineering completed in the same year were two aspects he considered deterministic. Likewise, he began his professional career as an engineer with the Sports Institute of Madeira, which is a department of the government of this Autonomous Region of Portugal. Although he could have obtained a leave of absence to dedicate himself fully to training, he preferred to maintain his professional career in parallel, just as he did when he was a student. Another event of great personal significance was his marriage, exactly half-way down the road, time-wise, from Atlanta to Sydney.

Two years away from Sydney, he achieved first place in the world ranking for the mistral class of windsurfing and had already been chosen to represent Portugal in the year 2000 Olympic Games. Meanwhile, he was European Champion in 1997, silver medallist at the European Championships in 1998, and bronze medallist at the World Championships the same year.

References

Abreu, M. V. (1998). *Cinco ensaios sobre a motivação.* Coimbra: Almedina.

Bloom, B. S. (1985). *Development talent in young people.* New York: Balantyne.

Buceta, J. M. (1998). *Psicologia del entrenamiento deportivo.* Madrid: Dykinson.

Burton, D. (1993). Goal setting in sport. In R.N.Singer, M. Murphey, & L. K. Tennant (Eds.), *Handbook of Research on Sport Psychology* (pp. 467–491). New York: Macmillan Publishing Company.

Crews, D. J. (1993). Self-regulation strategies in sport and exercise. In R. N. Singer, M. Murphey, & L. K. Tennant (Eds.), *Handbook of Research on Sport Psychology* (pp. 557–568). New York: Macmillan Publishing Company.

Danish, S. J., Petitpas, A., & Hale, B. (1995). Psychological interventions: A life development model. In S. Murphy (Ed.), *Sport psychology interventions* (pp. 19–38). Champaign: Human Kinetics.

Frankl, V. E. (1984). *Man's search for meaning.* New York: Touchstone.

Frankl, V. E. (1987, June). Le sport: phénomène humain. *Science du sport, documents de recherche et de tecnologie*, BU-2.

Freitas, J. (1996, May,20). Windsurf nao e' sacrificio. *Diario de Noticias*, p. 4

Hardy, L., Jones, G., & Gould, D. (1996). *Understanding psychological preparation for sport.* Chichester: Wiley.

Herrigel, E. (1997). *Zen e a arte do tiro com arco.* Lisboa: Assirio & Alvim.

Louganis, G., & Marcus, E. (1996). *Breaking the surface*. New York: Plume, Penguin.

Le Scanff, C. (1998). La préparation-entrainement psychologique pour les situation extrèmes : Application au sport de haut niveau. *Bulletin de Psychologie, 51* (6), 4 766–781.

Nideffer, R. N. (1993). Attention control training. In R. N. Singer, M. Murphey, & L. K. Tennant (Eds.), *Handbook of Research on Sport Psychology* (pp. 542–556). New York: Macmillan Publishing Company.

Nuttin, J. (1965). *La structure de la personalité*. Paris: PUF

Rotella, R. J., & Lerner, J. D. (1993), Responding to competitive pressure. In R. N. Singer, M. Murphey, & L. K. Tennant (Eds.), *Handbook of Research on Sport Psychology* (pp.528–541). New York: Macmillan Publishing Company.

Salmela, J. H. (1994). Phases and transitions across sport careers. In D. Hackfort (Ed.), *Psycho-social issues and interventions in elite sport* (pp. 11–28). Frankfurt am Main: Peter Lang.

Serpa, S., & Araújo, D. (1996). *Psychology of coaching: Concepts and Systematization*. Paper presented in the International Seminar of Sport Psychology (May. 31–June.1) Lisboa: Faculty of Psychology and Sciences of Education, Portuguese Society of Sport Psychology.

Singer, R. N., Murphey, M., & Tennant L .K. (Ed.). (1993). *Handbook of Research on Sport Psychology* (pp. 492–510). New York: Macmillan Publishing Company.

Suinn, R. (1993). Imagery. In R. N. Singer, M. Murphey, & L. K. Tennant (Eds.), *Handbook of Research on Sport Psychology* (pp. 492–510). New York: Macmillan Publishing Company.

Zaichkowsky, L., & Takenaka, K (1993. In R. N.Singer, M. Murphey, & L. K. Tennant (Eds.), *Handbook of Research on Sport Psychology* (pp. 511–527). New York: Macmillan Publishing Company.

Note: This chapter was sponsored by the Faculty of Human Movement (Technical University of Lisbon) and by the Sports Institute of the Autonomous Region of Madeira (IDRAM), Portugal

The text was translated from Portuguese by Edgar Potter

Identifying and Developing World-Class Performers

Robert M. Nideffer

Marc-Simon Sagal

Mark Lowry

Jeffrey Bond

The role of assessment in helping to identify and develop world-class performers has never been more important. The fact that the International Society of Sport Psychology (ISSP) has commissioned a book on the psychological preparation of elite-level athletes indicates two things:

1. That the challenges and pressures faced by elite-level performers are different or more intense than those faced by other performers;
2. That the role of the sport psychology consultant changes as the level of performance of the athlete changes.

This chapter will take a look at those assumptions, not just as they relate to elite-level performance in sport. We will begin by pulling together 25 years of experience and data that have been collected on elite-level athletes from around the world. Those data will show that even at an early age, elite-level athletes have more effective concentration and intra- and interpersonal characteristics than other athletes do. In fact, data collected at the Australian Institute for Sport

over the past 17 years indicate that over time (and with experience) these differences increase. It is a comparison of an individual athlete's scores on these performance-relevant psychological characteristics with normative data from world champions that provides the information needed to develop psychological skills training and intervention programs.

In addition to issues associated with the development of an individual's psychological skills, we will describe how the concentration skills of successful coaches differ from those of elite-level athletes. We will discuss some of the implications these differences have for the coach-athlete relationship.

Finally, the chapter describes some of the conflicts and breakdowns in communication that are becoming increasingly common in other high-pressure, high-performance environments. Helping coaches and athletes is not very different from helping managers and production personnel in today's highly competitive, fast-paced, global business environments maintain effective communication and teamwork. In fact, helping individuals perform under highly competitive conditions or in high-stress environments other than sport (e.g., business, and the military) is a logical extension of the services sport psychologists offer.

Elite-level Performers

In the early 1980s, the United States Olympic Sports Medicine Committee began funding an Elite Athlete Development Project. This project was designed to bring the sport sciences of biomechanics, exercise physiology, and sport psychology together so that athletes with a good chance of making an Olympic team could be provided with a comprehensive training program (Nideffer, 1987).

The Elite Athlete Development Project was initiated largely because the United States was losing its competitive edge. Countries like the U.S.S.R. and East Germany had begun spending more money on talent identification and on the development of athletes. As a result, the technical and tactical skills of athletes began improving dramatically around the world. As the level of competition began to increase, so did training loads. To be successful, elite-level athletes were having to perform at higher levels, were having to increase the consistency of their performance, and were having to perform much closer to the upper limits of their potential.

Today, elite-level sport is big business. What matters is the bottom line. The rewards for winning and the negative consequences of losing are formidable. As the pressures to perform increase and as the technical and tactical skill levels of the competitors even out, psychological variables begin to play a greater role in distinguishing winners from losers. An individual cannot become a world-class athlete in today's highly competitive environment without having both physical *and* psychological talent.

When it comes to training athletes in psychological techniques to control emotional arousal, distractibility, and focus of concentration, there is relatively little difference between work with elite-level performers and work with athletes performing at lower levels. As the data that follow indicate, however, the particular stimuli that interfere with an athlete's ability to concentrate and control arousal differ as a function of age and experience. Thus, the focus of performance-enhancement interventions is different at an elite level.

There are other, larger differences one encounters when working with elite-level athletes. For example, because the bottom line is so important and because psychological factors are so critical to success, psychological consultants are often asked to provide information that can be used in the selection process:

1. Will the athlete be able to fit into the existing team?
2. Does the athlete have the psychological skills required to play at the highest level?
3. Will the athlete be able to cope with the pressure of moving away from home to train?
4. Does the athlete have the level of motivation and self-discipline required to fully develop his or her talents?
5. How quickly can the athlete learn our system (how flexible is he or she)?

Elite-level performance requires intense training loads and personal sacrifices on the part of the athlete (e.g., the willingness to put sport above everything else including family and friends). Thus, consultants are often asked to help athletes deal with the emotional and physical consequences of these sacrifices *without* interfering with their performance. Finally, because there is very little balance in the life of an elite athlete, there is an increasing need for services designed to help athletes in transition make adjustments to new living conditions and performance challenges.

Assessing Performance-Relevant Psychological Variables

What are the psychological characteristics we need to assess in order to respond to the needs of coaches and athletes? Experience indicates a thorough assessment of an athlete's potential includes an evaluation of the following:

- The athlete's existing physical skills and tactical knowledge
- The athlete's cognitive and perceptual skills; that is,
    1. The athlete's information-processing capacity (ability to cope with complex and changing environments)
    2. The athlete's ability to be environmentally aware without becoming distracted
    3. The athlete's ability to analyze and problem solve without becoming overloaded and confused, and
    4. The athlete's ability to focus concentration appropriately (but not to the point that he or she fails to attend to critical task-relevant information).
- The athlete's *intrapersonal* characteristics, like drive, self-confidence, motivation, and competitiveness.
- The athlete's *interpersonal* characteristics, which include attitudes and behaviors that define how the individual relates to, and communicates with, others.
- The athlete's emotional stability, which involves assessing the individual's ability to control emotions that, if left unchecked, would lower performance.

Typically, the athlete's existing physical skills and tactical knowledge are assessed by the coach, not the sport psychologist. It is the psychologist's responsibility to assess cognitive skills, intra- and interpersonal characteristics, and emotional stability. How these areas are assessed varies from psychologist to psychologist. Many rely almost exclusively on interviews and performance obser-

vation. Although these are important parts of the assessment process, quite often, they are not enough.

At Enhanced Performance Systems, we use The Attentional and Interpersonal Style (TAIS) inventory to get athletes to provide information about performance-relevant cognitive and intra- and interpersonal skills and abilities. TAIS was designed specifically for this purpose. When TAIS is administered early in the consulting or training process, the inventory provides information that helps the consultant address performance-relevant issues more quickly and more reliably (Nideffer, 1976, 1993).

Defining Elite-level Performance

What constitutes elite-level performance in sport? The answer seems to depend on whom one asks, but how one chooses to define elite-level performance is not really what is important. The key is to define and describe the specific *level* of performance one is talking about. In this chapter, we will discuss several different levels of "elite" performance.

The TAIS data that follow have been collected from two different groups of elite-level athletes. The first group consisted of 4,541 individuals tested at the Australian Institute for Sport (AIS). Approximately 32% of the athletes were female. These AIS athletes ranged in age from 11 to 60, with a mean age of 22.9 years. The athletes were competing at a state, national, and/or international level in 44 different sports.

The second group consisted of 142 different athletes. At a minimum, each of these athletes had won an Olympic medal or a world championship in his or her sport or had been ranked in the top three in the world. In fact, over half of the athletes tested were multiple medal winners who had won several world championships. These athletes were from seven different countries and competed in 21 different sports. There were

119 males and 23 females. It is important to point out that the psychological characteristics of this group were remarkably consistent, independent of the athlete's gender, native country, or type of sport (closed skill, individual open skill, or team sport).

The Development of Performance-relevant Psychological Characteristics

Do the concentration skills, cognitive abilities, or intra- and interpersonal characteristics of elite-level athletes differ from those of nonathletes? If differences do exist, to what extent are they due to learning or training as opposed to innate/biogenetic predispositions? Although we cannot provide final and definitive answers to these questions, we are able to show that when data from The Attentional and Interpersonal Style inventory are examined cross-sectionally, there are significant differences in subject scores as a function of age. Not only that, but when the same subjects, in this case 776 AIS athletes, were retested 18 months later, the same pattern of changes occurred longitudinally that were seen in the cross-sectional data. This means that athletes' skills were continuing to develop over time.

In the data that follow, the 4,541 AIS athletes were divided into four groups based on their age (<17, 17–18, 19–24, >24). We began by contrasting TAIS scores of the youngest group of AIS athletes (N=907) with the scores of a group of normal adolescents from the United States (N=302).

AIS Athletes vs. Normal Adolescents

With respect to cognitive skills, scores on TAIS indicated that the AIS athletes under the age of 17 were significantly more focused and significantly less likely to become distracted and/or overloaded than were members of the normal adolescent group.

Intrapersonally, the athletes were more in control of situations, more willing to take responsibility, more self-confident, and more competitive than were adolescents in general. Interpersonally, athletes were more extroverted and more positive and supportive. With respect to emotional control, the athlete group was less behaviorally impulsive and less expressive of anger and criticism.

Changes in TAIS Scores of AIS Athletes As a Function of Age Level and Time Between Tests

This next series of analyses attempts to answer three questions. First, were there differences in the cognitive skills and the intra- and interpersonal characteristics of athletes as a function of age? In other words, were older athletes more or less skilled than younger ones? This question was examined by using a series of analyses of variance to compare the scores of the four AIS groups (<17, 17–18, 19–24, >24).

Next, when differences existed as a function of age, were they due to changes in individuals' scores as they aged, or were they due to some type of self-selection process? This question can be partially examined by looking at test-retest data. Fortunately, there was a group of 776 AIS athletes who had been tested on two or more occasions. The average time interval between testing was 18 months. If the same changes seen in the cross-sectional data were found in athletes who had been retested, that provides evidence suggesting learning was taking place. Thus, the concentration skills required for elite-level performance were at least partially learned. This question was examined by using a series of analyses of variance looking at various concentration and interpersonal skills as a function of age (4 levels) and test (2 test administrations).

Finally, it is important to look at particu-

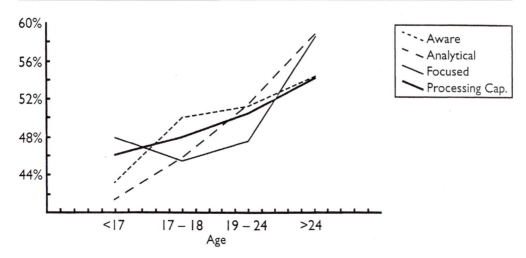

Figure 1.
Cognitive skills as a function of age.

lar TAIS scores in relationship to other scores. For example, when looking at cognitive skills, it is important to know if one skill is more highly developed or dominant than another (e.g., were athletes more focused than analytical?). To make comparisons between subjects' scores on different scales, it was necessary to transform the raw scores of all 4,541 athletes based on the entire groups' means and standard deviations, converting them to z-scores. It is these z-scores that were used in the statistical analyses.

Figure 1 shows the differences that existed in TAIS scores as a function of age. These data are based on scores from all 4,541 AIS athletes. As you can see, scores in the cognitive skills were different as a function of age. The slope of the lines representing the different concentration skills does vary, however.

To make it easier to understand the data and to get a sense for the magnitude of differences that exists between scores, we have converted standard scores to percentile scores. Thus, the percentiles shown on the left side of each graph indicate where the individual groups scored relative to the entire sample.

As Figure 1 illustrates, external awareness increased fairly constantly with age; the only difference in the figure that was not statistically significant was the increase that occurred between the ages of 17 and 18 and 19 and 24. Thus, analytical scores were significantly higher at each age level. With respect to the ability to focus, there is a decrease between the ages of 16, and 17 to 18 that approaches statistical significance ($p=.06$). It is conceivable that this drop in focus is associated with sexual development. In fact, scores on the scale measuring focused concentration did not increase significantly until sometime after the age of 24. Finally, as with analytical skills, athletes' scores on the information-processing scale increased consistently and significantly across all age levels.

Figure 2 shows the changes in the same four cognitive areas for the 776 athletes who were tested twice. As with the data for the entire AIS population, the scores for this group of athletes have also been converted to standard scores, then plotted as percentiles. The standard scores were calculated by using the means and standard deviations for the 776 subjects on the first test administration.

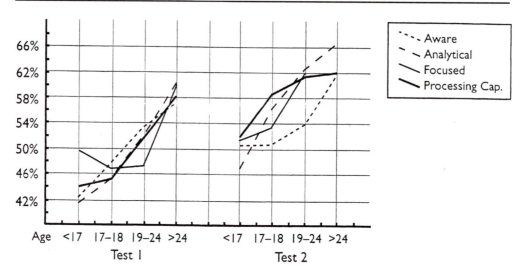

Figure 2.
Cognitive skills as a function of age and testing.

As Figure 2 demonstrates, the pattern of changes as a function of the age of the athletes was the same as it was for the entire AIS population. By looking at the two graphs, first test on the left and second test on the right, you can see the within-subject changes taking place.

The similarity of the data shown in Figure 2 to the data shown in Figure 1 strongly suggests that the differences we saw as a function of the age of the athlete were more likely to be the result of developmental changes than they were to some type of selection process.

The within-subject changes for these 776 athletes were highly significant. The absolute amount of change in subjects' scores over the 18-month interest interval averaged 6% on the scales measuring information processing, external awareness, and analytical skill. There was a 3% change in scores on the scale measuring focused concentration.

Figure 3 shows the relationship between the three different types of cognitive or attentional errors measured by TAIS and an athlete's age for the entire AIS sample. As you can see, young athletes were significantly

more likely to make mistakes because they were externally distracted than they were because they became too narrowly focused and underinclusive or because they became internally distracted. The reverse was true for older athletes. Past the age of 24, athletes were significantly more likely to make mistakes because they became overloaded, thinking too much, or because they became too narrowly focused and underinclusive.

Although athletes improved significantly in all three-error categories, the amount of change that took place and the timing of that change varied with the type of error. External distractibility decreased the most, and the changes that occurred were consistent and statistically significant across the four age ranges. Internal overload increased slightly, then began to drop. Not until the athlete was over the age of 24, however, did the drop become statistically significant. Finally, the tendency to narrow one's focus too much, becoming underinclusive and failing to attend to all of the task-relevant cues, began to drop significantly once the athlete passed the age of 18.

The same error patterns exist when we

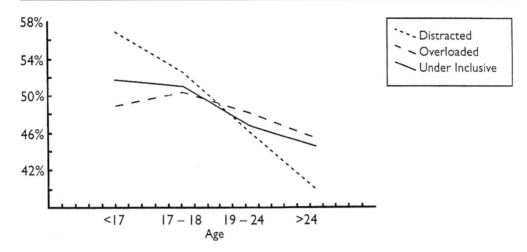

Figure 3.
Type of error as a function of age.

look at the test-retest data (see Figure 4). On average, there was an 8 percentage point drop in subject scores on the scales measuring external distractibility, internal distractibility, and underinclusiveness over the 18-month intertest interval.

Figure 5 shows the relationship between age and the entire 4,541 subjects' scores on four TAIS scales measuring intrapersonal characteristics. These include the athlete's need for control, level of self-confidence, competitiveness, and decisiveness.

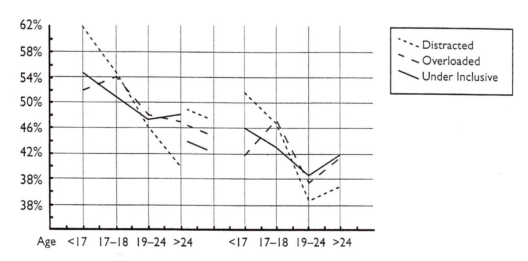

Figure 4.
Concentration errors as a function of age and experience.

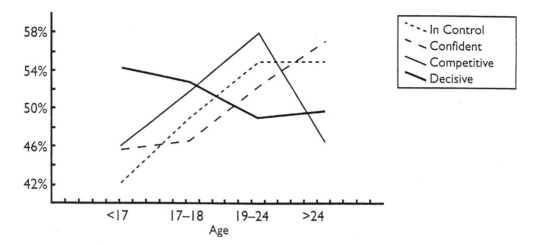

Figure 5.
TAIS intrapersonal scores as a function of age.

As Figure 5 indicates, the pattern of change in intrapersonal characteristics as a function of age varied. The TAIS scale measuring an athlete's willingness to take control of situations, as well as his or her feelings of being in control, increased up to the age of 24 and then leveled off. Confidence appeared to rise steadily, but this was due largely to the fact that 68% of the subjects were males. When we look at self-confidence as a function of sex, we find that for females, self-esteem increased slightly, but not significantly, up to the age of 24 and then began to drop.

With respect to competitiveness, there was a rise in competitiveness until the age of 24, followed by a precipitous and statistically significant drop. The fact that physical skills begin to diminish as athletes age may partially explain the rather dramatic increase that occurred in their ability to focus concentration once they passed the age of 24. Learning to focus may help to offset, at least temporarily, declining physical ability.

Finally, Figure 5 suggests that the scale measuring decisiveness dropped until the age of 24 and then began to rise again. The change from under 17 to the 19– to 24-year level is

significant. Because this scale is scored in reverse, a decreasing score means increased decisiveness and an increased willingness on the part of athletes to take risks.

As with cognitive skills, an analysis of the test-retest data revealed the same basic patterns described above. In addition, there was significant intrapersonal growth over the 18-month intertest interval. On the re-test, athletes described themselves as more willing to take control and responsibility, more self-confident, more competitive, and more decisive and willing to take risks. The absolute amount of change in subjects' scores averaged around 6% on the scales measuring control, confidence, and competitiveness, and 3% on the scale measuring decisiveness.

Figure 6 shows the relationship between age level and the TAIS scales measuring extroversion (enjoyment of others) and introversion (enjoyment of personal space and privacy) for the entire AIS sample. As you can see from Figure 4, younger athletes were significantly more extroverted than introverted. As the athletes grew older, however, this trend reversed itself. With age, athletes became more introverted (enjoyed personal

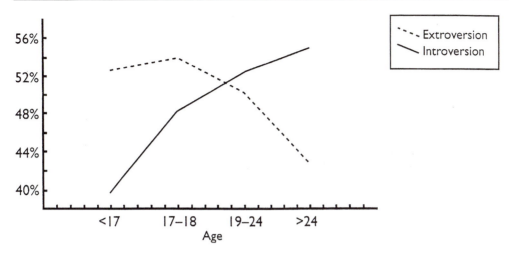

Figure 6.
Extroversion and introversion as a function of age.

space and privacy) and less extroverted. This change in scores was quite large (with introversion increasing by about 18 percentage points and extroversion decreasing by 12 percentage points). We believe this reflects some of the social sacrifices that individuals must make to fully develop their athletic talents. This same pattern appeared with the test-retest data.

Figure 7 shows the relationship between age and TAIS scales measuring expression of ideas, expression of anger and criticism, and expression of support. As athletes aged, there was a significant decrease in their expression of feelings. It did not matter if the feelings were positive and supportive or critical and angry. Interestingly, the significant drop in supportive feelings occurred several years

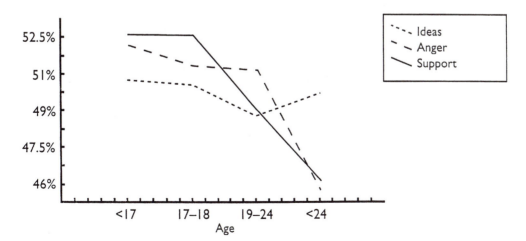

Figure 7.
Expressiveness as a function of age.

earlier than the drop in critical or angry feelings. With respect to the expression of ideas, there were no significant changes over time.

It is in the expressiveness area that scores for the 776 athletes who were tested twice differed significantly from the scores for the entire AIS population. Upon retesting, there were significant increases in the athletes' willingness to express thoughts and ideas, and support for others. The expression of anger dropped slightly, but not significantly.

Comparing AIS Athletes to World Champions

The data available show that elite-level athletes under the age of 17 tended to be more focused and less distractible than were their nonelite adolescent counterparts. They were also more willing to take responsibility, more confident, more competitive, more extroverted, and more supportive. As these athletes matured, significant changes occurred in their cognitive skills and intra- and interpersonal characteristics. These facts lead to two additional questions. First, given the changes, how do the scores of older AIS athletes compare with the scores of world champions? Then, how do the scores of both groups compare with those of the general adult population?

In this section, we used analyses of variance to compare the scores of older athletes at the AIS (1,946 athletes between the ages of 21 and 45) with those of the 142 world champions described earlier. For the purposes of these analyses, athlete scores have been converted to z-scores using the means and standard deviations for the adult population TAIS was standardized on. Thus, when percentile scores were reported, they told how the athlete groups scored in comparison with the standard norm group.

Figure 8 shows the scores for world champions and AIS athletes between the ages of 21 and 45 on TAIS scales measuring external awareness, analytical skill, ability to focus concentration, and amount of information a subject processes.

As you can see, it is the ability to focus concentration that distinguishes world champions (85th percentile) and AIS athletes (80th percentile) from the general population. Indeed, both groups were significantly more focused than they were aware, or analytical,

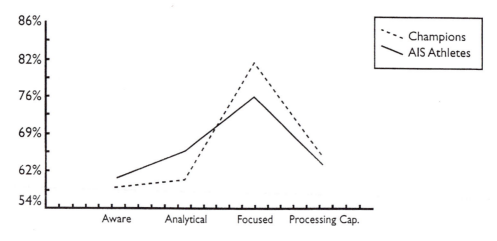

Figure 8.
Cognitive skills of world champions as AIS athletes.

or than they processed information. The five-percentage point difference that existed between world champions and AIS athletes with respect to focused concentration was also highly significant.

The only other difference between world champions and AIS athletes that is significant in Figure 8 was the difference in terms of their analytical skills. AIS athletes scored higher on the scale measuring analytical skills than did the world champions ($p=.009$).

When the two athlete groups were compared with the general population, the only difference that was not statistically significant was the world champions' score on the TAIS scale measuring external awareness. Thus, athletes in both groups had significantly better concentration skills than the average person did.

In terms of mistakes, both athlete groups were much more likely to make errors of underinclusion, because they narrowed their focus too much, than they were to make mistakes because they became externally distracted or overloaded and confused. This fits with the fact that both groups were dominated by a narrow focus of concentration.

World champions made significantly fewer mistakes in all three-error categories than AIS athletes did. When compared with the general population, both athlete groups made significantly fewer mistakes due to external distractions. Indeed, the extent to which the two athlete groups controlled external distractibility relative to the extent of control exercised by the general population was remarkable. World champions scored in the bottom 2% of the population on this scale, and AIS athletes scored in the bottom 3%.

When it came to thinking too much, becoming overloaded and confused by thoughts and feelings, world champions scored around the 25th percentile, significantly lower than the general population. AIS athletes, on the other hand, scored around the 50th per-

centile. The AIS athletes scored significantly higher than the world champion group on the TAIS scale measuring analytical skill. It may be that higher analytical scores increase the likelihood of thinking too much.

Both athlete groups scored higher than the general population on the scale measuring errors of underinclusion. World champions scored around the 54th percentile, and AIS athletes scored around the 60th percentile. This finding is consistent with the fact that both athlete groups were significantly more narrowly focused than were individuals in the general population. That focus and dedication obviously have some negative consequences (e.g., becoming too focused from time to time).

Intrapersonally, both world champions and AIS athletes had a significantly higher need for control and were more self-confident, more competitive, and less decisive than was the general population. The only surprise here is with respect to the decisiveness scale. This particular scale measures the extent to which individuals allow their concerns about avoiding mistakes to slow down their decision-making processes. It would appear that elite athletes were perfectionists, attending to details, practicing, and training until things were perfect. Under these conditions, performances were so well rehearsed and practiced that decision-making became automatic. Athletes were more cautious and slower to make decisions during training and when developing skills, not during the performance.

World champions had a higher (but not significant) need to be in control than did AIS athletes. In addition, world champions were significantly more confident, more competitive (85% vs. 80%), and slightly but not significantly more perfectionistic/less decisive (67% vs. 64%).

Interpersonally, both world champions and AIS athletes were significantly more extroverted than the average person, but not significantly different from each other (62% vs. 64%). AIS athletes were less introverted than either the standard norm group or the world champions (42% vs. 52%).

With respect to the expression of thoughts and feelings, world champions were much more likely to express support than they were to express either their ideas or their criticism and anger. When compared with AIS athletes, they were more expressive of both thoughts and ideas (50% vs. 38%) and positive feelings and support (78% vs. 58%). In comparison to the general population, both world champions and AIS athletes were more expressive of positive feelings and support, and AIS athletes were significantly less intellectually expressive.

A Service Provision Template

The cognitive and intra- and interpersonal characteristics that define world champions were consistent across gender, across sport, and across cultures. As you can see from AIS data, those characteristics were apparent at younger ages and continued to develop through the athlete's career. Using those characteristics, we can paint a picture or create a template that defines what a world champion should look like. That picture then helps define the services that are provided both programmatically and individually.

Athletes with world championship potential are not just more physically talented than other athletes. They begin their competitive lives more focused, less impulsive, and less easily distracted than their peers do. They do not become as easily bored by routine. They don't just want to do something well, they want to be perfect. They are more confident, competitive, and willing to take responsibility than their peers are. Further, they maintain a more positive attitude about things and tend to be more outgoing.

As they develop, they face special challenges. To continue to be successful, they must remain focused and dedicated to their sport. Their ability to focus is challenged by two things, and it becomes clear that a little bit of extroversion and willingness to be supportive of others goes a long way. At younger ages, the enjoyment of others undoubtedly helps to get world champions interested in and involved in sport. As the competition increases, however, the need to socialize and worry about the feelings of others, if too strong, can get in the way of the athlete's development.

Elite-level athletes have a period of adjustment during late adolescence and early adulthood, needing to work through relationship issues. Those who stay focused on their sport become less externally distracted, less extroverted, more introverted, and less concerned about supporting others. We are not implying these athletes are not outgoing or supportive. We are saying that there was a significant drop in scores in these areas for a very good reason.

The second thing that happens as athletes develop is that they become more skilled analytically. Here, too, a little analysis goes a long way. Most athletes have to polish and perfect their physical skills until they can perform them automatically, without conscious thought. This requires focus, dedication, and repetition. Athletes who are too analytical have a greater tendency to think too much and to overcomplicate things. Their constant analyzing and strategizing cause them to make too many changes and, this interferes with the repetition required for world-class performance.

The need to focus, polish, and perfect things, combined with a strong need for control, a high level of self-confidence, and extreme competitiveness can lead to management issues. As pressure increases, these characteristics begin to control the athlete and can interfere with his or her ability to communicate effectively or to listen to and trust the advice of others. What might be described as focused, when things are going well for an athlete, becomes stubbornness and inflexibility when things are going poorly. This focus leads to the errors of underinclusion we see elite athletes making. Often, these errors occur because athletes are making a conscious choice to ignore certain responsibilities (e.g., refusing to respond to the feelings of family, friends, or a spouse in order to remain focused on training). As pressure increases, however, the errors of underinclusion are much more directly tied to performance. Recall the last winter Olympics when a number of top speed skaters failed to realize just how much the clap skate would affect their sport? They focused so much on their own training and preparation that they failed to recognize a technical revolution that was changing their sport.

When we work with teams, organizations, or individuals, we assess them to see how well they match the template just described. Do the athletes have the characteristics required for elite-level performance? Does the coaching staff and the training and competitive environment support the development of those characteristics? We then design interventions to compensate for any weaknesses and to fill in the gaps. Even when things appear to be running smoothly, our experience and our assessment of the current situation allow us to anticipate and prepare for issues that will arise.

We work to minimize the conflicts and distractions that occur as athletes mature and as issues around dating become more important. We develop strategies to make sure that extroverted athletes stay focused by helping them select their friends and by making sure that teammates socialize with each other and remind each other to focus on the long-term goals. We anticipate problems due to over-analyzing and work to help athletes develop enough trust in coaches and other support personnel to turn many of the problem-solv-

ing responsibilities over to them, so they (the athletes) can stay focused on skill development and repetition. We help others understand the needs of the athlete and work with coaches to help them see how their cognitive styles and intra- and interpersonal characteristics can either facilitate or impede the development of the athlete.

Our research shows us that most college-level and Olympic-level coaches share many of the characteristics of world champions. Coaches and world champions share the same level of focus, need for control, self-confidence, and competitiveness. Thus, under pressure, they can both be extremely stubborn. It is the coach, however, who has the responsibility for managing that conflict in a way that maintains the trust of the athlete. Often, the coach needs the help of a psychological consultant to do that.

Coaches differ from athletes in that they tend to be more environmentally aware, more analytical, and better able to process information. These skills are critical because the coach has to be able to compensate for the extreme focus of the athlete. The coach has to be aware and politically sensitive. The coach has to see new developments coming, and the coach has to recognize when it is time to change. Athletes can afford to make errors of underinclusion; coaches cannot.

Performance vs. Management

The coaches we tested had the kind of cognitive skills found with entrepreneurs in business and with officers in the military. They were analytical enough in their thinking to be the leader and strategizer and focused enough to be "hands on" (worry about and attending to all of the details as well as to the bigger picture). It is becoming increasingly difficult, however, for coaches to fill both roles. Entrepreneurs in business can take a company only so far, and then their management style and their need to be involved in all of the details get in the way. The same thing is beginning to happen to many coaches.

The cognitive skills required to be a world-class manager are quite different from those required to be superstar as a performer. Managers have to be able to "see the big picture"; they have to be strategic in their thinking, flexible, and able to problem solve; and they have to know when to compromise. As the competitive environment the manager works in becomes more diverse, challenging, and technically complex, it becomes increasingly difficult for him or her to be both strategic and highly focused. Given this fact, it is not surprising to find that the dominant concentration style for CEOs in corporations consists of their ability to strategize and plan. Indeed, the least-used concentration skill for CEOs is focus. CEOs cannot afford to focus; they will lose sight of the future if they do. Instead, they have to be able to delegate, and they have to be able to rely on others in the organization to provide the focus

and follow-through, the attention to detail.

In sport, we are seeing this trend develop. It is already taking a team to provide all of the support services required to produce an elite athlete. Each member needs to be highly technically skilled in his or her respective areas (e.g., exercise physiology, nutrition, sport psychology, biomechanics, sports medicine). Within the sport itself, particularly in more complex team sports, we are seeing increased specialization within coaching staffs. Someone has to act as the coordinator, the chief tactician, etc. It is becoming much more difficult for one individual to be hands-on in all of the areas that are critical to help the athlete succeed. As those pressures increase, the head coach or manager begins to look more like the CEO.

What Business and the Military Can Learn From Elite Sport

We do a lot of work in many of today's rapidly growing, high-technology companies.

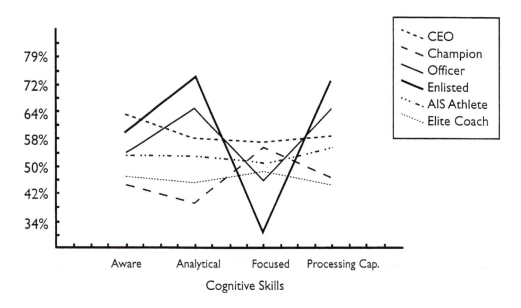

Figure 9.
Cognitive skills as a function of job.

We also do a lot of work for the military. Both in the military and in high-technology companies, those individuals who are responsible for the execution of a mission in the military (e.g., enlisted personnel) and/or for the production of a product in a company (e.g., engineering personnel and program managers) have to be highly focused and extremely dedicated. These individuals have to be attentive to details; they have to have in-depth knowledge and expertise that requires focused concentration.

Because those individuals who are responsible for the execution of a plan have to be highly focused and technically skilled, they need to be supported by managers (business) and officers (military) who, like today's coaches, have a broader focus of concentration, the kind of focus that leads to greater awareness of the competition and to an increased ability to strategize and plan.

Because success in business and on the battlefield requires the willingness to assume responsibility and leadership, a high level of self-confidence, and tremendous dedication, whether one is involved as a performer or a manager, conflicts between members of the team, in business, sport, and military can develop very quickly. It does not take much in the way of pressure and/or in terms of a difference of opinion to cause a breakdown in the communication and willingness to listen of two highly confident individuals.

Success in sport, business, and the military in today's highly competitive, global environment requires elite performers (athletes, engineers, enlisted personnel) to be more focused and dedicated than ever. In contrast, managers, officers, and coaches need to be more open and sensitive to change and more strategic in their thinking. The gap between the two groups in terms of their dominant cognitive styles increases the likelihood of a breakdown in trust and communication in high-pressure situations.

Sport psychologists help coaches and athletes maintain effective communication in high-pressure situations by helping them gain greater control over the emotions generated when everything is on the line and their ability to maintain control over the situation is threatened. It is greater control over emotional arousal that will allow an athlete, an engineer, or enlisted personnel to broaden his or her focus of attention, improving the ability to problem solve, to listen to others, and to compromise. It is greater control over emotional arousal that will allow a coach, manager, or officer to control impatience and to temporarily stop the analysis and problem solving, thereby becoming a better listener. It is control over emotional arousal that will help all of the members of the team increase their trust for each other and avoid taking things personally.

Implications for Psychological Consultants

The level of competition in sport, business, and the military is making it increasingly difficult to achieve world-class status. The performer and the manager will continue to see their respective bars raised, and though the cognitive skills required for world-class performance in these two areas are dramatically different, the psychological consultant will be called upon to help identify individuals from both camps who have the "right stuff."

The psychological consultant also becomes important from a developmental perspective by helping individuals create the types of training and work environments that will facilitate and support the development of the different individuals' skills and talents. Psychological consultants also have an important role to play when it comes to teaching the psychological skills that both groups need to gain even greater control over their ability to control concentration and emotional arousal.

Perhaps the most critical role that psychological consultants have to play involves finding ways to facilitate teamwork, cooperation, and trust. How does a general manager balance the need to win today's game with the need to develop next year's title contender? How do planners in the military balance concerns about the future against the lives that are being laid on the line today? How does the CEO of a company balance the need to move the company in a new direction because of changes in the competitive environment against the immediate operational issues that corporate producers are dealing with? The player on the field, the individual on the mission, and the engineer on the production floor are focused on today. The general managers, CEOs, and officers are focused on the future. Who's bridging the gap? What structures exist to ensure that the two groups understand, respect, and trust each other?

Organizations are already experiencing the issues we have described, and most of them do not have solutions. World-class performance *requires* the identification of exceptional talent and then good management and teamwork. There is a growing need for program managers and communications specialists—individuals who coordinate services (e.g., of sports sciences) and maintain the lines of communication between members of the team and levels within the organization. Depending on the size of the group you are working with, and the number of clients you have, you may be able to be that person. More than likely, however, you are going to need to be the one who identifies, trains, and supervises the person who can lead and manage others. These are individuals who work full-time within the organization and can carry your torch.

This is the role we find ourselves in at Enhanced Performance Systems. We are working less and less at the "end user" level in our efforts to help develop elite-level performers. We are increasingly system oriented and work to develop resources within the team, organization, sports-governing body, or military unit. We help in the identification and selection process to make sure the organization does not try to put square pegs in round holes or to turn production superstars into managers or coaches. We assist in the team-building process by helping organizations structure and train internal resources so they can maintain communication and trust and balance the needs they face today with the needs they will surely face tomorrow.

References

Nideffer, R.M. (1976). Test of attentional and interpersonal style. *Journal of Personality Social and Psychology*, *34*, 394–404.

Nideffer, R.M. (1987). Applied sport psychology. In J. R. May & M. J. Asken (Eds.), *Sport psychology: The psychological health of the athlete* (pp. 1–18). New York: PMA Publishing.

Nideffer, R.M. (1993). *Predicting human behavior: A theory and test of attentional and interpersonal style*. New Berlin, WI: Assessment Systems International.

Recommended Readings

Bond, J.W., & Nideffer, R.M. (1992). Attentional and interpersonal characteristics of elite Australian Athletes. *Excel* [Australian Sports Commission], *8* (2), 101–111.

Nideffer, R.M. (1989). Theoretical and practical relationships between attention, anxiety, and performance in sport. In D. Hackfort & C.D. Spielberger (Eds.), *Anxiety in sport: An international perspective* (pp. 117–136). New York: Hemisphere Publishing.

Nideffer, R.M. (1989). Psychological services for the U.S. Olympic Track and Field Team. *The Sport Psychologist*, *3*, 350–357.

Nideffer, R.M. (1990). Use of the Test of Attentional and Interpersonal Style in Sport. *The Sport Psychologist*, *4*, 285–300.

Nideffer, R.M. (1990). Using the Test of Attentional and Interpersonal Style with Athletes. In J. Bond & J. Gross (Eds.), *Australian sport psychology: The eighties* (pp. 149–160). Canberra: Australian Institute for Sport.

Nideffer, R.M., & Rembisz, R. (1996). Competing against the world: What Business can learn from sport. Available at: www.enhanced-performance.com/nideffer/articles/article 10.html

Expanding the Definition of Winning

Clark Perry, Jr.

Winning is an integral part of our society. Our worth is typically measured in a self-referent manner that compares our abilities to the abilities of those with whom we interact. We often define success in terms of outcomes accomplished on real or metaphoric battlefields. Funding from governments, sporting organizations, and corporate and private sponsors is typically predicated on winning performances. Paradoxically, I have experienced that the more we focus on winning, the less likely it is to occur (Perry & Marsh, 2000). Winning is an outcome that usually does not adequately describe the performance. What does it mean to have swum a 49.5-second, 100-meter free style in swimming or to have won a soccer game 3–2? In both cases, these numbers may mean winning performances, but the outcome does not describe the events that led up to that result. To achieve success, it is important to focus on the process that allows winning in conventional terms. In this chapter, I discuss how elite sporting individuals and teams achieve success by minimizing the focus on conventional winning. Expanding the definition of winning to allow for more experiences of success produces winning performances.

Conventional winning in sport is limited to the person or team that has gone the fastest, jumped the highest, thrown the farthest, or scored the most or the least points. Because of this focus, every other competitor has lost. How many people, outside of those immediately involved, remember who won the silver medal, got second in the World Cup, World Series, Super Bowl, or Grand Final? Success has long been recognized as a prime motivator, yet with conventional winning, very few actually experience success.

The Australian Institute of Sport (AIS) comprises a residential training center for elite athletes ranging in age from 10 to 28 years. It houses 200 athletes across nine different sports from developmental to Olympic level. An integral part of the AIS is the Sports Science and Sports Medicine Center, which houses the departments of psychology, medicine, physiology/biochemistry, physiotherapy/massage, biomechanics, and nutrition. Athlete/Coach servicing is the focus of the Center using a multidisciplinary approach. The AIS is primarily funded through federal government budget allocations with the aim being medals at international competitions. The AIS has been in existence since 1980 and is responsible for much of the improvement in Australian performances at Olympics, World Championships, and Commonwealth Games. Even though the aim of elite sport in Australia is winning, we find that this goal is quite paradoxical. That is, the more individuals focus on winning, the less likely it is to occur. The focus on process-oriented performance goals allows the athlete the opportunity to maximize success, by providing instructions on "how" that success will be achieved. It is the goal of the sport science team at the AIS to assist the coaches and athletes in setting, monitoring, and evaluating these process goals. Establishing a certain "philosophy" about winning creates an environment of excellence that allows the athletes the opportunity to compete in a more relaxed and confident manner. I highlight next some of the principles that guide our philosophy at the AIS.

Is it not true that everyone wants to succeed? The answer is yes and no. Many of us want to succeed, but also want not to. It is possible to be inhibited by success. Along with our obvious wish to make good, there may be a secret wish to sabotage the whole process. Somehow, there is a hidden reward in failure.

We can be inhibited about a kind of success other people take for granted—like speaking, which somehow turns into stuttering. Learning to dance for many was a daunting task during our youth. As much as we wished to be "mixing" on the dance floor, we were more concerned with embarrassing ourselves in front of others. So there we were, paralyzed, looking at one another polarized on opposite sides of the room. Elite athletes are not exempt from this type of thinking. "I am good, but am I really good enough to be a World Champion?" "Should I dare?" "Do I take the risk?" The consequence of not succeeding outweighs the potential joys of success. Therefore, it is "safer" to take the path to mediocrity.

Of course, lack of success at something does not always mean that we are inhibited. Most people who do not win Olympic Gold cannot blame it on a secret desire to fail. It *is* possible to set unrealistic goals. Here are five signs that may tell us the problem is *inhibition.*

1. **Repeated avoidance of a desired activity**. The athlete needs to perform certain exercises or training sets, but keeps finding a reason to avoid them (not a good day, other commitments). I've worked with athletes who talk all the right talk, but can't seem to get past the "I'll start that phase tomorrow." Tomorrow keeps being delayed until the next day, and the next day, and so on.

2. **Extreme self-consciousness**. The athlete is always watching him- or herself like an outside observer. This is not a bad strategy in learning and modifying technique, but such self-consciousness is self-defeating when it consumes the athlete's every thought: "How well do most other people perform this task?" "What will other people think of me?"

3. **The feeling that the athlete is consistently unlucky**. Circumstances keep thwarting these athletes. This was their time, but someone else does their best on the same day. The athletes have little sense of control. "I've trained great, but wouldn't you know it, the weather didn't cooperate." "The gods seem to always be against me."

4. **Extreme concern about the environment**. "The lighting at the venue isn't right"; "The field is in bad shape"; "The water temperature is too cold." The athletes keep making small excuses for not performing at their best.

5. **A sense that the athlete's body keeps getting in the way**. Just as an athlete is ready to compete, he or she starts to feel dizzy or has to go to the toilet. The athlete's legs feel heavy and tired. The athlete is prepared, but the athlete's body seems to feel otherwise.

Often these athletes need assistance in understanding why they are undermining their success. There is value in working with a sport psychologist to examine the etiology of this inhibition and develop strategies so that the athlete can overcome these self-defeating thoughts, attitudes, and ultimately, behaviors. One way to overcome inhibition is to help the athlete set short-term process goals and create opportunities for him or her to experience success. The athlete needs to persevere and push through the inhibition, especially if the individual is convinced that he or she is failing at it. Giving up reinforces a sense of incompetence; going on gives the athlete a commitment to success. This is true for athletes of all ages and levels, as well as coaches. For that matter, it is good advice for anyone interested in achievement.

Athletes who have given consistent, 100% efforts should never disparage their performances. They should be critical of elements of their performances that were under their control and learn from their mistakes, but stay confident and believe that they have the ability to change. They need to be the first and last people to please. This comes from setting difficult yet achievable process goals and using the achievement of those goals to judge a performance. Inhibited people are likely to think that others are laughing at them, thereby perhaps experiencing slight paranoia. Athletes must not indulge such paranoia by belittling themselves. In many cultures, it is unacceptable to talk about one's successes, but quite natural to discuss one's shortfalls, an interesting phenomenon considering that it does not impress other athletes or coaches. In fact, this behavior is more likely to alienate people. All of these attitudes reinforce the sense of unworthiness and diminish any kind of success.

"John" is a prime example of an athlete with inhibition towards success. He was always successful at whatever sport he tried—basketball, soccer, baseball, tennis—but as he reached late adolescence it appeared that basketball was where his true talents and de-sires lay. He was seen as the star player in his hometown and state, with a "can't miss superstardom" label. John was selected as part of an elite national training squad and relocated to a residential facility where the team could prepare for World Championships in 2 years. The first year saw mixed results for John; he had flashes of brilliance demonstrating great awareness and the ability to put the ball on the floor while maintaining an accurate, soft shot from anywhere on the court. At other times, however, he seemed to be completely out of sync; he made simple mistakes with little pressure from the opposition, moved to the wrong spot on set plays, gave the ball up when he was wide open for a shot, or forced a shot that wasn't there. His coach complained that John didn't appear to be willing to do the little things that were required to get to the "next level." He was carrying a bit too much weight, and it was starting to show late in games when fatigue would set in. John claimed to be committed to growing fitter and stronger, but when it came time for some extra gym work, something always seemed to come up—minor injury, illness, and other commitments. As a result, John was falling farther and farther behind. The coach also mentioned that John was a chronic complainer; the basketball shoes that the team wore didn't fit John right; the basketballs were getting worn, or the air in the balls was too much or too little; the temperature in the gym, too hot or too cold. I saw John at a training session one day and asked if we could go get a cup of coffee and have a chat about a few things. He agreed and commented that he actually had intended to come and see me anyway. Over a cup of coffee at a quiet café, John told me that he was finding it tough since coming to the center. Ever since he had played sports, he was the focus. His parents, coaches, and peers told him that he would be great at whatever sport he chose, and sports always came easy to him. Now he was finding that it wasn't that easy! He felt that he was preoccupied with the thoughts of not fulfilling everyone's expectations. "What if I give 100%, and it's not enough? I don't know if I can bear going home to all those people and telling them that I have failed."

As athletes attempt to succeed, it may help to recognize possible motives for *not* trying.

1. **Fear of arousing envy.** Without realizing it, many athletes associate success with greed. They are afraid to be seen trying to surpass their teammates, or sometimes even other competitors; they fear that they will be ridiculed as pretentious and trying to bringing others down. "How dare they think that at such a young age they could perform better than someone that has been a legend in their sport?" Athletes who feel this way probably also feel that people will, and ought to, hate them for trying to outdo the competition. Such athletes are inclined to be secretive about their ambitions and achievements. Compliments make them feel uncomfortable; it is as if the person giving the compliment had caught them doing something wrong. So they tend to deny that they have achieved much of anything. "It's nothing really," they say. "I was just lucky." How can people get mad at them if their success was all due to fate? The cure? They need to stop pretending that they have no aspirations. They should let the world know what they want and thank people if they praise them, no matter how uncomfortable such praise makes them feel. The athlete should admit being ambitious, should even tell a few people. Hiding ambitions can only make the person feel that he or she should not succeed. So the individual sees that he or she does not. It might be regrettable that others may be less successful, but sabotaging one's performance won't do them any good, just as pursuing one's own goals, assuming that all is done fairly, won't do others any harm either.

2. **Fear of ultimate failure.** Another common motive for sabotaging one's performance is fear that success will bring about demands that are greater than one can handle. Fear of ultimate failure is almost a fear of succeeding too well, of going so far that expectations will overshadow the athlete's capabilities. The athlete fears the great height because he or she does not believe that the individual can stay up there, and the fall back down will be too painful, too humiliating. Seldom does an elite athlete reach the top without considerable help from parents, coaches, support staff, and peers. With all this assistance, athletes often encumber themselves with a debt of responsibility. "If I don't perform well, I've let so many people down that have invested so much into me." This fear of failure ultimately becomes a self-fulfilling prophecy, as it mentally, emotionally, and physically prevents athletes from performing at their best. They should plan for one success at a time instead of anticipating where it will all lead. If the athlete believes that he or she has the ability and lets that belief be the prime source of motivation, the very effort will strengthen that belief, and confidence will grow, and because confidence itself is an asset, the athlete's chances of achievement will increase. As athletes strive and achieve, their fear of the great height will diminish. Athletes should regard this fear as an illusion of childhood, like the toddler's impression that his or her parents are gigantic. Yet, when the toddler grows to that size, it seems quite normal and part of a natural progression. Peter Sterling, former Australian Rugby

League star halfback, believes that preparation is the foundation of confidence:

If you've put in the work in the week before a game you can handle any situation. Preparation builds confidence. Our former coach Jack Gibson always said that if we'd done our homework well and stick to our tactics, we could give the opposition a copy of our game plan before the match and we'd still beat them (quoted in Writer, 1990, p. 110).

3. **Fear of independence.** Some athletes think that no one will care about them unless they are helpless or in trouble. "They must have such reasons for paying attention to me, or I will be lost, or overlooked." There can be some truth to this. Some people find their parents sympathetic only when they are sick or in some kind of crisis. When they are on their feet, their parents disappear. This is painful, but the alternative is more painful. Often, the way other people treat us is less of a problem and does less to our self-esteem than the way that we treat ourselves. If the athlete acts on the premise that his or her only attraction is as an invalid, then the athlete will promote a fear of accomplishment. Athletes need to find programs that foster independence. The key is a nonthreatening environment that encourages risk taking, teaches skills, and gives ultimate control of success to the athlete.

4. **Fear of losing identity.** It seems that some athletes won't be the same people if they succeed. Somehow becoming a top athlete will undermine everything that they stand for. Sexual stereotypes often contribute to these beliefs. Many men grow up thinking it's unmanly to have strong emotions, except perhaps, jealousy, lust, or revenge. Similarly, many women are taught not to use their minds or muscles, as they will be considered cold, threatening, and unfeminine. All kinds of inefficiencies result. The men are not as loving or creative as they might be; the women often shy away from science, business, or sport, as they are supposedly male domains. The reality is that no ability is incompatible with any other ability. Excellence of one kind never implies incompetence of another kind. Especially when it comes to a person's intellectual, emotional, and physical lives, these abilities can only enhance one another.

5. **Fear of losing goals.** If the athlete succeeds, then what is left? What will be his or her purpose in life? Some people constantly deny themselves things and experiences in order to save money, but somehow don't save it. What would they do for incentive if they had money? Others spend all their time and effort trying to lose body fat, but don't get lean. What would they do once they were fit? The prospect of success is terrifying in this set-up. Diversifying one's goals can ease this fear. Every successful life requires an endless sequence of challenges. There is always unfinished business. When someone runs out of obvious purposes, they need to set new goals. If people have nothing to strive for, they don't strive, and if they don't strive, they stagnate and wither. The great Australian cricket captain, Greg Chappell, was quoted as saying

People keep saying to me it must be great, now I'm retired, not to have all the pressure of cricket. They don't know what pressure is. Pressure to me is being a father, providing for a family, trying to run a business. In cricket the worst thing that could ever happen would have been to get dropped. I might never play another game of cricket, but I still would have had my family and my business (Writer, 1990, p. 108).

These other life interests that Chappell is speaking of demonstrate the need for a balanced approach to sporting achievement. If we have all of our proverbial eggs in one basket, we stand to lose everything in the event of a crash. This is the foundation of sound financial investment. Economists preach diversity when creating a wealth portfolio and tell investors to balance risk with opportunity. There is a need to spread investments in various sectors of the share market, property market, commodities, and cash. By balancing exposure, one is more likely to cope with certain downturns in the various markets. Why then do so many sporting people emphasize the need to become more and more selective as athletes become more elite? Athletes are told that if they are to make it in this highly competitive world of elite sport, they must focus solely on their sport. "There is no time to waste energy and resources on academic, recreational, social, vocational or religious interests. This is time that is better spent concentrating on your particular specialty or event." No! No! No! Nothing could be farther from the truth. Just as the wise financial investor looks for diversity in creating wealth, so too does the wise elite athlete look for diversity in the quest for excellence. This is not a quest for mediocrity. It allows the athlete the opportunity to take risks without the moribund consequences of ultimate failure. In 1995, ABC radio in Australia conducted a fantastic interview with four-time Gold Medallist in the discus, American Al Oerter. Until 1996, when Carl Lewis duplicated the feat in the long jump, Oerter was the only person to win four successive Gold Medals in a single event from 1956 to 1968 (see sidebar, taken from the interview).

I do not think that it is a surprise Al Oerter is regarded as one of the greatest Olympic champions of all time. It's apparent to me that he had his athletic career in perspective,

ABC: It was a surprising Gold Medal in '56, by the time you go forward four years to Rome in 1960 you were a red hot favorite. Was it a different feeling for you, more pressure?

Oerter: Well in 1956 we had a press conference immediately after the throw and since I had won a Gold Medal they asked me how I felt; "I feel good you know and in fact I feel so good I'd like to win four more." Not realizing I'd put myself in for sixteen more years worth of effort trying to get to the Olympics. But I lived to that and when Rome came up and when Tokyo came up and Mexico City came up I was just living to that promise I'd made to myself. I absolutely thoroughly enjoyed working for four years at a time. I used to have a calendar on the wall and it was 1460 days, three years and every one of those days I tried to work a little bit over 100% and when I did I crossed that day off as one step a little bit closer. It had nothing to do with Gold Medals, had nothing to do with competing successfully, but I flat out knew that when I got to the 1460th day I was ready!

ABC: After four Gold Medals, in 1968 you retired, as you look back over your shoulder, any regrets?

Oerter: No, because I was a single parent in 1968. I raised my two daughters by myself and if I had chosen to go to Munich it would have taken a great deal of time from them. I've always been a firm believer, although I'm not a preacher I don't mean to do such things, I'm a firm believer that if you are a parent you should take your parenting responsibilities seriously and I did.

ABC: After a couple of Olympic games out in 1972 and 1976, you did make a comeback in 1980.

Oerter: Yea my daughters were about to go away to college so I had plenty of time and I started in 1976 training for 1980, it was very low level but in '77 it became more intense. '78, '79 and in 1980 I was throwing the best of my life and I continued that and we obviously had a boycott, President Carter would not allow a team to go to Moscow but I continued until 1984 in Los Angeles. I would have made that team. I don't know if I would have won a medal, you never know such things, but I tore an Achilles tendon and never really had a chance to show myself off.

ABC: So in fact at age 50 you are still throwing the discus out over 200 feet. Would that be normal for a discus thrower or does it say something about your unique ability?

Oerter: Well I don't know if it says anything unique about me. I've always approached sport as just one of the things I do. When I started competing I didn't have a family in 1956. I didn't have a career as I was still in college. In 1960 I had a family. I had a technical career in computers and I maintained that career in all of those years and to me it was the balance between family, career and competing in the Olympic games that allowed me to compete comfortably. It was not a feeling of, I have to win, I have to do well to prove myself for income or whatever. Whatever I did in the games, I still had my family, still had my career and that was the balance that was necessary and that was true when I came back into sport. I never came back into sport to show what I was made of, or to recapture past glories or go through all that nonsense, those big ego trips that tend to trip up a lot of athletes. I went back because I truly enjoyed throwing, I enjoyed the training regimen necessary to throw well and that's what carried me through. Very simple. (Gavel, 1995)

and as he said, "It was the balance . . . that allowed me to compete comfortably."

Marsh & Shavelson (1985) have proposed a model of self-concept (see Figure 1). According to the diagram, self-concept is a multifaceted construct in which the particular facets reflect a self-referent category system adopted by a particular individual or shared by a group, or both. It is hierarchical, with perceptions of personal behavior in specific situations at the base of the hierarchy, inferences about self in broader domains (e.g., social, physical, academic) at the middle of the hierarchy, and a global, general self-concept at the apex. The hierarchical general self-concept—the apex of the hierarchy—is stable, but as one descends the hierarchy, self-concept becomes increasingly situation specific and, as a consequence, less stable. This is an excellent explanation for the danger in specialization. As the elite athlete removes facets from the hierarchy, self-concept becomes more situation specific and as a result more perilous. When the meaning of failure is totalistic—as is possible in this one-dimensional view of elite sport—the athlete is more likely to self-handicap and ultimately sabotage performance.

This is one of the reasons why at the AIS, athletes must either be enrolled in some formal education or pursuing a vocation. This philosophy is not a distraction to elite sport. Quite the contrary, we find that it improves the quality of the athlete's training. In relation to the Marsh & Shavelson (1985) model, it provides more facets for the athlete to judge self-worth, therefore increasing stability and promoting risk taking. As mentioned earlier, risk taking is the foundation for growth.

In an environment that promotes calculated risk, anxiety diminishes because the consequences of unsuccessful performances are examined in relation to physical, technical, emotional, and psychological readiness. That is, if an athlete does not perform up to

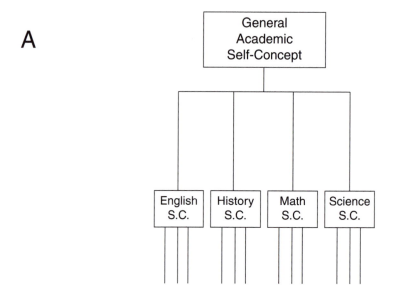

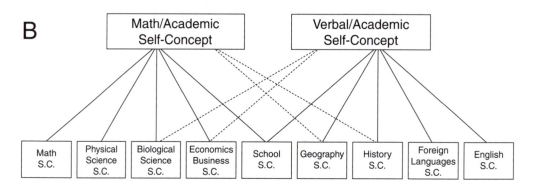

Figure 1.
(A) The academic portion of Shavelson, Hubner, and Stanton's (1976) original model and (B) an elaboration of Marsh and Shavelson's (1985) revision that includes a wider variety of specific academic facets (S.C. = self-concept). (From Marsh, Byrne, & Shavelson, 1988, pp. 366–380.

expectations, the coaches, support staff, and athlete/team review the preparation and performance in a holistic manner to ascertain where improvements can be made. Anxiety comes about because of a perceived lack of control. In this approach to sporting excellence, the athlete is responsible for his or her performance, not necessarily the outcome. Most outcomes are influenced by many extraneous variables—the weather, opponents,

officials, level of fitness and technique, and playing surface—over which athletes have little or no control on the day. Their level of fitness and technique can be developed in training, but come the day of competition, there's not much that can be done to dramatically improve their physical and technical readiness to compete. At competition, it comes down to what you can control and that is, *effort*, executing a plan that was rehearsed repeatedly in training. When an athlete is well-trained to compete, the performance is *allowed* to happen. That is, there is not much the athlete can do to improve performance, but there's a great deal he or she can do to worsen it. So in essence, the athlete needs to remove the pressure and release the person who has been training to, as Oerter would say, "show . . . off." One comment I have often heard from coaches is "All that stuff before was just training. Now this is the competition. Get out there and make it happen!" To me, such exhortations can add huge unneeded pressure. The reality is "at training is where you made it happen, you've come here ready to compete, now get out there and just enjoy yourself!" To me, this sends a message of control and confidence. If we do or don't get the outcome that we've been looking for, we'll go back to the drawing board and figure ways to improve together.

When we return to our basketball player, John, it became apparent to me that as he climbed the ladder of success, the journey became more precarious. Failure became an untenable option, so he was preparing to deal with that prospect by ensuring that he didn't get to the top. If he didn't risk everything, then he wouldn't lose everything either. John and I continued to work on his need to meet others' expectations, the origins of that need, and whether he wanted to continue with that sort of motivation. In a practical sense, we made sure that John had other interests outside of basketball. He enrolled in a course of study and started some part-time work that wouldn't conflict with his training. This provided him the opportunity to spread his self-worth beyond sport. With the assistance of the coaching staff, we helped John establish some clear goals that focused on his improvement as a player. They included physical, technical, tactical, and psychological skills. There were targets established with definite timelines, and John

was to focus on the process involved in completing these tasks. The result of this approach is that John could see how he was to improve and that he was in control of achieving these targets. As the weeks passed, John experienced more and more success, and this resulted in greater satisfaction and hence higher motivation.

The sports I work with at the AIS operate according to this general philosophy. I firmly believe that it has contributed to the international success that we have enjoyed over the past 10 years. More to the point, I'm proud of the athletes who have come through the programs, retired from sport, and diverted their passion to another life interest. As one of our athletes told me, "I'm not great because I'm a great athlete; I'm a great athlete because I'm great!" If every athlete felt this way we would not only have great performances, but also well-adjusted happy, contributing people in our community.

References

Gavel, T. (Executive Producer). (1995, April 10). *Grandstand: An interview with Al Oerter.* Sydney, NSW, Australia: ABC Radio.

Marsh, H. W., & Shavelson, R. (1985). Self-concept: Its multifaceted, hierarchical structure. *Educational Psychologist, 20,* 107–125.

Perry, C. & Marsh H. W. (2000). Listening to self-talk, hearing self-concept. In M. B. Andersen (Ed.), *Doing sport psychology* (pp. 61–76). Champaign, IL: Human Kinetics.

Shavelson, R. J., Hubner, J. J., & Stanton, G. C. (1976). Validation of construct interpretations. *Review of Educational Research, 46,* 407–441.

Writer, L. (1990). *Winning: Face to face with Australian sporting legends.* Chatswood, NSW, Australia: Ironbark Press.

Community-Based Sport Psychology

Barry Kerr

Introduction

Twenty years ago, I became involved in sport psychology after being encouraged by the manager of an Olympic team who believed in the contribution psychology could make to the mental preparation of athletes. At the time, sport psychology in Australia was in its infancy with scattered pockets of academics and practitioners applying their various skills and experiences to sport. The introduction of the Australian Institute of Sport and, later, state institutes provided coaching and sport science expertise to the more elite athletes of the country. Over time, sport psychology became progressively more appealing to sport participants, as well as to coaches and sport administrators, at a local and district level. As a clinical psychologist with no formal qualifications in sport science, but as a former player and coach of several sports, I accepted the challenge of assisting local sporting organizations and, later, Olympic and elite teams and individuals. Living in a beach resort area remote from tertiary institutions or, indeed, other practitioners, I realized the importance of promoting and developing the discipline within the limits of local resources. In this chapter, I intend to share some thoughts, models, and ideas that may encourage other practitioners in similar situations.

First Steps

Surf lifesaving is a national icon, a community service patrolling beaches with a competitive, sporting function that was used, traditionally, to hone the skills of lifesavers. I recall beginning my practice with athletes from local surf clubs and, from a very narrow knowledge base, worked with athletes using skills that I believed were transferable from my clinical practice. I am sure that the successes were matched by the mistakes that I made, but the experience of developing a repertoire of skills was a vast reinforcement for the effort made. Selection as a member of the state and Australian surf teams was my first, recognized experience as a sport psychologist. The motivation for my inclusion as a "secret weapon" came more from an enthusiastic organization than a practical reality. It became very clear that a disadvantage of being a "sport" psychologist was the title itself. With little introduction or induction to teams, athletes were ordered to consult me for a "talk." How often do I recall the response being, "There's nothing wrong with my head"? In addition, coaches from other sports may have felt threatened because of a "fear" that I would usurp their training or playing strategies. However, many coaches, particularly swimming, embraced the notion of mental preparation, and I believe this was because of involvement in American programs, which incorporated sport psychology. During my association with surf lifesaving, I attended the sixth World Congress in Sport Psychology in Copenhagen. The networking and discussions with other practitioners initiated a more directed search for "best practice" in the discipline.

In my opinion, many misconceptions about sport psychology still exist, and I believe they are based on unrealistic expectations and misinformation. Education about the complementary nature of sport psychology to coaching and performance enhancement can be achieved in several ways. Coaching accreditation programs are well in place in the community and usually have a psychology component. Most administrators welcome the offer of a psychologist to present a course or to assist in preparing course content included in the programs for coaches and for athletes. Local media welcome contributions regarding any aspect for sport, including sport science, particularly where the article demonstrates a positive aspect aimed at creating performance enhancement. I have written articles for local newspapers on stress in sport, the disabled athlete, and life after sport and several other articles for particular organizations, especially those involved with surf lifesaving. Similarly, local secondary schools or colleges with sporting programs appreciate the assistance of the sport psychologist working with their athletes. Before developing programs with teams or athletes, the need for successful negotiations with coaches is of significant importance to allay fears or threat of the role of the sport psychologist. A format for such discussions that I have found effective includes the following:

1. An explanation of how sport psychological principles can complement the role of the coach.

2. A discussion of general areas of concern regarding athletes on the team.
3. An outline of expectations the coach may have of the sport psychologist's inclusion with the team.
4. A joint program of functions and responsibilities relevant to the aims of the coach assisted by programs developed by the sport psychologist.

Each success promotes not only the credibility of the individual sport psychologist, but also the credibility of the discipline itself. Although the elite athlete will accept any assistance if it will promote his goals, I believe the most productive target population is children, particularly for the novice sport psychologist beginning a practice.

Children and Sport

Local communities offer an abundance of sporting opportunities for children ranging from participative activities to competitive events at the elite level. As an ex-teacher and child psychologist, I have been concerned that, in today's world, too much pressure is placed on children to achieve at unrealistic levels. In many cases, I suggest this problem applies to sport as well. Yet, involvement in sport has been one of the recommendations I have made as a solution to presenting clinical problems, as I believe sporting activities offer confidence building as well as developing interpersonal skills in an enjoyable environment. I recall instances of an Australian junior sprint champion being violently sick in a finals race because of pressure being applied by his coach and another boy being told, by his father, to sit alone at the end of the swimming pool because he didn't win every event. With children, it is important to de-emphasize winning and emphasize doing one's best so that winning will occur for the best performer on the day. A focus on doing one's best is preferable to attention being

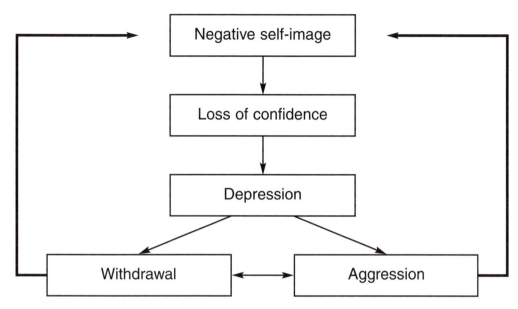

Figure 1.
A model suggesting the consequences for the development of a negative self-image.

given only to coming in fourth or last, an emphasis from which there may be deleterious reactions from significant others. If "failure" experiences persist with children, it is probable that they will develop a negative self-image and a subsequent loss of confidence. Figure 1 represents a possible model of the dynamics of a loss of self-esteem.

If a young athlete internalizes negative self-image, usually from pressure or failed experiences, he or she experiences a loss of self-confidence and motivation to continue with effort. Consequently, children can become depressed or, more likely, withdrawn, aggressive, or a combination of both. Once this condition is reached, any further effort that fails confirms the negativity. Whether the environment is that of the home, school, or sport, a cyclic pattern of behaviors can develop that become deleterious to a child's normal growth and development. In sport, coaches assume an immense responsibility for promoting healthy training and competition habits that demand attention to all as-

pects of the child's situation. Because most coaches and teachers have been successful in their respective fields, it is not unusual for them to focus on the "best" athletes to the exclusion of the "average" participant. I have seen many examples of training squads, in different sports, where there is little atmosphere and poor team spirit resulting in possible failure experiences with effects on self-esteem, for younger athletes. To remedy such situations, I would like to share strategies that I have found to be effective in building confidence and, in turn, create positive self-image and esteem in team situations.

Often, coaches and teachers have difficulty meeting the needs of all the athletes in a team or squad. In addition, there can be a tendency to perceive the training of an accomplished young athlete as taking more of the time and attention from the less capable, but equally ambitious, athletes. During training, it may be useful to set up a circuit to include alternate forms of activities rather than focus on the individual sport. Setting up volleyball, badminton, or cricket takes little time or equipment, and while the coach attends to one group of similarly accomplished athletes, others can achieve and be occupied by a recreational activity before their turn at training at the specific sport. This is particularly relevant to sports such as weight lifting, surf lifesaving, or gymnastics where the range of skill levels is wide but the target skill may be intense and completed in a short time. By setting up alternative activities, all athletes are occupied, and more focus can be directed to the needs of each group.

Most junior athletes are aware that institutes of sport exist and that they do not have access to such organizations offering a variety of scientific disciplines to assist them. Introducing the notion of a "camp" or "training workshop" held over one day or a weekend can involve young athletes in a pseudo-institute of sport for a short but meaningful time. I have found, in local communities, that many professionals are prepared to give their time to present, or teach, a topic of importance relevant to the sport concerned. Recently, I conducted a very successful tennis camp over 2 days that included presentations by a medical practitioner, a podiatrist, a dietician, a physiotherapist, and an optometrist (sport vision), as well as a visiting elite coach, who conducted skills sessions. Most important, the sport psychologist is the appropriate professional not only to facilitate the scientific program but also to speak to the parents (at least one present for each athlete) regarding the issues of stress, expectations, developmental levels of the children, and positive strategies of how parents may assist their children in a proactive way prior to, during, and after competitions. During the camp, an informal session allows contact between the coaching staff and parents in order to discuss their specific concerns regarding their children.

During the camp, a period should be set-aside for athletes to participate in decisions and expectations regarding the coach and the operation of the team or squad. A useful exercise is to devise a "contract" between coach and athlete. That is, "What do we expect of the coach?" whereas the coach may write the same regarding the athletes. Because the young athletes have been empowered to be part of the team's management, the subsequent discussions and decisions promote a sense of bonding as well as team atmosphere that will carry over into training and competition. Further, the election of a boy and girl captain and vice captain rewards those young athletes who have proven to be leaders in the squad. Other senior athletes are encouraged to "buddy" up with younger members of the squad for significant support and encouragement so that as many athletes as possible are actively involved in the conduct of interpersonal relationships within the team.

Coaches need to be encouraged to interact in a meaningful and more personal way with junior athletes. Sometimes this can be forgotten, not because of deliberate intent, but because of the intense focus on training programs. In a survey I conducted with a large swimming club, the athletes (aged 10 to 18 years) complained that the coach had no "interest" in them. Nothing could have been further from the truth, but the coach had forgotten that his squad was more than a group of sports persons. In fact, the children enjoyed being asked about school, other activities, and the like. There are, moreover, so many ways to say to a child, "You are wrong" without using the word "wrong." To de-emphasize winning and emphasize best effort are such necessary attitudes for children and adults to learn, because the "winning" in sport will be a result based on best effort. One elite coach with whom I have worked for 15 years has the goal, with his junior squad, of promoting a "good, healthy body as well as self-discipline." He places relatively little pressure on athletes to win, but trains very competitive and successful athletes.

Having "athlete of the month" has proven to be a useful strategy within teams to build confidence in junior squads because the coach is able to manipulate the choice of the athlete. A photo in the clubroom or a short article in the newspaper reinforces the efforts of all athletes in the squad. Other possible resources may include

1. Photo or advertisement of the sport in news agencies
2. Interview on local television
3. Notices or articles in the shop windows of local businesses.

I recall instances where the use of confidence-building techniques enhances the quality of young athletes' lives. For example, an intellectually disabled boy was a member of an athletic squad and was a sprinter with some ability. Although his competitive potential was limited, the enthusiasm and effort that he placed in his sport generalized to his schoolwork and home life. His parents remained excited as they watched their son achieve in his sport as well as interact, socially, with his peers of varying ages. The effect of this boy's inclusion in the squad was to motivate other members to emulate the effort and commitment the boy placed in his sprinting both competitively and in training. The coach often remarked that working with this atypical athlete challenged his techniques of training, which served to enhance his skills.

There is no question that sport can be an invaluable asset for the positive growth and development in children. Children can run, throw, or kick so that they are viable for some form of physical activity that can be used for positive effect. They can become addicted to their sport to the exclusion of other important aspects of their lives. This is particularly true for the teenager who participates in sport but is completing schooling. Balance must be kept, and sometimes, sport may need to be relinquished in favor of study. I have observed the opposite situation to occur where parents and/or coaches pushed children into sport and did not keep the appropriate balance in their children's lives. The focus of attention should always remain on only considering the best interests of children, including their involvement in sport.

Adult and Elite Athletes

Over the last 20 years I have been privileged to work with many olympian and elite athletes and have found that many are, necessarily, obsessive about their sport. Elite athletes, moreover, tend to be self-centered. They may need to be convinced that the efforts of the sport psychologist are directed at their needs, either personal or relevant to their sport. At times, being involved in the personal issues relevant to athletes raises ethical issues regarding a dual relationship, but in the same way, personal issues cannot be avoided. Therefore, it is essential that the sport psychologist and the athlete agree to a definitive and binding resolution on the conditions necessary for an effective relationship.

Borrowing from a model that I use in relationship counseling I challenge the athlete to enter into a partnership with me. Figure 2 represents a model of what is meant by focusing on the mutual benefits to be gained by athlete and psychologist.

This mutually satisfying relationship between athlete and psychologist begins with negotiating the expectations of each for the other. If discrepancies or disputes appear, it is important to find compromises or change the initial expectation so that both may be fulfilled and comfortable with the outcomes to be achieved.

Once resolved, the focus of attention remains on what is best for the partnership,

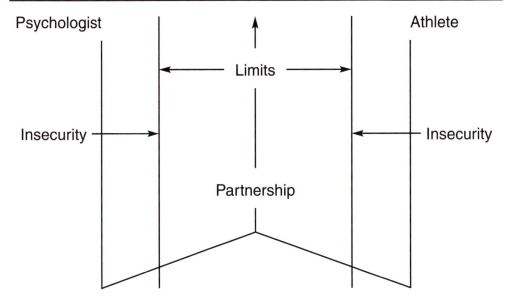

Figure 2.
Establishing relationship between psychologist and athlete.

and if there is equal "give" by both parties, the relationship will work perfectly. The partnership will remain effective and strong, however, only when the "give" by both athlete and psychologist remains within reasonable limits. Insecurity will be created if one or the other moves outside those limits due to badly constructed expectations or a power struggle. In such cases, I have experienced situations in which I have been initiating most of the input until the situation becomes untenable, and on occasions, the contact has had to be broken. Once a trusting and mutually acceptable relationship is established, mental preparation training programs will result in greater commitment and honesty to the mutual benefit of athlete and psychologist. If the focus of attention is to be on what is best for the partnership, then three conditions need to be fulfilled:

1. A commitment by both to put in the best effort for performance outcomes.
2. The trust that the other is equally committed to the task.

3. Changes necessary to effect the optimal relationship between psychologist and athlete.
4. I recall one elite athlete with whom I formed a partnership where each expectation for the other included
   1. Regular contact to arrange mental training sessions at mutually convenient times.
   2. Honest communication regarding training exercises with his coach and me.
   3. My commitment to him that I would attend the major competitions in which he participated.
   4. Commitment to seek compromise and resolution in case of disagreement or changes.

Over time, the athlete became unreasonably demanding although I was making all the effort regarding contact and appointments. In addition, I discovered that he had been lying to me about practicing mental plans during training. Contact with his coach revealed that similar situations were occurring and that conflict had infringed on their relationship. When confronted to resolve the conflicts, the athlete was dogmatic about his actions and was not prepared to be honest or compromise. The athlete dissolved his partnership with me as well as the one with his coach as he began contact with a different set of sport scientists and another coach. In retrospect, I regret having not confronted the athlete earlier when it became clear that he was not fully committed to the partnership and the insecurity in the relationship, as it developed, was inevitable.

Developing Mental Plans

When invited to be involved in a mental preparation program for elite swimmers in my local area, I became interested in the notion of "mental plans" as devised by Orlick (1986). I found that once credibility has been established, athletes like to be instructed authoritatively in all aspects of their preparation. Similar to a swim training program, athletes found the term "mental plans" appealing to them because it had connotations of proactive content and "sounded" appropriate. During initial consultations with athletes, I recorded a history of recent and present performances and administered a formal test. I asked the athletes about the techniques they used prior to competition. At all levels of competition, I found that the responses were similar: "warm up and stretch" and little pertaining to mental preparation. At the same time, some athletes also described feelings of "nausea, a sense of helplessness or a desire to run away" as they stand behind the blocks before competition. As well, distractions such as the crowd, swimming against more elite competitors, or pressures from coaches/parents tended to exacerbate the earlier sensations of distress. It was clear to me that the experience of such emotional reactions must relate to a possible diminution in optimal performance.

The use of cognitive strategies prior to, during, and after competition not only can be useful in restructuring the intrusive thoughts mentioned above, but also can be positive regulators of arousal with subsequent performance enhancement. Athletes can be trained to perform a set of tasks, or rituals, and in doing so, they are actively involved in creating a positive mental set to offset distractions. Precompetition strategies typically involve the use of progressive relaxation techniques that have been shown to be useful and productive in such situations. However, in my experience, self-hypnosis has proved to be an even more powerful technique because of the nature of the technique together with the dynamics by which it operates. I am aware that the literature provides controversy regarding the efficacy of hypnosis in sport, but I have found it an invaluable tool in clinical practice as well as an equally effective core technique in sport. Because hypnosis is typically used in clinical practice for stress management, ego strengthening, and desensitization, I believe it is an ideal technique in sport for the same purposes.

Disregarding the academic arguments for or against hypnosis, my experience has shown athletes warm to the use of the technique, with enthusiasm, and in fact, I have never found an athlete who rejected the technique or was not susceptible to suggestion using hypnosis. Like all skills, hypnosis needs to be taught and practiced, so that the outcome is the athlete's ability to practice self-hypnosis. Self-hypnosis, in turn, can be applied to other strategies, which require an altered state of consciousness to be completely effective, to create pre-event readiness. Figure 3 represents the model used in the intervention that swimmers found so useful.

One technique referred to in the diagram refers to "tree it," which was a term developed by Orlick (1986) after he worked with

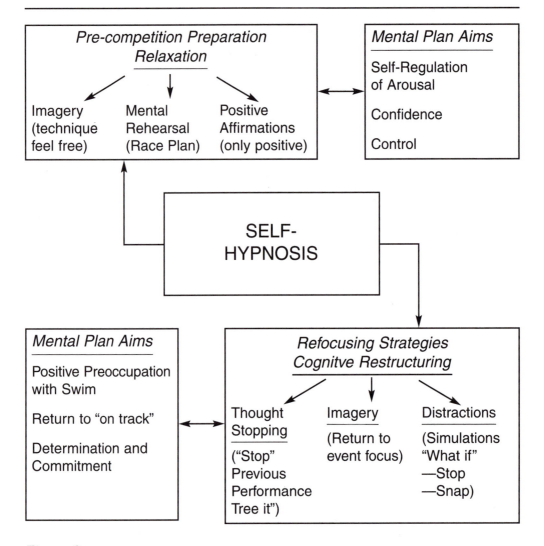

Figure 3.
Pre-competition warm-up strategies.

teams of rugby league players in New Guinea. Rather than display anger, joy, or other emotional responses where conflict may have been a possibility, at the end of the game, players were conditioned to run to a tree and "touch" it to return emotions to nature. That is, the players were able to let go of all emotions experienced in the game in a symbolic manner. Orlick (1986) called this ritual "treeing it" and suggested that it had considerable relevance for precompetition strategies in all sports. In practicing mental plans, it is useful to locate a point where the athlete can "tree" all other thoughts and focus only on her- or himself and the sporting space (the swimming lane). For the swimmer, this may mean touching the door of the dressing room or the diving block of the pool. Similarly, I have found it effective to suggest to golfers that they consider the competition as 18 games of golf of one hole each, rather than as 18 holes of golf. Concluding each hole, the golfer may slap his golf bag to signify the end of that segment of his game be-

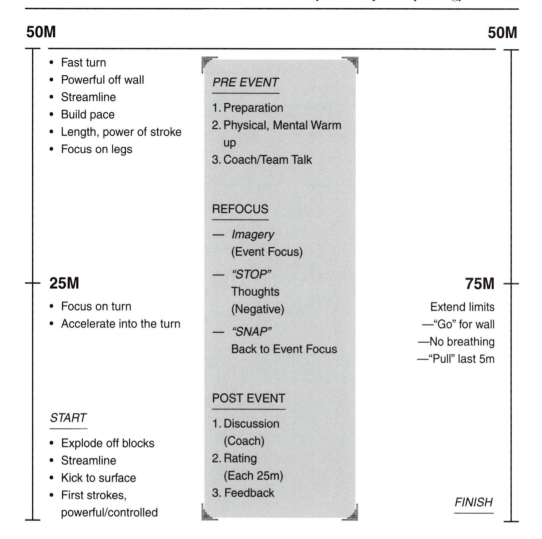

50M   **50M**

- Fast turn
- Powerful off wall
- Streamline
- Build pace
- Length, power of stroke
- Focus on legs

PRE EVENT

1. Preparation
2. Physical, Mental Warm up
3. Coach/Team Talk

REFOCUS

— *Imagery*
   (Event Focus)

— *"STOP"*
   Thoughts
   (Negative)

— *"SNAP"*
   Back to Event Focus

25M   **75M**

- Focus on turn
- Accelerate into the turn

Extend limits
—"Go" for wall
—No breathing
—"Pull" last 5m

POST EVENT

1. Discussion
   (Coach)
2. Rating
   (Each 25m)
3. Feedback

START

- Explode off blocks
- Streamline
- Kick to surface
- First strokes, powerful/controlled

FINISH

Figure 4.
A race-focus plan (100 meters).

cause he can achieve nothing further by perseverating on the difficulties of the previous segment without its becoming a distraction. Similarly, elite weight lifters warm up in a room adjacent to the lifting platform, so as they enter the competitive arena, they learn to touch the doorjamb of the warm-up room, signifying their focus on beginning their pre-event strategies and rituals.

Using self-hypnosis to facilitate the technique of mental rehearsal is the most powerful and impressive technique to be learned. It is important, almost essential, that athletes be instructed in how to mentally rehearse using perfect technique and trying to attain personal best performance. With a group of swimmers, this technique was used with considerable success. However, to create a better "picture" of the rehearsal, it was useful to create a race-focus plan that the coach and I jointly devised. In the 100-meter freestyle event, the coach defined exactly what he expected should be the focus of attention at points at either end of the pool and

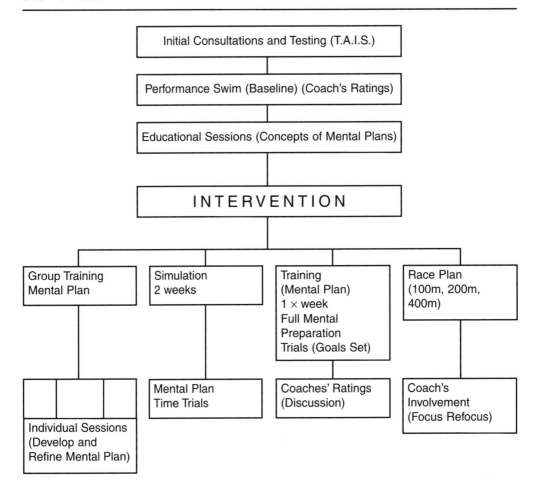

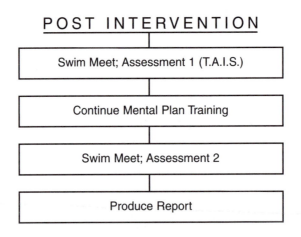

Figure 5.
Development of an intervention.

halfway down its length. A sample profile of the race focus for the 100m freestyle event is reproduced here as Figure 4.

Mentally rehearsing perfect technique and following a race-focus plan were practiced at training, in groups, and in individual sessions. Using this technique, many athletes could mentally rehearse their actual personal best times within one or two seconds.

Performance simulations during training, augmented by the coach's ratings of performance, were also effective. This was particularly so for young athletes and some elite, disabled athletes for whom a change in "safe" environments and different venues caused distress. At present, I have just completed a program of desensitization with a group of young athletes competing in national age championships at a venue in another state. Experience has shown that many athletes were overawed by the large crowds, the noise, and the differences in organization, or they were homesick, which worsened their natural feelings of tension. For local teams of many sports, it was useful to simulate the competition atmosphere by using the available resources. For example, parents, employees of the swimming pool, and other squad members acted as a noisy, distracting crowd while referees, timekeepers, and starters were in place to set up a simulated atmosphere similar to the real event. Athletes needed to be encouraged to practice the precompetition strategies within this environment and perform as if it was the actual event. Such simulations should be part of training programs; for the squad in this project, the simulation occurred twice a week leading up to a major carnival. In addition, it is important that the coach maintain his own ratings of performances so that he or she can monitor, assess, and advise on techniques as well as performance outcomes. For the coach, such evaluations have significant implications for further training modifications.

Finally, to integrate these techniques into a successful program, the model presented in Figure 5 is suggested as a possible intervention strategy compatible with many sports at the community level.

Related Issues

Although some of the techniques developed in the sporting environment enhance performance, I have used them effectively in clinical practice. Mental rehearsal, affirmations, and self-hypnosis are typical features of stress-management programs used with clients. Also, sport psychologists may be requested to be involved in atypical situations such as trauma counseling or interventions with problems encountered by athletes within their normal daily lives. In the past, I have been involved in the debriefing of athletes, coaches, referees, and administrators in situations involving death. The death of an elite "iron man" lifesaver in a car accident and the drowning of a young surfboat rower in dangerous surf led to debriefing interventions with other athletes, referees, administrators, and families. In the case of the young surf lifesaver who drowned in heavy surf contesting the national titles, the debriefing proved effective in reducing the effects of the tragedy, but the intervention was not completely satisfactory because of the large number of people involved. In Australia, the national titles in surf lifesaving represent the largest number of competing athletes other than the Olympic games, and it is reasonable to believe that all personnel participating were affected by this atypical tragedy.

At the request of the executive of the surf lifesaving organization, I was involved in the debriefing of the senior executive, chief referee, and several of the beach referees who were responsible for the conduct of the titles. Consequently, the decisions regarding the continuation of the events in very heavy surf was at their discretion. After the tragedy, intense media criticism followed, with commentaries accusing the officials of irresponsible behavior and decision making because of the conditions that prevailed on the day. It came to my attention that several of the key personnel had reacted with behaviors that were atypical but distressing to their families. Common responses were reported to be

1. Bad dreams and flashbacks.
2. Dizziness and palpitations.
3. Sleep disturbance and mood changes.
4. Increased alcohol intake, aggressive reactions to family, and a reluctance to attend work.

Different people have different reactions to stressful situations, and the symptoms described may be indicative of other conditions. However, because these reactions occurred some days after the tragedy, it is reasonable to consider that the men had experienced a critical incident stress disorder. The debriefing sessions were designed to allow the following outcomes:

1. To reconstruct the actions of the personnel involved, reasons for decisions, and reinforcement of such decisions to recreate a complete plan leading up to the tragedy.
2. To obtain a report from each member about his or her reactions to the event at the present time to be verbalized at the meeting.
3. To give the group an opportunity to ventilate feelings and reactions regarding the entire situation. Typically, group members were supportive of each other, an attitude that assisted each from the sense of being alone.
4. To explain stress and the physical and psychological reactions to stress.
5. To discuss strategies that would reduce or eliminate the effects of the stress reaction by
6. Talking about the experience

7. Attending to the overindulgence of alcohol
8. Continuing normal work and home activities
9. Accepting that they may feel "bad" but, with time, the negativity will fade or disappear.

Although the results of this debriefing were satisfactory, the lesson learned was that a contingency plan needed to be in place for future events. It was resolved that professional counselors and appropriate resources would be available during major carnivals in case an incident involving death, personal danger, or acute discomfort occurred.

Conclusion

Community-based sport psychology has grown as a productive source of involvement for practitioners over many years. Theory, research, conferences, and workshops continue to provide important forums to modify and improve the practical aspects of the discipline. Practitioners need to avail themselves of every opportunity to learn new skills and adapt theoretical concepts and principles into practical strategies. In this way, they can remain current with contemporary theories and practices. However, in reality, athletes and coaches are interested only in practical and performance outcomes, not in academic dialogue. For this reason, I applaud the important aims of this publication, as I believe it is long overdue for practitioners working outside universities or sports institutes. Further, although the models and suggestions made in this presentation may seem simplistic, I hope they may offer something to the young sport psychologist beginning practice as a springboard to individual initiative and ideas always welcome in community-based sports.

For me, the most significant reward from being involved in sport psychology has been its interaction with clinical practice. I believe that the line between sport and clinical psychology is blurred in that so many techniques and applications of one are transferable to the other discipline. In sport, we aim for performance enhancement and the development of mental plans whereas, in clinical practice, we devise strategies for a better quality of life or therapeutic outcomes. It seems that the techniques are, often, the same, but the applications may be different, and this is only contingent on the context under consideration.

In the case scenarios presented relevant to crises, the techniques and applications are the same. Finally, sport psychology has an immensely important future in Australia for promoting healthier, productive environments not only in sport but also in education, organizations, and businesses that continually seek goal-oriented and motivated outcomes.

Reference

Orlick, T (1986). *Psyching for sport*. Champaign, IL: Human Kinetics

Reflections on Sport Psychology Practice: A Clinical Perspective

Noam Eyal

Introduction

I write this chapter following several years of experience in psychological consultation to athletes from a wide range of branches, ages, and quality groups. My first encounter with sports psychology occurred during my work as a clinical psychologist. Having a background in competitive sports, I was curious to find out how my feelings as an athlete are integrated in the psychological theories regarding consultation for athletes. The distance from this point to actual practice, concurrent with the clinical work was short. Of all the questions that occupied my thoughts, from the beginning of my work up to this day, one key question stood out: What place does the psychologist have in the sports culture? What is the real reason for athletes to invite the psychologist into their intimate world and at what, or whose, expense? In other words, what is the Point of Archimedes from which the psychologist can, or is asked to, affect the psychology of the athlete?

A similar question occupies the mind of the clinical psychologist practicing psychotherapy. A partial answer is provided when one has to choose the course of training in which one will specialize, such as family consultation or psychoanalysis. Usually, the psychologist meets with people who have turned to him or her of their own accord after

preferring this psychologist to the others. Hence, these people accept the therapeutic approach and the other conditions set by the psychologist as the basis for consultation.

The situation is usually different when it comes to the issue of the bond between the sports psychologist and the athletes. Many athletes are treated by a psychologist chosen for them by the coach, trainer, club manager, or national association. In the world of sports, it is acceptable for the psychologists to offer their services to the athletes—as occurs in the ball teams that employ their own psychologist. Because, in this case, the athletes cannot select a psychologist of their choice, it is highly reasonable that some resentment may develop. The natural suspicion as to the psychologist's ability to maintain proper ethics, having his or her livelihood dependent on a manager or coach, must be factored in as well. The situation is different, of course, in the circumstance of personal and private consultation chosen by the athletes themselves. Additionally, the therapeutic mandate given to the sports psychologist is limited to specific aspects of the athlete's personality to begin with (according to certain naive points of view). The psychologist is asked to assist in areas specifically associated with the sport demands of the athlete: control of stress associated with the competition, improvement of the ability to concentrate under strenuous conditions, and development of drive under conditions of burnout, to mention a few classic situations. Over the years, I have discovered that the public label tagged on the sport psychologist brings some of the athletes to reveal the distress that they carry with them to therapy by focusing on one of the classic issues of sports psychology. Athletes who have turned to me regarded my attention as if it were directed towards sports issues only. When I made it clear that the issues raised in the room do not necessarily need to touch solely on issues of sports, the style of the talk directed at me changed as well. The athletes allowed themselves to distance themselves from their athletic identity and to observe it from their overall identity. I understood that if I did not clarify this issue in advance, merely defining myself as a sports psychologist would block the option for some athletes to express themselves freely without internal censorship, a fundamental condition for the success of any type of psychological consultation.

Some of the athletes with whom I have consulted were interested in discussing their competitive careers only and in acquiring specific skills in psychoregulation, and I respected that. Many others, however, claimed that they had never experienced any difficulties under stressful competitive conditions, during long and boring training sessions, or from disrupted attention. It was clear to me that the athletes had a tremendous need to talk about themselves—sometimes without saying a word about an important competition awaiting them the following day. When I allowed for this, their overall feeling improved, and they experienced better athletic achievements. The athletes taught me how to treat them, and the consulting style I have crystallized is unlike anything I have done in the past. This is not the clinical psychology I am familiar with

from dynamic psychotherapy either.

The world of sports has rigid rules of survival. Sometimes, these are unpleasant for the psychologist, and I will elaborate on this topic later. The psychologist continuously needs to adjust the style of work to these rules, without losing the uniqueness of the psychology profession. It is possible to do this by setting a specific therapy setting for each athlete, for instance, according to the branch of sports, its special requirements, career status, timing, and reason for seeking therapy, but primarily according to the "type of psychological listening" required by the athlete. This is a key term in my perception of the consultation and the most important element for finding and crystallizing the Point of Archimedes in the therapy of every athlete.

My principal thoughts regarding these quests are found in the following pages.

The Specific and Nonspecific Contribution of the Sports Psychologist to Athletes

The search for and attribution of hidden psychological motives for competitive success or failure are prevalent among competitive sports enthusiasts. The interest in the personality characteristics of the great athletes has become almost as popular as the preoccupation with their physical abilities. Common psychological descriptions are given much consideration, and this trend is expressed well in the media and popular sports literature. Seemingly, these are ideal conditions for the invitation of many psychologists to consult single athletes and professional clubs, but the increasing popularity of the "Psychology of Competitive Effort" is creating its own dynamics. It has become clear that various professionals, who are not at all psychologists, offer psychological assistance to the athletes under various disguises. Doctors, physiotherapists, masseuses, biomechanics, nutritionists, and managers—all operate regularly as a supportive staff for the athletes. They discuss the athletes' difficulties with them, calm them down, motivate them before competitions, and offer them advice. The majority of athletes, being young, are not aware of sports psychologists and, therefore, have difficulty appreciating the differences between a psychologist and a nonpsychologist. Some athletes and coaches receive help from a nonpsychologist as a comfortable outlet that allows them to avoid the embarrassment associated with seeking help from a psychologist. On the other hand, the professional supporting staff often uses psychological means in their relationship with the athletes because this is an important source of power. The provision of psychological services is useful in strengthening the bond with the athlete and increasing the chances that the athlete will continue receiving professional services of the supporting staff.

The more psychology and psychological consultation are perceived as being more important than before for athletic success, the greater the threat they pose to the influence and position of the club's traditional expert veteran service providers. Because of this, I have encountered, more than once, various objections to my entry into the club in the capacity of a psychological consultant. Various experts from the supporting team express this by avoiding referring athletes to psychologists or by referring them in a discouraging manner. Of course, some clubs accept the psychologist with interest and support, and even with enthusiasm. According to my experience, they are the exception. The more professional the club or athlete and the greater the success, the greater the competition among the various professionals over the psychological closeness to the athlete and the tendency to distance him or her from the sports psychologist. The psychologist must deepen the understanding of how to position him- or herself in the professional setup of the club to successfully face this type of internal struggle and have a positive influence on the athletes. Similar considerations exist when facing an individual athlete in the setting of the private clinic because he or she is assisted as well by professionals from additional areas. The psychologist must convince the athlete or the coach as to his or her unique contribution and the qualities that make him or her different from the other professionals offering alternative, nonspecific psychological services.

My personal experience points out two primary approaches through which the psychologist can clarify his or her contribution. The first is based on convincing the sport professionals that physical training and exercises have an analogous mental aspect; that is, that the determining psychological qualities are nothing more than skills that can be perfected by exercise and study, in accordance with the athlete's needs and limitations. This goal is achievable by suggestive techniques. The athlete is an object to be convinced. The greater the perception of the "convincer" as being highly reputable and the tools of convincing more scientific, the easier it will be to have the athlete crystallize a truer self-perception in his or her attitude regarding his or her ability. In other words, the convincing tools that the psychologist places in the athlete's hands are the psychologist's contribution to competitive success. In this sense, the psychologist positions him- or herself in the forefront of the "succession of convincers" of the sports world. Everybody, beginning with the coach and professional staff, through the slew of aids to the media and fans, try to convince the athlete that he or she needs to and can rise above. The psychologist, on his or her part, observes the athlete's performance and crystallizes an opinion as to the reasons for the athlete's inadequacy. Later on, the psychologist listens to the athlete's complaint, if one exists, and jointly crystallizes a psychoregulation plan. This approach is relatively easy to market in sports because of its conceptual closeness to a trainer-trainee or teacher-student relationship prevalent in the authoritative sports world. The psychologist brings a modular knowledge charge, and he or she, better than anyone else, knows how to adapt it to the changing needs of the athletes. This, however, is not a specific contribution. The association with the "succession of convincers" enables the psychologist only to elaborate the suggestive approach, which is prevalent in the world of sports. The psychologist's contribution will be important, but under no circumstance will it be specific.

The alternative to this approach is fundamentally different. Although the first approach is based on cognitive theories and enables a clear-cut teacher-student relationship between the psychologist and the athlete, the noncognitive psychological theories refer to consultation in a different way. They assume that the athlete has been driven to a career in competitive sports out of character-based needs of which he or she, for the most part, is unaware. When the athlete fails, an internal conflict is possibly created or sharpened either between clashing needs (the aspiration for power versus the need for stability and fear of failure) or between the athlete's "internal" world and the reality in which the athlete lives (fantasies of self-exposure on the background of a closed religious community). A prevalent example for this would be an athlete's maturing and a higher level of character organization development with a lessening of the narcissistic needs for admiration and adoration by the spectators. This may significantly lessen the motivation to compete in general and before spectators in particular. In this case, there is no use trying to "convince" the athlete, because it is unclear what he or she is unconvinced of. If the

athlete gets the opportunity to speak freely and without guidance, and the psychologist avoids identification with the role of an athlete (taking a convincing emotional stand as to what is right to do as an athlete), only then, maybe, will the athlete be able to understand what has gone awry in his or her professional life at this specific moment. Clearly, taking such a stand puts the psychologist in a totally different place in comparison to a psychologist who exercises suggestive approaches. Being disassociated from the "succession of convincers" in the sports world, the psychologist makes it undoubtedly clear as to the specific contribution of the psychologist in comparison to that of the other people talking to athletes.

There are, at least, three possible fundamental approaches to the establishment of a connection with the competitive athlete:

1. Every complaint made by the athlete, including personal problems, receives attention through guidance: what the athlete should do to restore the desired balance of his or her character as an athlete.
2. Every complaint receives the attention of the psychologist in a way that is unconditional to the individual's being an athlete. The person applying may discuss any issue he or she chooses without any guidance or direction from the psychologist as to the topics worthwhile or necessary to discuss.
3. Listening to the athlete's complaint is determined by changing data. Sometimes the listening is unconditional, and sometimes the athlete is guided to discuss issues that are of high priority on the psychologist's choice list (e.g., a club's demand of the athlete).

Although the first two approaches to the establishment of a connection are well defined, as are their advantages and disadvantages, the third requires a renewed definition with each meeting. It is very possible that in the case of lengthy therapy, the unconditional listening will be replaced by suggestive guidance or vice versa, and this possibility will be brought to the athlete's attention. It is highly possible for serious ethical problems to emerge: The athlete must be convinced that the psychologist, who is suddenly offering guidance and convincing, was indeed unconditionally listening to the athlete earlier and is able to revert to that type of listening as soon as possible. If the athlete conceives the psychologist as just one more person—such as the coach or doctor—who knows from a subjective position what is right for the athlete, the athlete's ability to speak freely is blocked.

There is a sharp paradox here: How is it possible to ask someone to speak freely if he or she knows that you are not listening freely? In such a case, a strong tendency develops to tell the listener what he or she wants to hear. From this point on, the psy-chological therapy ends and a pedagogic therapy begins. Therefore, it is likely that a third approach is almost impossible, at least theoretically. On the other hand, the complex situations in the sport world require one psychologist to cover all the psychological needs of the athlete.

The ideal situation in which the athlete can simultaneously use various psychological services provided by more than one psychologist—private or group consultation, learning psychoregulation—is utopian. Even if this is desired or possible, there is no time for it, and it only adds much confusion to that already existing.

In the following examples of consultations, I will try to demonstrate various approaches to the establishment of a therapeutic bond between the psychologist and the athlete. I will present the course of consultation followed by a discussion on the considerations that have guided me.

Case 1

B. was in her early 20s when she came under my care. She was well-known from a very young age as the national champion in a branch of personal sports that requires great precision and patience. Because she also excelled in international competitions, she was invited, for the first time in her career, to a world tour of professionals. Her request for psychological help was made approximately 2 months before the beginning of the tour with no clear complaint. B. "only" wished to improve her concentration skills under stressful conditions in order to be more successful in the competitions. It was difficult to find signs of any conflict during the diagnostic process, because, among other reasons, B. cooperated only partially and refused to expose all sides of her personality. I taught her the basic techniques of psychoregulation: guided imagery (Weinberg, 1988), autogenic training (Schultz, 1932) and goal setting (Locke & Latham, 1985). B. responded with overt indifference and cooperated with correct politeness. I thought it right to draw her attention to this, but her behavior did not change, and her explanations for this behavior were apologetic but without any guilt feelings whatsoever.

After several weeks during which she kept all the meetings on a regular basis but with little progress in psychoregulation, I became convinced that B. was seeking advice to receive something else. I assumed she was not aware of her wish and I decided to "confront" her (Kernberg, 1985). This is a well-determined therapeutic move with the goal of creating an inner confrontation between the patient's defensive mechanisms and the element causing the anxiety by the therapist raising a specific issue deliberately.

Upon termination of a routine session, I announced to B. that I had decided to end the therapy because I had no help to offer her. I asked her to set the date for our last meeting. B. appeared to be in shock, but said she would come to the last meeting. She did not arrive and did not notify anybody of her intentions. This was 3 weeks before her planned trip, alone, on the professional tour. The following morning, I called to find out why she missed her last appointment. B. sounded very confused and said that something terrible had occurred. She asked for an appointment as soon as possible and appeared as scheduled. I saw before me a person in the midst of a panic attack: sweating heavily, pale, hands trembling, stuttering, and drinking water continuously. She had difficulty speaking coherently but said that her car had broken down in the middle of the highway on her way to my office, for the last appointment that she did not keep and to which she referred as our last meeting. Her car's engine just quit, and B. found herself helpless on the highway shoulder, in the dark with no one stopping for her. Then and there, she experienced a panic attack for the first time in her life. She was overcome by a huge fear regarding her pending trip abroad and her life in general. She said she was scared of the mere thought that the therapy was about to end and did not know how to handle her anxieties. The deterioration in her condition affected her training as well, and she was unable to carry out basic elements of her sports activity successfully for 3 days. She felt that all her grandiose fantasies about taking over the sports world were crashing down and she was losing her self-confidence. B. said that she totally identified with her car's ruined engine when no one was stopping to offer her assistance. Her coach was perplexed and rebuked her for the bad timing of her breakdown.

I listened to her and when she was done, I chose a paradoxical response. I cheerfully reacted: "Excellent!" B. was flabbergasted, as I planned. I told her that the true reason for her seeking therapy—the enormous anxiety overcoming her—had finally surfaced and that now she could be treated. I asked, "What would have happened had this occurred abroad with no psychological help and with you truly alone?" B. burst out in tears and asked to resume therapy with no delay. I offered to meet her five times a week, alternating the location between my clinic and the training field where she would exercise the basic skills of her sports activity *in vivo*. We constructed a list, jointly, of these skills in an estimated hierarchy based on level of difficulty of execution. The goal was to build her self-efficacy (Bandura, 1977) through systematic desensitization. B. left the session with a "to do" activity list of tasks ranging from very simple to complex ones. She requested to begin exercising the simplest task that same day. In the first week, B. failed to perform even the simplest task properly. Because she was overcome by paralyzing anxiety, every type of coordinated activity failed and exacerbated the anxiety further. There was a necessity to distance her from her regular training arena, replace basic accessories that she used, and make many additional improvisations, their sole purpose being to enable her to perform any physical activity without experiencing anxiety. An indication of her initial ability to perform the basic skills in her field of sports appeared only in the second week. During the third week, she began advancing up the skill hierarchy we established at the beginning of the process. Concurrently, we carried on very intensive therapy focusing on her termination of the therapy that symbolized the end of the first part—the dependent part—of her career that would end on the eve of her travel abroad on the professional tour.

The goal of the therapy was to have B. crystallize a better understanding of the meaning of maturity and of getting out and experiencing the big world. B. felt that "being big" was a dangerous move that exposed her to anxiety that meant "I am not as strong as I thought." Her gradual improvement in executing the basic skills of her sport activity helped to process the experience of failure as a mishap that might be corrected and lead to growth into the adult world. Eventually, the athlete went abroad as planned. We agreed for her to contact and inform me of the results of her first competitions. I did not hear from her during the following 2 years, until she resumed therapy. The media reported her to be very successful.

Elaboration

B.'s therapy is very typical of the sports psychologist's work. He or she is seemingly asked to assist in guidance or suggestive consultation, and no one will complain should he or she leave it at that. Sometimes people will complain if the psychologist tries to do more than that, but careful listening enables one to hear the athletes express a wish they themselves are unaware of. B. came to the therapy sessions with a vague feeling she was not ready for professional competition. Her obstinate objection to treating the signs of tension directly using psychoregulation techniques presented a signal that there was a need to break through her repression regarding her unwillingness to compete. Her refusal to accept know-how for the treatment of the concentration and tension installed in her hands the feeling of continuous, although ineffective, control. My announcement of my intention to end the therapy turned the order of events on its face. From that moment on, she experienced a loss of control, and then the feeling, up to this moment hidden in her subconscious, overcame her. The anxiety attack was exacerbated while she was standing next to her ruined car engine on the highway shoulder. This anxiety attack could have occurred, at that time, following any other mishap in her life. The great symbolism in the automobile (Auto—me, myself in Latin) broken down on the way to the last therapy session just exacerbated the panic, as happens so often when a strong conflict is repressed. Only then did B. understand her motivation for seeking psychological help—insignificant to her up to that moment.

From that point on, her cooperation in the daily sessions was perfect. B.'s therapy was based on the third approach to the establishment of a connection, which I have proposed in the introduction. A complicated integration was made between a clear suggestive approach (systematic desensitization) and the approach—in this case, a specific one—of unconditional attention (short-term dynamic therapy), indeed around a single focused issue (parting) which was crystallized jointly with her (Malan, 1976; Mann, 1973). In my opinion, had I not confronted her strange indifference, the anxiety would have erupted during the professional tour competitions, when the pressures increased. Alone, with no professional support, it is doubtful she would have recovered from such a breakdown. Such events occur often and may traumatize an athlete, causing severe damage to his or her career and possibly its abrupt ending without a true understanding of what ensued. Such an event might have a devastating effect for many years on the behavior and reaction to various trying situations completely unrelated to sports.

An interesting phenomenon that took place during this case relates to the reactions of the coach and other professionals who work with the athlete. An approach of an athlete to the psychologist on the eve of an important competition usually results in hostile reactions on the part of these elements: "You mean we are not good enough to help one moment before the big test, unlike what we were up to now?" This approach exacerbates, of course, the athlete's conflict regarding exposing his or her deepest anxieties in the presence of a psychologist. Indeed, B.'s coach blamed the psychological therapy for the eruption of the anxiety attack. His helplessness in trying to give B. effective advice was very frustrating for him. He tended to accept the doctor's advice and treat the athlete with anxiolytic drugs, but her rapid improvement changed his approach towards the whole issue of psychological consultation.

Case 2

Psychological work in a professional sports team exposes the psychologist to professional internal conflict during a large part of his or her meetings with the team and the professional or managerial staff. Part of the conflict is associated with the psychological consultation itself, and the other relates to the impact of the events on the psychologist's own personality. That is, the intensive dynamics that characterizes a sport team heavily covered by the media and involves many talented players does not leave the psychologist distant and self-assured as to his or her position in the club. One day, the psychologist feels wanted and liked and the next day—rejected and forgotten. The psychologist is dragged into many trial situations that he or she must withstand as part of the overall highly competitive atmosphere that characterizes a professional club. Such an organization operates according to almost set virtual rules accepted by everybody as an established, obligatory tradition. The purpose of these rules is to settle the interpersonal relationships and define the goals expected from the various function holders: managers, coaches, players, and medical staff. Of all the various professionals assisting the team, the psychologist is one of the most recent to join the tradition of the sports club. In most clubs, the place of a physiotherapist and masseuse has been guaranteed for many years now, for better for worse, not so with the position of the psychologist. Many coaches dispute the mere necessity for a psychologist in the team setup. Statements such as "Professional athletes must overcome their mental problems on their own" or "Talking to a psychologist is a type of pampering that invites weakness and not self-sacrifice" are prevalent. Worse than that, one sometimes hears, "I (The coach) am the team's psychologist." At times when a coach or management employs a psychologist, they do not know where to position that professional in the club hierarchy. Where should the psychologist physically be during training or a competition? Whom should he or she be talking to at a given moment, and to whom must the psychologist present the information he or she accumulates? The common complaint towards the psychologist is "You know all the problems, but you do not provide solutions." In an organization where the remaining days until the next competition are the last grace period, the holding back of possible information that is allegedly known to the psychologist (Is a key player acting out an injury?) is perceived as a lack of loyalty to a particularly suspicious system.

The psychologist's first assignment in the entry process into the club is to find his or her place in the existing setup. Usually no one will assist the psychologist in achieving this, primarily out of ignorance as to how the process should occur. A clear and defined hesitation in finding one's place will distance the psychologist to the margin of the circle of influence, a location from which the ability to influence is low. From that point on, the path to ineffectiveness and expulsion from the club is short. When the team is successful, the pressure on the psychologist is low. He or she might be perceived as unnecessary, though even the managers with a highly developed sense of thrift will hesitate to discharge a psychologist and by that rock a successful system.

This is not the case with a failing team. Then, the guilty parties are sought after, and the psychologist is asked difficult questions regarding his or her contribution. The psychologist is highly tempted to demonstrate successful psychological assistance to one athlete or another. The problem is created by the psychologist's entry into the internal competitive circle that continuously exists between the various club staff members: "I am also close and important for the athletes' success." If the psychologist is able to avoid such competition, he or she creates a stronghold that, with time, will prove itself to be of high importance for the club's internal balance: The psychologist—a reliable address within the club for consultation and the sharing of feelings (especially negative ones). In other words, the psychologist must find or form within the club a Point of Archimedes from which he or she will be able to influence most of the people, without being involved in the internal competition. The psychologist must prepare for times when he or she will be attacked personally. The psychologist also must avoid becoming an object of envy due to his or her influence and closeness to the players, coaches, or managers. The less the glory of success attached to the psychologist (as opposed to his or her immediate and full proximity to crisis situations), the stronger his or her position and influence.

Freud named the psychologist's entity "Absenteeism" (Freud, 1912), and Bion (1961) described the psychologist's position as "lacking desire" (something for him or herself) or memory (settling of accounts with previous events and their results). The psychologist is required to perform "containing" (Winnicott, 1971) of the overflowing emotions at times of stress, erosion, and catastrophe (difficult defeats, losses in the last few seconds, injury of the team star, resignation / firing of the team coach). He or she is the person who needs to perform "holding under pressure" (Casement, 1985) for large parts of the club. To demonstrate these thoughts, I will present a crisis event that occurred in a professional basketball team towards the middle of the regular league season.

I had worked for this team as a consultant to the coach, players, and sometimes the club managers since the beginning of the season. Part of the psychological consulting included a regular weekly discussion with the players alone. The mere existence of such a forum, closed to the coach and the other staff personnel, was an innovative idea for all. Many objected to it, and its continuation was constantly in doubt due to various disturbances. I insisted on continuing the discussion meetings despite being harshly attacked by some of the players (who preferred to sleep in the extra hour), the coaches (who feared being part of the issue discussed, thus weakening their position), and the managers (who aspired to know every word being said in the club). The insistence on keeping the team forum, where the players talked about themselves, proved itself at a later stage of the season when most of the club systems collapsed. The club, thrown into a losing streak, a period of coach changes and injury to key players, became involved in quarrels with the fans and with the fickle sponsor.

Even when it all seemed to be falling apart, the team continued to meet on a regular basis despite the external turmoil and the difficulty of remaining a team on the parquet. This nucleus of "sanity" was the base for a wonderful recovery later on. The conversations were carried on to allow the expression of the players' every rising thought or feeling. The team had a developmental assignment: to become a cohesive team. The main idea, according to which I suggested guidance to the team, was described by Fairbairn (1952): To turn an arbitrary collection of people into a working group, they must perform a difficult psychological transfer from "destructive dependency" one on the other (insisting on the individualism in the team and mutual exploitation in order to realize the egocentric aspirations) to "creative dependency" (the ability to give and receive without the feeling of taking advantage or being taken advantage of). Such a psychological transition enables cooperation under stressful conditions and acceptance of the coach's authority as the representative of the law and order in the group. The players in the group understood the idea, but, as expected, had difficulty implementing it. They insisted that everybody else give up their egocentric aspirations whereas each of them demanded to be the exception and receive special treatment. Many issues on the team's minds were treated in these discussions, and a fertile dynamics of teamwork was created. Despite this, the team was unable to perform its best for many months. The best players in Israel played on the team, which was reinforced by two excellent NBA retirees. Salaries were paid on time, and the home audience was large and warm. The team was named "The Dream Team" by the media, and the expectation from them flew sky high. Losses occurred in the last seconds of the game to opposite inferior teams as well. The team failed to demonstrate one quality game. The result was increasing pressure on the players and team stars who tried winning the games alone. The teamwork faded away, and the coach was helpless. There was continuous discussion on replacing him, and an atmosphere of a severe crisis was created, the essence of which was the expectation that the coach would be replaced.

I invited the players for the weekly discussion early in the morning, a time at which most were usually still asleep. It was Saturday—Sabbath in Israel—a wintry and rainy day. The streets were empty, and on my way to the club, I wondered which of the players would be absent, using some lame excuse and totally ignoring the team's serious condition. All arrived on time, except for one of the foreign players. In most of the sessions, I allowed the players to suggest the subject for discussion whereas I provided the reflections and interpretations and was responsible for the setting. For this discussion, however, I had prepared a defined message (a message discussed in previous sessions) that I wanted the team to assimilate even at the expense of straying from the regular path. This is an unusual step in the psychodynamic setting. I made that decision because the club was in a complete leadership crisis. The players rejected the authority of the coach and management and intervened when somebody tried to take charge. This was clearly "destructive dependency": A good shot to the basket by one player caused envy and anger among the others who kept the ball from him later on. There was the necessity to provide the players with a convincing interpretation of their condition with the hope that having such knowledge would prove to be effective. The players took their regular seats in total silence, which was very unlike them. I told them about the Roman Empire and the rule of the governors in the various provinces. I stressed the weakening of the Caesar and the whole empire due to the governors' ambition and their desire to succeed the ruling Caesar. I described how the empire lost many territories and resources and much influence over small tribes and weak states due to the redirection of resources to internal struggles.

Then I described the Roman custom to show the unity of the empire through the parade of Electors, the carriers of the "bundle of twigs" (*faschio*), which symbolized the endurance and durability of the united many versus the collapse of the single individual. When I mentioned the single individual, I took a single twig out of my bag and asked the team star to try to break it with me. After doing so easily, I took out a bundle of twigs (chopsticks) and asked him to break them. I turned to him, after he failed to do so, and said, "You look like a single twig when you play alone, but when you are all together, you and the others are unbreakable." Then I added the need for difficult and frustrating personal sacrifice. Without giving up some of the personal fantasies, it is impossible to enjoy team success.

The players sat in complete silence for a long time. Then the team star said he would like to ask for the team's help. He asked them to help him to be more aggressive by having someone begin an offensive that he would join. This strange sentence caused a wave of reactions from the players, the main point being "This is our problem. Every one of us expects the others to sacrifice themselves. Every one thinks only of himself, and that is why the team is stuck." All thoughts involved offense and not defense. The players did not discuss the twig metaphor, but turned directly to each other asking for help and mutual coverage of their weaknesses. I let the players process the message in their own way and ended the session. All the players participated with unusual enthusiasm during the training that followed immediately after the meeting. In the days that followed, the players began asking for assistance from one another in various basketball maneuvers. The communication between them was less sharp and more to the point. The team won eight consecutive games and finished the season among the top teams of the league. The coach was eventually replaced, but following that team discussion, it seemed that the players were more interested in seeking the teamwork than in breaking somebody's authority over the club.

Their type of game pointed at a transition to "creative dependency": spontaneous self-sacrifice with no demand for immediate return, and pleasure taken from each other's success.

Elaboration

This event has several significant meanings. The effectiveness of such psychological intervention and its timing can be discussed at length. I would like to stress a different element, which is the psychologist's ability to find a place in the influential circles within the club and his or her unique position as an influential element in critical moments. It seems to me that such an event demonstrates how finding his or her place in the Point of Archimedes keeps the psychologist in an influential position over the athletes even when the rest of the systems collapse. The psychologist is asked to remain as the last provider of assistance, especially when serious mishaps are occurring in the function of all systems. In such moments of crisis, the psychologist's duties and the resources available to him or her become objects for rude attacks. Session appointments made with the athletes are canceled because "additional training is more important." Negative information regarding players provided by the psychologist is used to "shake up" players. The psychologist's pay is withheld because his or her "work had no results anyhow." The psychologist must function despite these attacks, being the last element representing the right order and common sense. In this case, my struggle, for months, to maintain the team discussion forum in opposition to all the objections enabled me to activate the last Point of Archimedes remaining on the players. This after threats, fines, and reprimands were of no help to the team management and the professional staff. It is important to state that following this discussion, the importance of the "team discussion" for the players lessened. Such discussions were held less and less, and my job focused on personal consultation.

It is my opinion that the team has gone through a developmental phase that will continue to be expressed in a dialog between the players outside the team forum. The expression of the development of "creative dependency," in the framework of a team of athletes, must occur especially through exercises in the specific branch of sport; the main issue is cooperation during training spilling over into competitions. On the other hand, continuous "destructive dependency" that does not allow for development of the team, benefits greatly from the discussion dynamics, as was in this case. I felt the need to gradually decrease my contacts with the team and enable them to continue and crystallize opposite the coaching staff—which was changed—in the course of training and competing. The players continued to mention the "twig bundle" metaphor, one to the other, in a sarcastic way, for a long time after the discussion presented here. In this sense, the team found a common language, born in the team discussion and matured on the parquet.

Case 3

S. is one of the best known and admired basketball players in Israel. This athlete is blessed with a radiant and charismatic personality with the ability to capture the heart of the spectators wherever he plays. The basketball player specialized in tilting the balance in close games with a last-second basket. In the course of a relatively short basketball career, he won many games with individual operations that commonly ended with the buzzer; some of these contests were critical games such as cup finals. He starred in various international games in the framework of the national team and was known throughout Europe, but this player also was known for his instability. For extended periods, he suffered health problems, fatigue, and lack of motivation with no clear medical explanation.

My work with him took place in the course of one playing season, in an elite team in the first league. We were bonded throughout the game season by a continuous therapeutic bond in the form of a regular weekly session and lengthy telephone conversations when he was out of town. The nature of the therapeutic bond was psychodynamic supportive (continuous clarification of personality conflicts from his past with a strong emphasis on quick organization in the present). His team won most of its games but suffered instability: Three coaches were replaced, key players were injured and replaced, and a consolidated team was not formed. The event I will present enabled a turn in S.'s course of therapy. At the end of the game season, the team was in second place in the league with one home game remaining to ensure this ranking for the play-off. The team led safely throughout the game. Two and a half minutes before the end, the advantage stood on nine points, S. lost three consecutive balls, and with two seconds remaining, the rival team had two penalty baskets with the possibility for a changeover and lead by one point. The atmosphere in the home arena was somewhat traumatic. The coach went down to the dressing room angry and shocked. The fans threw coins and pillows and threatened to break onto the court. All the team's players were paralyzed with fear. S. left the court and sat on the bench, holding his head between his hands and waiting for the game to continue. Everyone kept their distance from him. One could feel the waves of hatred towards him from all corners of the arena. When the game restarted and the team was one point behind, S. walked on court and positioned himself approximately six meters from the opponent's basket. Being known as a "shooter of victory baskets," he was surrounded by three opposing players, much taller than he was. The ball was passed to S., who caught it—overcoming all the other hands anticipating the move—jumped, and shot the winning basket with the buzzer. The ecstasy was absolute. During the following hours, S. was under controlled excitement. This was the situation in the 3 days following the game. On the fourth day, a notice arrived about S.'s being hospitalized due to a breakdown in his health expressed as severe fatigue with no physiological findings. I met him in his home because he refused to go out or accept any visitors. It became apparent that he was suffering from perception disturbances, pain in various parts of his body, noticeable anxious depression, and signs of developing basketball phobia. S. contemplated the option of not returning to the game. Because he did not see any connection between the game several days earlier and the deterioration in his health, I offered to have him enter a hypnotic state in order to pinpoint the cause of his suffering. Under hypnosis, S. reconstructed the dramatic events of the last minutes of the game in relative safety. He described the moments of terror and loneliness he experienced before the winning shot: hard feelings of guilt that his mistakes would hurt the team, the deep disappointment he was causing his fans, and from the understanding that he must shoot the winning basket under such difficult conditions. He described the development of a dissociative experience that began as soon as the ball was passed to him. It was clear to him that the ball was moving directly towards his hands in a ballistic curve without his even noticing the guards who were trying to block him. The basket itself seemed to be within reaching distance so that all that was necessary was for him to reach out and lay the ball gently in the ring.

All time and distance dimensions disappeared while the environment was perceived as silent with no movement or disturbance whatsoever. The dissociation faded away immediately afterwards. S. was scared of the mere occurrence of such an event without understanding its meaning. It was clear to him that he experienced a very frightening experience that did not allow the return to everyday life.

His usual cognitive situation seemed to him suddenly to be fragile and completely unguaranteed. Clinically, I could estimate that the entry into a dissociative condition under such immensely stressful conditions caused a massive anxiety attack that worsened with the approach of the next scheduled game. Additionally, S. needed to go back on and play before he could feel his personality returning to its normal level of organization. During the following couple of weeks, S. almost did not leave his home. During the games, he sat on his team's bench with his condition fueling various rumors, being the key player and loved figure that he was.

I selected a new type of therapeutic intervention to confront the current crisis. The therapeutic goal chosen was to create a reconstruction of the complete mental experience, which was fractured in the transition between altered states of consciousness that S. had experienced.

We met daily in his home for 2 to 3 hours. S. advanced within 2 weeks from a total refusal to leave his home to a routine training schedule. The reconstruction of his self-confidence included massive reference to his past successes through watching videos showing the highlights of his career and the daily exercising of physical skills: light running, various strength exercises, and eventually basket shooting as well. Three weeks later, S. returned to playing. S. did not return fully to his usual ability until the end of that season (one month), but it was clear that he had recovered from the mental crisis into which he had been thrown.

Elaboration

Several questions arise from this event. First, what was the healing element that helped S. return to himself and possibly prevented his early retirement from the game? It is safe to say that S.'s almost total seclusion from the outside world during the period following the described event ties his healing considerably to the therapeutic work done with him. In addition, our being already involved in a therapeutic process from the beginning of the season enabled a rapid reference to the crisis. Because the team secured its place in the play-off, the management and the coach approved my request not to place the acceptable pressures on the player to return to training soon. In my opinion, the main healing element in the therapeutic intervention was the interpretation of the content of his words as they came up in our prolonged discussions. The basketball player, an intelligent and especially sensitive guy, grasped his breakdown as the betrayal of the body over the personality, therefore being afraid to return to normal life in which he would have to compete again with a traitorous body. The new interpretation given to his condition described the experiences in a different way: "You needed to enter an altered state of consciousness in order to succeed in something especially complicated. The right thing happened to you, but now you are going through the withdrawal process. You are unfamiliar with the experience and, therefore, afraid. If you do not want it, it will not occur again in the future, but should you want it, you will already be experienced and less vulnerable."

This message works repeatedly and enabled the reconstruction of the moments of loneliness opposite a hostile arena, which presented the trigger for the dissociation. We examined the option that the events did not occur by accident and the loss of balls by the player during the last minutes of the game is related to something else—S.'s subconscious need to create an almost lost cause that only he can save.

The character lines of this player supported this supposition. He always searched for special high-risk situations; only then did he feel vibrant and interested in the game. A mere win bored him. S. knew that he was playing for a home audience and that the whole club was expecting him, in his first season with the team, to exhibit his unique ability to win in a close game. Up to that game, which was the last home game in the regular league and therefore maybe in the whole season should the team fail to ascend to the play-offs, he did not "supply the expected goods," and this was sort of a last chance to prove himself. This understanding sharpened a dull image for the player regarding himself: "You tread a fine line and challenge fate—the only way you are able to receive satisfaction." Following this insight, the basketball phobia disappeared, taking with it the fear of reexperiencing the dissociative experience. S. began to conceive this as his unique skill and began contemplating aloud that it might be interesting to experience it again before a supportive audience. One year later, he was playing for a team where he received the total admiration of the fans. During the final second of the cup finals, S. shot a winning basket in a single operation overcoming all the opposing players alone and endowing his club with the national title for the first time in its history. S. told me he had experienced a dissociation identical to that which he experienced one year earlier and that was the only way he could overcome the full defense anticipating the move. There were no negative side effects in this case in the days that followed the event. The experience of an altered state of consciousness was no longer a frightening experience as it had been one year earlier. The basketball player learned something new about himself, and this internalization allowed him to dare to perform this skill once again in the most important moment of his career.

These events raise an additional question regarding the psychologist's function in a professional sports team. A leading player happens to go into a psychological crisis, and the club pressures the athlete to return and function soon. The psychologist is mobilized to contribute to the effort of convincing the player, but an athlete who has had such an experience, like the one described here, will have difficulty returning and functioning normally if only out of fear that the player will lose his or her place in the team make-up, be fined, or simply slandered in the sports circles. The athlete will have difficulty continuing functioning unless he or she is provided with a tolerable significance to the new situation. The psychologist can recruit various psychological techniques to blur or "close" the emotional event, but by doing so, he or she blocks the possibility of important development of the player's personality. A crisis event might turn from a frightening experience, which is not understood, into a unique skill that will express itself in better achievements, as occurred to S. one year later. This type of transition is possible only if the psychologist encourages the athlete to understand the event and not run away from it to suggestions of tranquilization, despite the various pressures to return the player any kind of function. Obviously there is a certain price of temporary detachment from him- or herself and his or her function as an athlete, and the player is expected to continue contributing to the team's success, immediately, and not in the future, because the development of the athlete's career is not of interest to his or her teammates. A professional conflict is raised here: To whom is the psychologist obligated?

1. The club's interest: May the personal price paid by the athlete be whatever it may be, the player must mobilize himself or herself for the good of the club that is paying him or her (and the psychologist) to perform for the good of the team. Professional athletes are requested to pay a high personal price, even experiencing a high level of pain. If the psychologist does not contribute to the immediate self-sacrifice of the athlete, he or she might be risking his or her position.

2. Obligation to the athlete's personality: Every person who seeks psychological help expects to receive therapy that is most suitable for his or her personality and not for any type of interest represented by the psychologist. Events occur in a competitive career that might follow the athlete for the rest of his or her life. The athlete expects to receive help that will make it easier to confront physical and emotional stress with the help of professionals who accompany the player throughout his or her career. A psychologist who does not operate according to this principle is betraying this basic trust of the athlete.

It seems to me that the club holds the right to examine jointly with the psychologist his or her ethical limits and select the right person based on his or her answers. As long as there is no specific demand for this, the psychologist must act according to the psychological Hippocratic oath: At least do no harm in the immediate or future term to the person seeking help, who sees in the psychologist an objective person who does not fear for his or her personal and professional status.

Case 4

Dreams are the high road to the unconscious (Freud, 1900). This determination by the father of the psychoanalytic method is true regarding competitive athletes as well. Circumstances exist, within the therapy session, in which an athlete describes a dream and tries to analyze its meaning. Not every athlete understands the association between the dreams and the deeper, elusive but authentic part of the personality. There are circumstances in which such an understanding is formed and has the ability to enrich the therapy. The athlete gains a new source of knowledge regarding the primary motivations influencing his or her career, successes, and failures. An event from an athlete's therapy session that has gone through such a process is described here.

A. came to me at the age of 17 following a 5-year career as an excellent long-jump athlete. He was very successful in local competitions and was preparing for the junior world championship. However, his performance was faulted by instability in major competitions. He commonly disqualified himself and was unable to reproduce his ability in competitions. He also missed many training sessions due to illnesses and injuries, and the medical team attending to him had a feeling there were psychological elements contributing to this, as major competitions approached. I accepted him for therapy on a weekly basis that lasted for approximately one year. I found what Kernberg (1984) called "narcissistic components" in his personality, which caused A. to suffer from low self-esteem, substantial envy at other athletes' success, compulsive occupation with self-care, graceless exploitation of acquaintances and fosterers, great arrogance, and lack of true emotional intimacy towards those surrounding him (Kohut & Wolfe, 1978). For him, his sports career was a high purpose, which must be catered to, at all times, by every one of his acquaintances. Any deviation from this immediately brought on blatant and offending comments. Under the cover of "the winner" hid a very concerned personality, concerned for his body's health, collapse under the pressures of the next competition, the advisability of devoting one's self to an unprofitable career, and the toll on his schooling. The preoccupation with these troubles caused him to fail in important competitions. A. was unaware of the relation between his failures and the inefficient organizational level of his personality.

When he applied for therapy, he asked me to teach him stress-reducing techniques that he heard were successful with other athletes. Following the diagnostic stage, I offered A. psychotherapy. A. was offended and claimed he did not need this. I explained to him that psychoregulation would not help in his case because his anxieties were not at all related to the external pressures exerted on him but to the imbalance fixed in his personality, which increased when he faced a challenge. The conquest of this imbalance might force him to sharply confront the feelings of low self-esteem. A. was faulted with a self-failing behavior, in order to avoid such an internal conflict, that should be the focus of the therapy. A. was reconciled, and his therapy turned out to be effective because part of his behavior and some of his feelings changed for the better. He became successful in competitions at which he had failed in the past, and it seemed that he was on the high road to success in the junior world championship.

Approximately 2 weeks before leaving for the championship competition, A. came with the following dream: "An unfamiliar stadium . . . packed with spectators . . . I disqualify all my jumps and I am graded last. There is not even a rank . . . the team doctor calls me over very aggressively and says to me: 'I told you not to come here . . . it was clear to everyone you would disqualify all of your jumps.'" A. was greatly shaken. He said that the dream diminished all his self-confidence just before the trip and that maybe he should not go at all, being still unprepared. This was the first dream he brought with him to therapy, and therefore it required very careful treatment. I asked him about his associations regarding the dream and its exact timing. He said that on the evening before, he again had an argument with his coach, who blamed him for not exerting himself during training. He admitted this was true, but justified it by saying he feared injuring himself from overexertion as had occurred in the past just before competitions. Suddenly he silenced up and then surprisingly stated that the doctor in the dream was "speaking in your voice," referring to me, and sitting in the couch just as he had done in the therapy room here.

This phenomenon of the dream-work is called "Condensation." It deals with the masking of an unconscious wish in a disguise, which has a better chance than that of the original form of penetrating the psychological defense mechanisms and reaching consciousness. I raised the supposition that A. was ascribing the thoughts of his disqualifying his jumps to me and therefore could travel to the world championship. On the evening he heard his coach blaming him for not preparing properly for the competition, A. dreamt that a person was sitting on my couch saying the things said by his coach, the content of which was failure. A. reacted by asking me what my true opinion was and whether he should cancel the trip. It is important to state here that one of the rules of psychodynamic therapy is that the expression of opinion on the part of the therapist might block the free expression of the consulted, among other things, because the athlete will fear the therapist's criticism should their opinions not coincide. When I mentioned this to A., he blew up in rage and said he needed my opinion regardless. At this point, I interpreted his words as another way to avoid taking responsibility over his life and passing it onto people who were close to him such as his coach, his doctors, friends, or psychologist. Because his self-esteem was so vulnerable and he feared criticism, he refused to make his own decisions as to what he wanted more. As a result, he was unable to focus his efforts in one main area, recognizing the fact that one must make concessions in one area to achieve something elsewhere. A. wanted to be a successful athlete and an outstanding student; he also wanted to work nights to earn spending money. All these plans created a self-failing behavior, the awareness of which was achieved through the therapy. At this time, on the verge of a world championship, he understood something new about himself, but had difficulty relating to this understanding as to something of his own. He preferred to leave this new knowledge with me.

A. was fuming with anger: "You need to encourage me before such an important competition. Instead, you are undermining my motivation." He settled down with great difficulty. Outbursts of rage characterized him when he felt he was unable to steer his interlocutor to give him what he wanted. I explored with him whether he believed that I needed to recommend that he ignore the interpretation he himself gave to his dream. A. left the session quiet and pensive. One week later, he returned and informed me of his decision not to participate in the world championship. He realized he was not interested in traveling despite the great pressure placed on him. He said he was greatly shocked of his deep need to receive my approval for the trip. He said, "You will not jump with me, so why should you decide for me?" It became clear to him that he himself did not believe in himself and was totally dependent on the admiration and encouragement of his various acquaintances. Within several days, he lost all interest in the event for which he had prepared throughout his full career. A short time later, he decided to totally quit competitive sports, to join the Israeli Airforce Flight School, and to become a fighter pilot, a goal he achieved 2 years later.

Elaboration

This incident demonstrates one of the overt fears of the competitive sports professionals: The application of an athlete for psychological help that results in quitting the sport competitions. Many athletes who start out competing in competitive sports fall out of the cycle of competitions over the years. There are many reasons for this, and many athletic talents feel "lost." Coaches and other professionals are concerned that the athlete's in-depth study of the activity, to which they have devoted their lives, will decrease their willingness to adhere to the hard task. These concerns worsen when an athlete turns to receive psychological consultation. The psychologist is expected to help the athlete to develop and realize his or her potential. In other words, the psychologist is expected to convince and encourage the athlete more effectively than the others do.

What happens when the consultation work brings the athlete to lose interest in continuing his competitive career, as happened with A.? Did I betray his trust? Should I have convinced him to the best of my ability not to give up the once-in-a-lifetime opportunity?

Some psychologists will probably disagree with me on this issue. They may claim that the sports psychologist's duty is to focus on qualifying the athlete for maximal effort in training and competitions by providing psychological techniques and encouragement in places where the intrinsic motivation is fading. Is ignoring unconscious contents (that actually become conscious through the dream, and are, therefore, bothersome and require some sort of attention) not associated with so many competitive events in which athletes experience unusual and frustrating phenomena, such as peak ability in training versus inferior performance in the determining competition? Or could it be related to recurrent injuries very close to or during the competition, tardiness, inappropriate operation of the equipment, violation of regulatory rules leading to suspension from the competition, and other self-failing behaviors? These phenomena are usually associated with a "loser" image or an inability to withstand the pressure. Are these phenomena not expected when one receives many signs and signals from the athlete's or sports team's collective unconscious? Is the athlete able to confront the pressures successfully when a significant part of his or her personality is not ready for the competition? Sometimes, indeed, yes, but in many cases this is a failure waiting to happen. Indeed, there is only one winner in the competition, and that is the athlete who arrives physically and mentally better prepared than all his or her competitors are. Why help an athlete cover up inner conflicts (instead of trying to understand them) and, in so doing, drive him or her to competitive failure resulting not from inferior physical ability but from being psychologically unprepared? What is the public responsibility towards public financial support used to finance expensive training and travel to competitions, which, in this case, are doomed to failure in advance?

These questions are embarrassing for all the decision-makers in competitive sports and especially embarrassing to the sports psychologist who often knows more than the others regarding the athlete's inner reality do. My experience as a clinical psychologist consulting athletes, among others, has helped me to establish the following approach: Any referral of an athlete that is not on an acute basis (such as a request for some tips regarding the participation in next week's competition) requires a personality diagnostic evaluation. The goal of the diagnosis is to come up with a prognosis that can determine the chances for improvement or change in those personality traits that enable the development of a competitive career. The determination of the therapeutic method depends on this evaluation and the time available for the therapy. If help can be offered by psychoregulatory means, the internal conflicts are limited. If there is a need for personal intervention that requires the use of psychodynamic means, the athlete (and sometimes his or her coach or parents) needs to be informed of the possibility that, at the end of the therapeutic process, the athlete may need to examine his or her motivation to compete in the future. Additionally, there may be a temporary or continuous ill effect on the athlete's ability to train or compete because of a certain regression in his or her personality during the course of therapy. Professional therapy assists a person in arriving at decisions about problems of which he or she was previously unaware. An athlete might discover that his or her will to compete is a neurotic symptom, just as compulsive vomiting is a neurotic symptom of a bulimic disorder.

Because the goal of therapy is to make the person's neurosis easier to bear, an athlete may discover that his or her personality no longer needs competitive sports as a way of life, even if that athlete is greatly talented. Such a discovery was the lot of the long-jump athlete. He left competitive sports very calmly, which supports my hypothesis that convincing words would not have cast in him the mental powers necessary for a competitive athlete at a world-championship level.

It is important to inform the people involved in the athlete's career (parents, coaches, agents, etc.) of the details regarding the possibility of the loss of interest in competitive sports, because it is their responsibility to choose the type of psychological therapy they feel is the best for the athlete. Many people choose to live their lives totally ignoring vast parts of their personality, but because the competitive career promises financial success, glory, and college grants, it is a consideration that bears much weight. On the other hand, the desire to prevent big disappointments that can be predicted with great certainty and with deep personal repercussions presents a consideration that bears much weight as well.

Case 5

Z. is one of the best soccer players in the country, a senior player on a leading and dominant team. In his past, he was a successful player on a European team and is recognized throughout the continent. His success began when he was very young. He was, therefore, invited to participate concurrently in the junior and adult teams of his club, the team of the military unit in which he served, and the national junior and adult teams. For years, he almost never rested from activity for more than 2 to 3 days. He participated in many games and trained under firm coaches who demanded maximum exertion from him. Z. developed a reputation as a hard-working athlete who did not turn down a coach's demand even when his health betrayed him. The heavy workload caused him to suffer chronic pain, which he ignored with the help of painkillers. Z. learned to overcome injuries that made others rest for long periods. At the age of 25, he suffered an injury in one of his knees during a game. Following a difficult surgical operation and prolonged rehabilitation process, he regained his athletic fitness. Then, he suffered an identical injury to his other knee. For several years, he alternated between states of health and injury while undergoing complicated and painful surgical procedures. Every time he regained fitness, he was injured severely again.

Z. came to me as a last resort. The local sports world and the media were already mourning his career. Hence he thought, "Psychological therapy cannot do more harm than good." He had no request, complaint, or question for therapy. On the contrary, he had clear requests from the other professionals from whom he received medical assistance during rehabilitation. I found out that he was assisted by no fewer than 17 different types of supporters, among them three orthopedists from three continents, two physiotherapists, a chiropractor, a shiatsu and acupuncture healer, a masseuse, a healer, a crystal healer, a dietitian, a nail healer, a personal coach, and a rabbi. He used the ample free time he had as an unemployed athlete to consult with these people. I also found out that his other consultants did not limit themselves at all to their individual areas of expertise, but each supplied as much psychological consultation as he or she dared. Nor did Z. himself limit them to their areas of expertise. He became confused trying to follow the many different instructions he received because they often contradicted each other. There was no coordination between the various healers and consultants. No one was interested in knowing if Z. had consulted anyone else, and therefore, they were unaware of the distress Z. was in. Overwrought from the overwhelming amount of advice and recommendations, he always arrived at or was in a hurry to some sort of consultation session, without seeing the grotesqueness of his situation and his subjection to the status of "a patient." Because he was very well known in Israel, and an item for journalistic articles, any publication regarding his distress brought forth additional experts who offered other types of free therapy. With his help, I tried to focus on the type of therapy he considered requesting from me, which was not already being given to him by others. Additionally I initiated a process that rendered psychological consultation from people who were unauthorized to do so illegitimate.

Z. did not know what he wanted, either from any one of his therapists or from psychological therapy. I decided on a staged course of therapy. The first stage was to reduce the possibility for disturbances of the therapeutic process between him and me by reducing the conflict created between him and his various consultants. It was obviously necessary to somewhat cut down their numbers and focus only on their areas of expertise. I asked Z. to describe in a diary all that happened in his consultation sessions during one week. We discovered that the athlete was reconstructing, together with each of his therapists, the events during which he incurred his injuries. He described his various feelings in great detail again and again, without remembering what each of his consultants contributed during these sessions. In other words, Z. described typical side effects of a post-traumatic stress disorder (PTSD; DSM-IV, 1994): a renewed traumatic experience expressed by the compulsive need to reconstruct aversive events, marked reduction in any type of significant activity, narrowing of the emotion, a very low stimulus threshold for pain, and psychogenic pain (as was discovered later).

Z. created a "support group" composed of various consultants from whom he expected listening and palliation more than anything. As we found out, neither he nor they were aware of this. Their difficulty in understanding his intentions frustrated him and exacerbated his condition. He searched for abreaction (emotional relief) in opposition to the instructions to suppress his experiences, which came from those surrounding him and his therapists, who urged him to forget the past and concentrate on the future.

The professional literature (Brett & Ostroff, 1985; Dasberg, 1976; Freud, 1921) and clinical experience show that attempts to suppress trauma are relatively comfortable for the present but might drive the affected person to chronic pathology. When the patient tries to reconstruct the traumatic events, without an appropriate reaction from those surrounding him (e.g., through the unprofessional assistants), a personality conflict occurs (between the need to provide an understanding and the attempt to suppress). This conflict reduces the ability to cope and steals a great amount of mental energy from him or her. It was clear to me that Z. would not be able to progress with the psychological therapy if he would continue the discussions with so many people. Yet, it was not at all easy to dissociate him from people with some of whom he had developed a dependency over several years. However, there was no alternative to lead him out of this therapeutic maze without ending the majority of these ties. In an unusual move, on my part, after receiving his permission, I contacted most of the therapists in order to get an impression as to those with whom I could sustain professional cooperation. Eventually, I selected five people, including an orthopedist, physiotherapist, dietitian, chiropractor, and personal coach. The team gathered for a meeting under my direction and in the presence of Z.

This meeting had important results. The various therapists discussed openly their difficulty in containing the flabbergasted Z.'s emotional distress. I translated the general message into a request of the team for each to deal with his or her area of expertise and leave the emotional part for the psychologist. Z. understood that the team supported him implicitly but requested to discuss the matters only with the psychologist, in a suitable therapeutic space, that would enable him to be understood in the most appropriate manner.

Indeed, from the time of the meeting on, there was a significant change in Z.'s rehabilitation process. He gradually thinned the group of therapists and consultants without being asked to do so. A month following the above-mentioned meeting, he reduced the number of his therapists to 12. Three months later, the number was seven, and in the last months of his rehabilitation, he consulted only four people. This team reconvened once every several weeks to discuss the progress of his recovery.

After the creation of a suitable therapeutic space for psychological therapy, it was possible to enter the second stage. A thorough diagnosis was made regarding his psychological condition. This evaluation revealed that despite the elapse of several years since his first injuries, and not few months since his last surgical operation, Z. had yet to develop the personal phenomenon of chronic reaction following a trauma. He was still in the acute stage where the post-traumatic anxiety and the attempt to suppress it are recognizable. The therapy was directed to locate the "traumatic nucleus," the most difficult event in terms of the significance attributed to it unconsciously by Z. because clarification in a discussion did not bring significant progress. I asked the soccer player to view videotapes of the games during which he was injured, something he had avoided persistently throughout the years. Z. agreed reluctantly. He arrived shaken at the following meeting. He said that after watching his third injury, he was flooded, more than ever, with feelings of severe anxiety. He recalled the details of his evacuation to the hospital, crying bitterly, convinced that this time he would not "make it." Despite his rehabilitation following a difficult surgical operation, he felt just as he did during those same moments. "I will never make it. . . ." "I cannot suffer anymore; therefore, I will always be injured." Z. refused to recognize the success of his recovery and feared he would be injured repeatedly without the ability to tolerate additional treatments. He developed a phobia (focused anxiety) of returning to playing soccer despite the fact that it was clear to all members of the rehabilitation team that he was fit to play. He also developed a performance anxiety and had difficulty integrating himself into his team's game.

After reviewing the course of his career and the "soul player" image attached to him—that of one who is willing to sacrifice himself for club and country with no complaints—we established together the following therapeutic message, which we have been processing for a long time: "You were injured repeatedly because you did not recognize your physical limitations and overloaded yourself. Now you know where to draw the line between what is allowed and what is not, and you will be able to stand up and face any coach and club and refuse to play when injured or exhausted. The need for everybody's admiration will not be achieved by total self-sacrifice but through a quality game and the aid of appropriate periods of rest, preventive medicine and immediate care when needed."

All the supporting medical team personnel contributed to the assimilation of this message, each in his or her area of expertise. The physiotherapist taught Z. agility and flexibility exercises. The personal trainer taught him to perform a long and personal warm-up exercise that suited his new condition. The orthopedist explained to him the practicality of the (few) limitations that applied to him. The chiropractor set up a weekly therapy to prevent sensitivities in his back, the source of his problems, and the dietitian taught him weight control in order to prevent extreme weight gains that would increase the load on his knees.

Following 10 months of psychological therapy, the soccer player returned to regular activity and stunned everybody with his excellent ability.

Elaboration

Z.'s therapy marks one of the edges of the professional legitimacy, in which the psychologist is allowed to offer help to an athlete who approaches him or her. To stray beyond this range poses a threat to the psychologist's ability to return further down the line and take his or her place in treating the symbolic (the patient's need to understand himself better) and not the concrete (the patient's demand for suggestions) in the athlete's discourse. In the absence of a different professional element, I had no choice but to take upon myself the overall therapeutic responsibility in the selection and organization of the rehabilitative team suitable to the soccer player's needs. This is a common scene in the area of psychomedical services. An athlete with a multifocal complaint finds him- or herself in several concurrent different therapies, the goal of which is to cover the objective or subjective needs of the athlete. Each consultant may supply a recommendation that might contradict a different recommendation supplied to the athlete one day earlier, a recommendation that seemed, so far, logical to him or her. Therefore, it is no wonder that Z., like all the others, developed inner conflicts when the orthopedist did not see any harm in a full training session whereas the physiotherapist demanded personal training, the chiropractor requested a week's rest, the personal trainer scrutinized the athlete for continuing to be afraid and being spoiled, and the dietitian pressured him to reduce the percentage of fat and to increase muscle mass with the appropriate training regimen (and we have not yet mentioned the spiritual and alternative consultants who offered abundant conflicting suggestions). Athletes such as Z. usually follow the advice given to them by the last consultant they met the same day.

In the circumstances under which the therapy is not provided under one professional roof, with full coordination of all therapists and consultants, or when it is known that the athlete is being offered help by additional elements other than the medical team, the primary element capable of achieving therapeutic integration is the psychologist.

After achieving the first stage of rehabilitation as described above, the psychological process included several months of discussion therapy 2 to 3 times a week. The moment the soccer player found himself within the "therapeutic space" (a clear and stable framework with set rules and total freedom to say all that is on his mind, which receives full unconditional listening; Winnicot, 1971), significant changes began to occur in his ability to suffer pain, as well as in his self-confidence, his ability to dare and risk powerful kicks and brave rough tackles and to apply a continuous effort.

This is where Z. was saved by the outstanding inner powers that he has been blessed with, and that were still within him even after all the years of suffering. He lost his confidence in the surrounding support system that is so important for the athlete's success. Only when order was restored with the help of the coordinated team of consultants was he able to discuss, in therapy, the psychological crisis he experienced regarding the loss of confidence in himself and in the support system surrounding him. Eventually, Z. once again became a soccer player of an international caliber as he was before his injuries.

References

Bandura, A. (1977). Self-efficacy: Toward a unifying theory of behavioural change. *Psychological Review, 84,* 191–215.

Bion, W. R. (1961). *Experiences in groups.* London: Tavistock Publications.

Brett, E. A., & Ostroff, R. (1985). Imagery and post-traumatic stress disorder: An overview. *American Journal of Psychiatry, 142,* 417–424.

Casement, P. (1985). *On learning from the patient.* London: Tavistock Publications.

Dasberg, H. (1976). Belonging and loneliness in relation to mental breakdown in battle. *Israel Annals of Psychiatry, 14,* 307–321.

DSM-IV (1994). *Diagnostic and statistical manual on mental disorders.* Washington, DC: American Psychiatric Association.

Fairbairn, W. R. (1952). *An object-relations theory of the personality.* New York: Basic Books.

Freud, S. (1912). *Recommendations for physicians on the psychoanalytic method of treatment.* Standard edition, 5. London: Hogarth Press.

Freud, S. (1921). *The mass psychology and the analysis of the self.* Standard edition 5. London: Hogarth Press.

Freud, S. (1900). *The interpretation of dreams.* Standard edition 5. London: Hogarth Press.

Kernberg, F. O. (1984). *Severe personality disorders: Psychotherapeutic strategies.* New Haven: Yale University Press.

Kohut, H., & Wolfe, E. (1978). The disorders of the self and their treatment: An outline. *International Journal of Psychoanalysis,* 59, 413–425.

Locke, E. A., & Latham, P. G. (1985). The application of goal setting to sports. *Journal of Sport Psychology, 7,* 205–222.

Malan, D. H. (1976). *Frontier of brief psychotherapy.* New York: Plenum.

Mann, J. (1973). *Time limited psychotherapy.* Cambridge, MA: Harvard University Press.

Schultz, J. H. (1932). *Das autogene training.* Stuttgart: Thieme Verlag.

Weinberg, R. S. (1988). *The mental advantage: Developing your psychological skills in tennis.* Champaign, IL: Human Kinetics.

Winnicot, D. W. (1971). *Playing and reality.* London: Tavistock Publications.

Reflections and Insights From the Field on Performance-Enhancement Consultation

Kenneth Ravizza

Early in my career after conducting a relaxation and imagery session with a group of athletes, the coach confronted me and said, "Ken, I know all this relaxation and imagery work is important, but I really don't care if they can relax in a quiet comfortable environment. I want them to relax in the midst of performance when the pressure is on." Like most coaches, that coach wanted something practical, and his comments prompted me to begin to integrate performance-enhancement skills into specific task-relevant performance cues. This approach of integrating the mental skills into existing practice and performance procedures has become a critical aspect of my work.

Many coaches and sport psychology consultants view mental training as something that happens once a week for an hour, and then they get to the "real" stuff when they go to practice. However, a successful mental-training program must be reinforced by the coaches and integrated into practice and performance. This integrated approach provides athletes the opportunity to develop, refine, and practice their various performance-enhancement techniques. The continuing emphasis on practicing the methods allows them to be more effective in pressure situations.

My intention in this article is to share some practical realities of working with coaches and athletes. Two additional cues that are intricate parts of my approach are the role of a personal philosophy and the holistic nature of my approach. I have discussed these topics in detail elsewhere (Ravizza, in press), and they are, therefore, excluded from the scope of this article, in which I will discuss the approach that I have developed in working with elite athletes over the last 25 years. I will address the ideal working relationship with an athletic team and the way I integrate performance-enhancement skills into direct performance-related cues.

The chapter has four sections:

1. The basic parameters to my approach (i.e., educational approach, proactive perspective, the importance of collaboration, and receptivity to learning from coaches and athlete),
2. A discussion about gaining access and implementing programs,
3. Methods of enhancing quality practice including the importance of awareness, and
4. Some of the critical lessons I have learned.

Program Parameters

Educational Approach

My approach is educational in nature and focuses on the mental and emotional aspects of performance enhancement. I am not a psychologist, so when serious psychological issues become apparent, I make referrals to a network of professionals I have developed confidence in over the years. This also means that if the coach is looking for someone to address psychological issues (e.g., eating disorders, drug issues), then I am not the appropriate person. It is extremely difficult to be responsible for the serious psychological and drug issues and to be effective on performance-enhancement issues.

I believe mental skills can be developed like physical skills. Some athletes have "natural" abilities with the mental game, but most athletes must constantly refine and develop their mental skills to effectively meet the multitude of situations they confront. I have watched athletes go from being at the top of their game to aging and losing physical skills. For example, I have seen numerous athletes who never had a problem with confidence be flooded with self-doubts at the Olympics. As Dan Gould stated so clearly, "At the Olympic Games confidence is fragile" (Gould et al., 1998, p. 9). I have worked with some teams for 5 to 10 years. I remember one older player telling me that when he was in his prime, the mental game was not that important because his talent was so strong. Toward the end of his career, he needed to use his mental game to harness that wealth of wisdom he had gained from his years of experience and use it to his advantage to make up for his deterioration in physical skills.

The foundation of my educational approach to performance enhancement provides the following three components: (a) accurate and relevant up-to-date information, (b) the opportunity to develop specific mental skills, and (c) support in learning the skills on a daily basis.

Respecting the Athlete's Knowledge Base

The practitioner must be knowledgeable of the research data and be able to make the research meaningful for coaches and athletes. The psychologist should provide accurate information concerning the importance, development, and refinement of the performance-enhancement skills. In conveying information to athletes and coaches, the consultant must remember that elite athletes already have a very successful track record in their sport. One should provide accurate information concerning the importance, development, and refinement of performance-enhancement skills. For example, when I work with a Major League Baseball player, I am working with someone who is the top $1/10$ of 1% of all the people who play baseball in the world. As a colleague once said, "When you work with Olympic and professional athletes, you are really working in the area of 'abnormal' psychology." It is difficult to talk about "level of significance" with such an elite group. It is important to listen to the coaching staff and athletes about what they currently do they believe is effective and work from that starting point. In many cases, coaches and athletes already do many of the tasks that we talk about, and the consultant's role is to provide a structure or framework for these existing techniques. This framework helps athletes make the required compensations and adjustments in pressure situations.

Thus, my role is to translate technical, research-based, theoretical information for that athlete and/or team. It must be practical, relevant, and effective for that situation. It cannot be information for the sake of knowledge alone. My goal is to interpret information in a manner that is effective for that athlete and that unique situation. I want to equip the athletes with skills to deal with the variety of situations that they confront so that they can become their own best expert. As an educator, I have to assess where the athlete is starting from and move him or her toward the desired outcome. These athletes may not reach the ultimate goal, but at least I have helped them move in that direction.

A female gymnast I was working with was one of the most negative people I had ever worked with. I kept emphasizing positive self-talk and affirmations, but we were just not connecting. I was providing her with important information, but she was not hearing me. I was not making it "meaningful" to her, and I definitely was not speaking her language. Then one day, I walked in the gym and said, "Mary, it looks like today is not going as bad as yesterday." Her face lit up, I was speaking her language, and presenting my comments in a perspective that was meaningful to her. We definitely connected. She tended to have a negative orientation and I had to start from there. The technical information could now be processed. Then my goal was to help her move to a less negative approach.

I have become a "realist" in my work; to think one is going to help everyone change from a negative to a positive perspective is unrealistic. For some athletes, this negative perspective is what works for them. There will be resistance to changing unless this attitude is no longer is effective. As consultants, we provide information, and we must learn the art of making it meaningful to the coaches and athletes. Sometimes the athlete must fail before he or she is willing to consider any new information or methods to improve.

Developing Performance-enhancement Skills

In the second component of my educational approach, I teach athletes performance-enhancement skills. I begin by teaching self-regulation skills, and I start with relaxation techniques. Once athletes have acquired these skills, I have them practice relaxation with various distractions such as tapes of crowd noise or coaches screaming in practice. I then have them learn to stand in a centered, balanced position and carry the ability to relax to a standing position. The next stage is to have them explain their pre-performance routine, then practice being centered and balanced as they execute that routine. For example, in tennis, the player develops a pre-serve routine, and this routine is incorporated on a consistent basis as part of the performance execution. The final stage is to have the athletes be in control and trust their ability as they execute their performance. Thus, athletes learn to build confidence in their self-regulation and concentration skills so they can cope better with adversity.

I want the athlete to develop the self-regulation skills, but these skills must be directly related to performance. For example, the athlete who has difficulty performing when the pressure is on must learn to be in control of herself or himself before trying to control performance. Similarly, a javelin thrower who excels in practice but tightens up in competition needs to realize that self-control contributes to body control, which leads to skill control (Ravizza & Hanson, 1994). In the competitive arena, breakdowns are manifested in the mechanics. Often, the coach attempts to fix the mechanics when the underlying issue is anxiety.

When athletes first learn the mental game, many focus so much energy on the mental aspects of performance, and specifically the pre-performance routine, that they forget to actually compete. As performance-enhancement consultants, we seek to get the athlete to the start of the performance with the best opportunity for success, by being ready and focused, and then to perform.

During the performance, the athlete should be equipped to use concentration and refocusing techniques as needed. I help the athlete make the transition from the general ability to relax, to the ability to relax in the performance situation, by having performance-specific cues to focus on.

Supporting Change

The final component of the educational approach is to support the athletes as they make the transition to integrate mental skills into every daily practice routine and in the competitive arena. This support is critical because athletes must continuously compensate and adjust as they learn what works for them. As with any new skill, the athletes must remain patient as they work through the learning process. The support can be from my comments, the coach's feedback, and sometimes just the act of my being physically present, without even saying anything. Many athletes have informed me that sometimes when they see me, it serves as a reminder of the things they need to do. I serve as a "trigger" for the athletes to remember their mental game.

Proactive Approach

The proactive season-long approach has proved to be the most effective in my work. I want the coaches and athletes to understand that the mental aspects of performance are critical parts of performance. The performance-enhancement approach is based on the concept that the mental and emotional aspects of performance are essential components of what it takes to perform at an elite level. The proactive orientation is totally different from the medical model "problem" orientation of traditional psychology. I do not want to wait until things break down and then "fix" them.

The weakness of a medical model, or "problem" approach, is that players who talk with the sport psychology consultant are frequently typecast as "messed up." Early in my career, I was introduced to the team with the coach's saying "If you are screwed up, then talk with Ken." I have worked with some coaches who say all the right things, but in reality when that coach observes athletes talking with me, it is viewed as a sign of weakness, as compared to the perception that these people want to be great, and they are willing to do whatever it takes to achieve their goals.

The proactive approach also promotes program implementation before the season starts because once the season starts, everything intensifies. Professional football coaches have a "bomb-shelter" mindset once the season begins. Time, energy, and the player's attention become a high priority, and the basics of strategy and skill execution are the highest priority. As a performance-enhancement consultant, don't fool yourself that your program takes priority over the basic needs of the coaching staff's game preparations. For me, the performance-enhancement program is everything, but to the coaching staff, it is one small part of the total program. Thus, before the season begins, I want the players to know the importance of commitment and responsibility, the ways in which stress impacts performance, mental preparation strategies, effective thinking for that sport, concentration and imagery techniques, and self-regulation. Athletes need to develop these skills before the season so they can implement the necessary techniques when the pressure is on. For this reason, I like to start with five 1-hour presentations that cover the basic framework of the program. After the players have the basics and some experience with the various techniques, they are equipped with some methods for coping with adversity when it strikes. This approach helps me because I know that they understand the techniques, so when the teachable moment occurs, I can help them apply the skills that were previously just abstract concepts.

Collaboration With the Coaching Staff

In working with teams on a season-long basis, it is critical to earn the coach's respect and trust. My approach is a collaborative approach, and the goal is to work together with the coach(es) to develop, refine, and reinforce the mental game. As I mentioned earlier, many coaches view mental-skills training as something that athletes do off the field, and then they go perform. It is critical that the mental aspects of the game, including skills, are reinforced by the coaching staff in practice, as well as during the competition.

Athletes learn physical skills through repetition. It is the same with the mental skills. When I first began my work, I approached the athletes like students in a class where you present the material, ask if there are questions, and move on. I learned that in sport, I had to keep repeating myself because performance knowledge is different from academic knowledge. Learning a sport skill involves constant compensation and adjustment. The athlete takes one step forward one day and two steps backward the next. There is a great deal of frustration especially at the elite level, where the improvements are so subtle.

When I first worked with a team on a season-long basis for successive seasons, I worried about what I would do the second year because I had "said it all" the previous year. Then I read a story about the great American football coach Vince Lombardi (Dowling, 1970), who, after winning the Super Bowl, was criticized because the following preseason, he began practice by working the basic fundamentals. He was asked why he would do this with such a great team, and he responded, "The players forget a lot during the off-season" (quoted in Dowling, p. 9). It is the same for mental training, but it is also important to remember that each player has changed from the previous season. The expectations change, and the player's role on the team changes. Something that used to upset me was working with a player for three years and having the player come up in the third year to say, "Ken, I finally understand the importance of being focused." Better late than never! Therefore, just because a consultant presents the information and believes the players may understand it, that does not mean that they are necessarily able to incorporate it in the pressure situation. They may understand it intellectually, but for it to be of any use, they must develop an experiential understanding of it, so that they can use the information when the pressure is on. They need to become their own best experts.

In order to build this type of collaboration with the coaches and players, it is critical to gain support at all levels. Initially, the coaching staff must understand and support the importance of the mental game and the applicability of these concepts and techniques in a manner that is consistent with their current approach. This requires taking the time to clarify the concepts and techniques so that everyone is comfortable with them. The staff should feel they have had an opportunity to modify my basic approach, vocabulary, and methods to integrate it into that staff's approach (Halliwell, Orlick, Ravizza, & Rotella, 1999).

It is important to build support for the program at all levels of the organization. Strength and conditioning personnel and athletic trainers have an impact with the athletes, and it is critical that they understand and support the performance-enhancement program. I always work closely with the strength and conditioning staff because the off-season conditioning is an excellent time to work on daily goal setting, pre-performance routines in the weight room, and various concentration methods. The conditioning staff appreciates and values a more focused and committed athlete. I find the athletic trainers appreciate my support for the athletes as they help the athletes go through the frustrating aspects of injury recovery. Some athletes have benefited from imagery skills to complement the healing process, as well as to visualize practice sessions, so that they keep their mental game sharp and are at least doing something to feel a part of the team. It is also critical for the injured athlete to have someone to share the emotional fluctuations that accompany injury recovery. In addition, we have to realize that we are infringing on the athletic trainer's territory because we are "helping" the athlete, and this is the traditional role of the trainer. I found that many athletic trainers provide more than just physical expertise. They also provide important emotional support. The trainers are in a unique position because they are not directly involved in team selection or playing-time decisions. This makes them a safe outlet for the athlete to share things with. When all the people involved with the team understand the program, they are less threatened by it and more likely to support what a consultant is trying to do.

Another reason this type of collaboration is important is that I cannot be at every practice or every game. The coaching staff has to reinforce the concepts and techniques in my absence. If the athletes hear the information only from me, its effect will be limited. If they hear it from the coaching staff, they know it is valued. This is why I also encourage the coaching staff to be present at the mental training sessions because the players see that the coaches value the program. Also, this allows the coaching staff an opportunity to view the athletes in a totally different situation. Occasionally, the situation may arise where there may be some sessions in which the players have concerns about the coach's being present. In this situation, I just tell the coaches we need to meet without them this particular time.

Receptivity to Learning From Coaches and Athletes

Elite athletes and great coaches use many of the techniques that we address in the academic study of sport psychology, often without much thought. Athletes realize that to perform they cannot be too analytical because it will get them thinking too much. As stated earlier, the role of a performance-enhancement consultant is to provide a structure and framework for the mental game. Showing how the various components of the mental game work as an integrated whole provides the player with a broader understanding of when and how to use mental skills in a variety of pressure situations.

I have always worked from the perspective that the elite athlete knows what works for him or her, and my job is to help that individual refine and develop the mental skills. I want the information to originate from the athlete's personal experience, so it is relevant to that individual. Sometimes we think we have the "secrets for success," but elite athletes already have many of these skills, or they would not be performing at that level. When the knowledge comes from the athletes, it is their knowledge, and they can take ownership of it.

Pat Summit, the University of Tennessee women's basketball coach, expressed the importance of ownership and accountability when she stated,

> The more responsibility they are given the more committed they will be to a project, and the more they then make it their project. When it's theirs, they feel more accountable for its success or failure, and they do whatever it takes to help it succeed. It becomes "our" team instead of "my" team. Responsibility

equal accountability equals ownership. And a sense of ownership is the most powerful weapon a team or organization can have. (Summit & Jenkins, 1998, p. 37)

To promote this perspective, I ask athletes questions (i.e., when you perform well, what do you do to mentally prepare? When you lose control, what are the early warning signs?) These types of questions (Orlick, 1996) help the athletes become more aware, and they help provide feedback about what is effective for that athlete. Such questions also have helped identify what is effective, particularly when the pressure is on. Most important, talking with the athlete directly allows me the opportunity to build a working relationship based on trust and respect. It also allows the athletes to know I respect their wealth of experiential knowledge.

A technique that I have found effective with elite athletes is to ask them what their mental game is like when they are performing well. Some people say if they start to think about it, they may lose that ability to perform. My response is that when they perform, they are eventually going to lose it, so we should get the information on it now. I have also found that an athlete's discussing the mental aspects of the performance (focusing, mental preparation, etc.) is not quite the same as his or her thinking about the technical aspects of mechanics execution. If the athlete overanalyzes the mechanics, then problems are likely to occur.

One method I use when athletes are performing well is to set up a meeting and have them talk to me about their mental game as I tape the session. Then later in the season, when they are struggling, we meet and just listen to the tape. The players quickly realize they are not doing certain things now that they were doing earlier. What seems to make the difference is that the information is not coming from me; rather, they are listening to themselves, and what better authority is there? In addition, when they are struggling, everyone is giving them information, adjustments, and a multitude of strategies to try. This definitely contributes to a loss of concentration and intensity because there are now so many ways "to fix" the issue.

The educational, proactive, collaborative elements have served as the background to my approach. As I noted earlier, I have been fortunate to learn a wealth of information from the coaches and athletes I have had the privilege to work with. I have spent a multitude of hours observing and consulting with athletes. In the next section, I will discuss some of the important factors in gaining access in working with coaches and athletes.

Steps to Gaining Access

To gain access as a performance-enhancement consultant, I have to know the sport and the types of pressures that those athletes confront both on and off the playing venue. This type of sport-specific information helps me earn the trust and respect of coaches and athletes, which are prerequisites to having any impact on their performance. It also is important to understand the context of the situation in which I will be delivering my program so I can adjust it as needed. In some cases, the context that I anticipate I will be working in will help me to determine if I want to make the personal commitment to that team and/or situation.

Know the Sport

As a consultant, you have to learn the sport. There are major differences between each sport and the demands made on the athletes. For example, open sports (soccer) vs. closed sports (curling), contact sports (hockey) vs. noncontact (tennis), team vs. individual, time (swimming) vs. judges (figure skating). All of these sports have inherent differences. In designing an educational program, the consultant must be aware of the inherent differences of various sports and adjust his or her efforts to meet these demands (Ravizza, 1988).

Although a background in athletics is important to your success, it is not essential to have played the sport to be effective with athletes in that sport. You must, however, learn the nature of that sport. Two sports that were unfamiliar to me were field hockey and water polo. I read books, sport journals, watched videos, interviewed performers, and observed practices. For example, I quickly learned that water polo has three components: swimming, wrestling, and basketball. I also never realized water-polo players are some of the most highly conditioned athletes. All of this sport knowledge is so important in talking with elite-level athletes.

For example, when we discuss arousal and its effects on performance, it is one thing to address the "inverted-U theory" and quite another to talk to field hockey players about how, in practice, they should be relaxed while making a stick-stop when the ball comes 12 inches off their stick; but, in the game, they may be trying too hard, the shoulders tighten up, and the ball comes 16 inches off the stick, which impacts the timing of the pass. This type of dialogue lets the athlete know that you understand the demands of the sport. This gives you additional credibility because you speak the athlete's language and the information you present is applied immediately.

It is also important to understand the subculture of the sport and design your program to meet those needs. For example, the country-club golf culture is completely different from the hockey locker room. I have had the privilege of learning from a multitude of coaches and athletes. Just as coaches have to pay their dues climbing through the coaching ranks, sport psychology and mental training consultants have to pay their dues

working with and observing athletes. I volunteered for many years before I began to ask for payment for my services. From an athlete's perspective, a master's degree or a doctorate does not mean you have "practical" knowledge. Elite athletes expect and know whether someone has the experience . . . they can smell "garbage" better than most people can. Thus, you must know the subculture, information, etc. that you are presenting, or you will be wasting the time of the coaching staff and athlete alike. I was fortunate at my university to have direct access to coaches and athletes and was able to learn by observing and asking questions. I remember one player saying to me, "Ken, you are always asking me questions. What is your question today?" One question that yields a wealth of information is to ask coaches, while they are observing practice, "What are you seeing?" This really gives me their perspective and educates me to a completely new perspective. If I can gain a better understanding of what the coach is seeing and looking for, that awareness can only help me in my work with the athletes.

Earn Trust and Respect

Two teams I have worked with provide prime examples of earning this type of respect and trust. The first was early in my career when the baseball coach at my university wanted to learn more about the mental game (Ravizza, 1990). We met every Wednesday morning for one hour for 10 weeks. I shared my educational approach; he expressed his needs and concerns and taught me about the mental aspects of baseball. This type of "checking-out process" helps the coach lower the risks of handing over control over certain aspects of the program. The coach must have confidence in the consultant as a person and the material the consultant presents before he or she surrenders any control. If the coach does not check the consultant out at the start, the lack of trust will become an issue at some point. The surrender of control is one of the major reasons coaches are reluctant to have any consultants work with their teams. This is especially critical with the mental and emotional aspects of performance. As consultants, we forget the coach has been working diligently for endless hours to prepare the team, and the thought of having an "outsider" come in and "get into a player's head" is disconcerting to say the least.

The second team I worked with was a major college football team. When the coach first contacted me, he emphasized that another coach had referred me, which is how most of my consulting opportunities have occurred. I have never had a coach check out my academic resume and my publication record. After numerous conversations with the head coach, he gave me access to his 10 assistant coaches. I gave an hour-long talk to the staff that focused on the importance of the mental game. After my presentation, the head coach discussed my presentation with his staff and the feasibility of my working with his team. I then conducted a follow-up session to answer questions and address specific needs. Once the staff was supportive, the next phase was to give a presentation to 20 key players. During this meeting, the head coach observed my presentation and his players' verbal and non-verbal reactions to the material. After the talk, the head coach solicited feedback from the players. The final phase was to address the total team (100 players) and have them give their feedback to the coach. By this point, the program had gained support at all levels, and I could refine it to work in the context of that unique situation.

This is the ideal type of evaluation because it allows me to know they truly want, value, and support the program and fosters my own personal commitment to that particular team. Going through this process also gives me an opportunity to assess if this is a group I want to work with. When I make a commitment to work with a team, I must make a total commitment and bring my passion to the consultation process.

I emphasize to the coach that we need to spend the time at the start truly getting to know each other as people and then to understand the concepts and methods involved in implementing a program. Regarding these types of presentations, it is critical to present material in a language that coaches and players can understand. Be careful not to use an abundance of overheads, Power Point presentations, or the traditional methods we cherish in the academic environment. The presentation needs to be practical, and the coaches and players have to feel it was worth their time to listen. One sport psychology consultant was invited to talk with a group of elite-level coaches; but his attitude was so condescending and irrelevant that 10 minutes into the presentation, the coach who invited him stopped the talk, asked him to step outside, wrote him a check, asked him to leave, returned to the room, and apologized to his coaching colleagues.

In all my years, I have never been asked to give research references. Athletes and coaches are pragmatic, and the manner in which a consultant presents his or her material is more important than all the technical information. For example, I seldom give research references because the coaches and athletes are not interested in research data but in practical application and various stories and examples of how the information has been used. I cannot emphasize enough the importance of giving practical stories or examples. This is why it is important for young practitioners to work with athletes at any level so they gain practical experience (Halliwell et al., 1999). Elite athletes can definitely distinguish academic knowledge and book knowledge from the real world of sport.

Understand the Context of the Situation

Throughout my career, I have worked in a multitude of diverse situations, which I will refer to as "context," that range from working with individual athletes to working with teams and helping coaches provide the performance-enhancement program. I have also worked on the short "quick-fix" approach and on a season-long basis. In this article, I focus on the ideal situation of working with teams on a season-long basis. From the ideal situation, there are various contexts in which certain components of my approach, and the program as a whole, may have to be adjusted to meet the needs of each unique situation that I confront.

To be effective, I have to learn the context of the situation that I work in. By context, I mean that I first have to determine if the program can be effective. This determination is influenced by the support received from the coaching staff as evidenced by such things as the amount of time provided, the schedule of the time provided, and the amount of reinforcement the program receives from the coaching staff. Another way to determine the support for the program is how long I have to wait for phone calls to be returned by coaches and management's staff. In my 15 years with the Anaheim Angels, I have had to work with six different head coaches and four different general managers. Each placed a different value on the importance of the mental aspects of performance. For example, one coach said, "I am a big believer in the mental game," yet when I asked him for a half-hour meeting with the team before practice, he claimed there was just not enough time to do it. Another coach, who was supportive, would ask, "When is the best time to do it, because I want to be certain they are fully focused when you talk with them?" Even though I was working with the "same" organization, it is obvious that the context had changed, and I needed to adjust my approach accordingly, because the context impacts program effectiveness.

In the next section, I address two major aspects of my work. Awareness training serves as a foundation to my approach, and it is developing these skills in practice that is going to help the team perform to their potential. I have found that most coaches are very interested in whatever can help them enhance the quality of their training.

Awareness and Quality Practice

Awareness is essential for athletes to make the adjustments required to perform at the elite level (Ravizza, 1998). It is my assumption that increasing the athlete's awareness can speed up the athlete's learning process because the athlete is actively involved in it. The best opportunity to develop this awareness is in one's practice and training.

Awareness: A Critical Foundation

We shall not cease from exploration

And the end of all our exploring

Will be to arrive where we started

And know the place for the first time.

—(Eliot, 1971, p. 59)

Awareness development has been central to my approach. If athletes are going to learn from their experience, they have to be more aware of their experiences. So often, the athletes are working hard, but they are doing the wrong work, or they are totally "mindless." This mindless state may be great when one is "in the zone," but there are awareness and conscious thought that go into the preparation. This awareness is an integral part of the holistic approach. The athlete is not just a body, but also a total functioning human being.

As athletes perform, their awareness changes from the conscious level to the more automatic level. This is similar to Zen philosophy where one has to be in control so one can let go of control and where one has to be aware to let go of awareness. When the pressure situation arises, it can be more effective "to try less than to try to do more," which often results in unnecessary tension and excessive trying.

Some athletes are hesitant to get involved in sport psychology because it gets them "thinking too much," which leads to "paralysis by analysis." If the athletes lack awareness, however, then they can overexert, lack focus, etc., but because they are not aware, there is not a problem from their perspective. A performance-enhancement specialist has to be careful because some athletes will overanalyze and this pulls them from the actual playing of their sport.

Traffic Control

In the book, *Heads Up Baseball* (Ravizza & Hanson, 1994), we compared performing an athletic skill to the task of driving a car. When driving, we come to a signal light and have to check the color. If it is green, then we go. With athletic skills, I want the athlete to occasionally "check in" and, if all is well (green light), then keep going. D. Newburg (personal communication, December 16, 1998), a performance consultant, stated that the key to performance is to control "your response to the response." We are going to respond to the pressure, but we need to respond to that reaction and not just mindlessly allow our emotions to pull us along. For example, when athletes experience pregame pressure, they need to recognize that response (shortness of breath) and respond to it (regulate the breathing). If the light is yellow, then the athletes need to quickly process the information and decide what to do. If the light is red, then they have

to stop, or they will crash. I find many times when the athlete performs poorly and crashes, it is often because they were spinning out of control and didn't even recognize it. The most pragmatic aspect of the signal light analogy is the green light. When things are going well, just go. This allows those athletes who are hesitant to reflect on performance learning to become more conscious only when there is a need for it. Another benefit of this traffic-light analogy is that it provides a vocabulary with which coaches can address the athlete's experience and enhance their self-regulation skills. I call this "traffic control." I want the athletes to recognize their signal lights. A person's signal lights are unique to that individual. The signal light enhances the athlete's awareness of his or her experience. What do I experience, think, and focus on when the lights are green, yellow, or red? For example,

- Green—total involvement, clear thinking, present focus, just doing.
- Yellow—negative self-talk, frustration, lack of commitment, excessive trying.
- Red—belief in the negative self-talk, things speeding up, rapid breathing, anger.

These are examples of emotional states that athletes experience during performance. It is important to recognize that there are differences among individuals. Not every athlete would necessarily agree with how these mental and emotional states are classified. This awareness is a critical first step to gaining control.

The signal-light concept is also used for the athlete to anticipate the potential stressors of the upcoming competition. What are the yellow lights for this competition: venue, opponent, umpire, travel, teammates, family, injury, etc? Thus, the athletes are prepared, have contingency plans, and are ready for the potential distractions and obstacles. We practice how to deal with adversity by simulating game situations (crowd noise, bad calls by officials), and the players and coaches must practice coping with them. Even though a simulation cannot replicate the intensity of competition, some aspects of the simulation are very similar to real competition, and participants have to focus on those aspects. This can only help the athletes' confidence because they have anticipated potential distractions and have practiced coping with them.

Thus, proper preparation involves much more than just visualizing positive thoughts; it includes preparing for adversity. This has been another change in my work. When I started, I was using my work on peak experiences to serve as my foundation (Ravizza, 1977). This concept of being in the zone, or the flow state, drove my work. Then one coach I was working with said to me, "I am tired of hearing about the zone. That type of performance occurs once a season. I want these athletes to know how to cope with adversity." It took me a few years to truly understand what this coach was telling me. Basically, peak performance is not about performing perfectly or being in the zone; it is about learning to deal with adversity by learning to compensate and adjust. Thus, if you only have 70% of your confidence, then take that 70% and do battle. Stop worrying about the 30% that is not there. When the athletes take what they have and compete with it, they are more likely to perform on a consistent basis.

Development of Awareness

When I work with coaches, I encourage them to ask athletes more questions about their performance instead of always telling them what to do. So rather than telling the tennis player "to get your arm back farther," the coach asks, "How far back is your arm?" Reflection on this question will require that the

player become aware of the arm and how far back it is. It will also provide the coach with an opportunity to assess the athlete's awareness level. This point, made by Gallwey (1974), encourages coaches "to say less and notice more" and is very important for sport psychologists who too often use some technique to "fix it." This is particularly critical for the young consultant who has all the theoretical knowledge and current techniques but tries to help too soon or provides too much information. I remember in my early years when I saw a situation where I knew I could help. The coach pulled the team together for me to talk with, and once they were close, I started sharing all my wisdom, but they were not paying attention. D. Wolfe (personal communication, November 11, 1980), the coach, said, "Stop, Ken. Get eye contact." In a sense, I was out of control, and it took someone else to make me aware of it.

The athlete's lack of awareness becomes a challenge when a coach informs me that a particular athlete is not being honest with himself or herself about performance. An example of this occurs when the athlete is trying too hard and is in the yellow light zone, but does not even recognize it. I find that such an athlete is not dishonest, just unaware. We can develop this skill, rather than questioning the athlete's values and ethics. Such an approach makes the situation more manageable.

Thus, the signal-light analogy has been very productive in my work, especially for elite athletes who know they do not need to be aware when things are going well, but do need to know when they are losing that focus so they can compensate and adjust and get back on track before they really get out of control. I believe this is one of the reasons why athletes are hesitant to become involved in mental training or sport psychology, or both. They are afraid they will think too much, and some highly educated athletes fear they will overanalyze their performance.

Another tool that has helped me check on the athlete's awareness, and more specifically his or her listening skills, is after talking with an athlete, to ask what he or she has heard me say. I have been shocked at what the individual heard me say. This is why it is important to occasionally ask," What did you hear me say?" This has helped me to clarify my points and keep the information short and simple. The KISS principle, "Keep It Simple, Smart," is crucial, especially in the mindset of competition (Halliwell et al., 1999).

Quality Practice

When I began my work, I focused the vast majority of my energy on the "The Big Game." Today, 5% of my attention is on "The Big Game," and 95% of it is on today's practice. I am not certain that I can help the team win the big game because there are so many extraneous factors involved (injuries, the officials, etc.). However, I do know I can help increase the quality of practice. The mental skills can help the athletes by having them be more focused and prepared. In some sports like figure skating, the athletes train on their own for certain practice sessions. I emphasize the need to practice better than their competitors do. This requires setting goals for practice and having a plan or something they are working on when they do the skills. This intention will provide a level of intensity because there is a clear purpose. For example, when soccer players warm up, there is a certain point where each kick has a target and the athlete is not just mindlessly kicking the ball. Rather, they focus on the target, and the kicks are more game like.

Coaches are more excited to learn about methods of enhancing the quality of practice because there is not as much at stake as compared to big games. In addition, they know that quality practice is critical to quality performance. In 1992, the NCAA mandated that college coaches reduce practice time so the student-athletes would have more time to focus on academics. As a result, many coaches said, "Ken, we just don't have the time now for mental training." In contrast, Dave Snow, the head baseball coach at Long Beach State said, "Ken, now I need you to get more involved in our program. Because we have less time, we need the players even more focused in practice" (D. Snow, personal communication, September 12, 1992). Coaches are very interested in what mental training can do to help athletes achieve a higher quality of training. Many people in our field claim they have some secret to winning the big game. Practitioners have to realize that this is an insult to the coaches who have diligently worked with the team to reach their goals. I know that for me, I do not have any secret, but I do know that the mental game has to be practiced on a daily basis if it is going to be effective in the pressure situation.

Segmentation

One way to enhance quality practice is to have the athletes learn methods of segmenting their academic, social, and personal lives from today's practice. We discuss matters such as practicing at 3:00PM, and what the athlete can do to mentally prepare for practice so that when it starts he or she is ready and focused to get the most out of it. When I worked with the coaches at Harvard University, they mentioned that many athletes brought their academic problems to practice. One method or symbol they used to help separate academics from practice was a bridge the student-athletes crossed that separated the academic buildings from the athletic facilities. Athletes were encouraged to leave their academic problems on that side of the bridge and take advantage of practice time to set those problems aside. After practice, with a fresh perspective, they could re-address those academic issues.

The act of getting dressed for practice is another symbol to segment school, personal, or work activities from sport. On a "yellow-light" day, the athletes can symbolically acknowledge and release their pressures for that day as they get dressed. For example, when they dress for practice, taking off the sweater represents not worrying about a math exam, and shedding the pants may represent setting aside an argument with a friend. Each item of clothing represents something from the day that needs to be "put away." Then as the athletes put on the practice clothing, lace up the spikes, and walk to the venue, they can focus on routines that can be used to set goals for the day, adjust their energy level, and do whatever else is necessary to be ready for practice. There are times that the athlete needs to put meaning into some of the routines that they do—"The time is now; the place is here."—Because each day they choose to take a step forward toward their dreams, remain the same, or take a step back. A step forward is not always being successful, but they can fail and learn from their failure.

Learning to Have Good Bad Days

Practice is also a wonderful place for the athlete to work on their compensation and adjustment skills. The athlete and team have to learn to perform through adversity. So, if practice is not going well, consultants should focus on specific tasks that can be done to turn it around. For example, if the athletes are having a rough practice, they can turn it around for one minute instead of trying to turn it around for the whole practice. Once the athletes turn it around they need to learn what they did to turn it around, (communicate more, direct their attention on the ball, instead of their worries) because this is what they need to do in the competition to turn it around. Just turning it around is not enough . . . they have to know what they did

to turn it around. This will provide them with "something to go to" that is task relevant and that has been effective in the past. Peak performance is about compensation and adjustment. Like everything else that is done in competition, it has to occur in practice. For example, with Coach Snow's baseball team, we have a drill in which the players imagine they just made an error, and they practice turning it around by establishing a routine to recognize the error, release it, refocus on the task, and move to the next pitch. Thus, because errors happen in the game, we practiced compensating and adjusting from the error. As this is practiced, it becomes more refined and simplified so when adversity hits, the athlete knows how to "turn it around" and has practiced it. Thus, the athlete has to learn to have "good bad days" in practice because when the final score or time is posted no one cares how the athlete felt or what distractions there were; the athlete must perform.

Lessons Learned

In the next section, I share some of the lessons I have learned that have helped me negotiate the often turbulent and uncertain waters of consulting in the area of performance enhancement.

Confidentiality

When I work with a team, I do not provide specific information to coaches or management. This is the best way to be unsuccessful because once you break confidence, every player on the team will know about it. I do not want to be involved in team selection or playing time because if the players know my input is considered, they are going to tell me what they think I want to hear. If I am involved in team selection, I have a responsibility to let the athletes know my position. Any information that I do share with the coaching staff is general information, unless I obtain the player's permission to be more specific.

If I believe there is something the player shares with me that I think would help the coach in working with the player, I will ask the player's permission to share that information with the coach. About 90% of the time, the players are willing to have me share the information. I remember my first year in Major League Baseball. I worked with the team before the game, and then I watched the game with a friend. During the game, I talked with my friend about my work with the team. I spoke in very general terms, no names or specifics. The next day, a player I worked with asked me what I was doing talking about our work together while I was watching the game. His wife, whom I had not met, was sitting behind me and heard me talking. She assumed I was talking about her husband. From this I learned "Be careful when at the venue. You never know who is watching or listening."

Helpful Hints for the Young Practitioner

As young practitioners, you cannot do what I do; it took me 20 years to learn and refine my approach. You have to be yourself, and you have to bring your self to the consultation process. Be careful of only hearing the athlete's perspective. Attempt to get the coach's perspective, or what I call a "reality" check. Sometimes I made the mistake of being too nice so the athlete would like me, but there are times when you have to be strong and assertive and let the athlete know your perspective on the issue. Some athletes will not want to hear it, and you may lose your working relationships with them, but if you are not strong, you are going to have only a limited effect. For example, one coach said to me in the early phases, "I don't want 'I'm okay, you're okay.'" I have found certain athletes respect you more when you

are assertive and let them know what you think. This is part of the "art" of doing the work, and it develops over time.

Keep the Faith

It is important for young practitioners to realize that they are not going to have an impact on all the players and coaches. This is where the textbooks are misleading. When I read the literature in our field, it sounds as if coaches and athletes are waiting for us with open arms. This is not the case, and not every major team and organization would have mental training and sport psychology consultants working with their teams. On some teams, assistant coaches feel threatened by the presence of a performance-enhancement consultant, and they will actively subvert your work.

In addition, the context of the situation you work in is going to have an impact on what percentage of players is going to get involved. I generally have one-third who will get involved, one-third who will get involved when they have problems, and one-third who will have nothing to do with the process. As mentioned, these percentages will change based on the context of that specific situation (i.e., the amount of demonstrated support you have from the coach). One phenomenon that often occurs is that the player who needs it the most will have the most resistance to the program. Sometimes you have to be patient and wait for the teachable moment. My relationship with teams has varied from being totally accepted and an intricate part of the program to implementing a program from a distance. At times, there is uncertainty in my position, and often it is by design. The best example is Olympic teams where there is a strong likelihood of becoming caught between the different perspectives of coaches, the National Governing Body, and the players. I work with all three groups as they resolve the natural progression of conflicts that must be overcome.

I have worked diligently with some athletes, and they have not appreciated my efforts. At the time, this hurts when you make a total commitment, develop and implement a program, and receive little recognition or appreciation, but this is where the consultant has to be clear on why he or she is doing the work. If you are expecting athletes or coaches to acknowledge their work with you to the media, you may be waiting a very long time. I attempt to stay out of the media, as I want the athlete and coaching staff to take the credit. Coaches can become irritated after they have done so much of the work, and a consultant steps up to get the credit. This does not help future working relationships. I want the athlete and coaches to receive the credit because they are the ones who have earned it.

As performance-enhancement consultants, we do not attend all the practices and competitions. We are part of the staff and team, but we are often not in the inner circle on a daily basis. I believe this type of working relationship is one of our strengths because we come in and move away, a flexibility that provides us with a fresh and insightful perspective. Many coaches appreciate the information and insights I provide by not being in the midst of the action all the time. The negative side of this orientation is that you often are not an intricate part of the team. There are times you are an outsider, and it takes a while to integrate back into the culture.

Remember That Patience Is a Virtue

One aspect of consulting that is not discussed enough is patience. Many consultants make the mistake of trying to do too much. There are times to be almost invisible and not do anything unless it is critical. I remember when I first began working with a gymnastics team. I was invited to accompany the team on a road trip. When the team returned,

the coach talked with the team about having me travel with them. The coach said, "I'm not certain it was worth the money to bring Ken with us since he didn't do much." At that point, the team captain said, "That is what we like about Ken—he doesn't do anything unless it is needed."

Sport psychology consultants can be ineffective if they try to do too much too soon. An intricate component of the art of effective consulting is to be patient and I would suggest to the young practitioner to do less rather than trying to do too much. As consultants, we do not want to become stressors to the coaches and athletes. For this reason, I suggest that the practitioner clarify his or her role and the expectations of all parties. Another technique that I have found effective is to let athletes and coaches know that they can say, "Not now, Ken!" I can handle it. I do not want them to worry about my feelings; they have enough to focus on. At moments like these, I have had to learn to not take things personally.

Provide Post-competition Support

Be patient after the competition in talking with coaches and athletes. This is especially the case after poor performances. There is very little we can do to help. All we can do is be there when they are in pain as this demonstrates that we care. I dislike being in the locker room after a tough loss, but we have to do it. I am there, I am available, and I wait for the coaches and athletes to come to me. I also have found that directly after competition, many coaches are so mentally exhausted that it is not a productive time for substantive interaction. Of course, if the coaches want to address certain issues, I am available.

Establish a Support System

Another thing that has helped me is having a group of colleagues and coaches to whom I can reach out for support (Halliwell et al.,

1999). This support can be technical, emotional, or philosophical. At times, I become so involved in the situation that I lose perspective. I remember that when I first began working with professional baseball, Bruce Ogilvie was a mentor who shared so much with me. He informed me of the joys of doing the work as well as the pitfalls. He mentioned that he had been released from teams many times and that I should be prepared for that. He expanded on this, saying that sometimes management did not formally terminate a program—they just didn't return his phone calls. There have been times I just wanted some feedback—"What happened? What was the mistake?"—but in the sport world, this type of feedback is the exception. This is so because, in one sense as consultants, we are a commodity just like the players. In my 15 years with the Angels, I have been released, sent to the minors, and rehired. It was not until I had these experiences that I could truly be empathic with the athletes and understand the uncertainties they constantly confront.

My peers have helped me to be more effective by providing me with that fresh perspective or that needed "slap on the head." I have had the privilege of developing and implementing mental-training programs with other sport psychology consultants. I worked three years with Wes Sime and the University of Nebraska football program and two years with Bob Rotella with the U.S. Olympic Equestrian team. It is truly exciting to share ideas and receive feedback from someone who is right there with you. I think one of my greatest assets has been my use of colleagues to support me in my work because without their support, I would not have been able to be as effective as I have been. I have also used people in my support group to provide services for selected athletes and/or teams.

Performance Enhancement in Various Fields

Throughout my professional career, I have worked with four major groups in the area of performance enhancement: students, athletes, business and community groups, and health-related practitioners. Much of my work has developed from my university position where I have taught stress-management courses for the past 20 years. This has provided me with a broad view of performance issues in many different areas. I have consulted with numerous business groups and community organizations from law enforcement to health administrators and from physicians and nurses to business leaders. My experiences and the knowledge I have gained from my sport consultations have helped me develop methods that are basic and effective. The great thing about sport is the athlete receives immediate feedback on his or her performance. This type of instant feedback has helped me modify and refine my methods and approach.

I remember talking with a group of recreational softball coaches about mental preparation for performance, concentration strategies, playing the game one pitch at a time, and performance evaluation. After my talk, a gentleman came up and said that he was a surgeon and that he was relating everything I said to surgery. He said taking one pitch at a time is similar to taking one stitch at a time during an operation.

When I was a graduate student, I took a tennis class with Tim Gallwey, author of *The Inner Game of Tennis* (1994), who began the class by asking the group two questions: "How many of you are here to improve your tennis?" (Most people raised their hands.) and "How many of you are here to improve your awareness?" (Very few people raised their hands.) At that point, he went on to explain that the class was going to teach us to improve our awareness because that was something we could use in all aspects of life.

If my only concern is helping the athletes perform their sport skills better, that perspective is rather shallow in my opinion. However, if the athlete can understand the role of commitment and passion in performance, set goals and establish a plan to achieve them, develop routines to mentally prepare for performance, learn to focus, regulate his or her intensity level, and learn to evaluate the performance, then that athlete is more likely to use these skills in other aspects of his or her life. These are life skills, not just sport skills.

The advantage of working in the field for years is hearing athletes I worked with 10 years ago say, "Ken, when I was an athlete I used some of the stuff you shared with us, but now I use it even more in my job and with my family." This is one of the things that truly has made the work worth doing. This particular athlete said, "I wanted to call you because when I was a gymnast and you were working with us, I wasn't really into it. But today I used it in my job as a firefighter when I went into a burning building and saved three people's lives." He continued, "Ken, I could hear your voice as I was in the pressure situation." These types of reports are why I am proud to be an educator who helps athletes refine and develop their mental skills.

I also think many business people are active in conditioning, playing sport, or following a team. People generally can relate to sport, and sometimes it is more effective and less threatening to use an analogy or example from sport to make a point. For example, an athlete has to deal with poor officiating whereas a salesperson has to cope with a difficult supervisor.

Closure: Ending the Working Relationship

The issue of closure has been a difficult thing for me in my work. I personally grow frustrated when I work with an individual athlete, and I think the individual is genuinely committed to working through the issue, but then he or she never arranges the follow-up sessions. At this time, what I do is tell the athlete that after the first session, I want the athlete to decide if he or she thinks it is worthwhile and then make a commitment to at least two follow-up sessions. This enables the athlete to determine if it is worth the time and experience. It helps me, when I know it is the athlete's last session, to bring closure to the relationship and give the individual some final essential points that he or she can take away.

Closure is an even more difficult issue when I am working with a team. If coaches do not want the program, they often do not provide any feedback on what went wrong from their perspective. They just move on and sometimes won't even tell a consultant that his or her services are no longer needed. For me, this is very difficult to deal with because when I work with a team, I invest my knowledge and passion into it, and I at least think I deserve to be told why the program was terminated. This feedback is critical if I am going to improve as a consultant. I remember that after working with the Angels for 5 years, I was sent a letter informing me that my services were no longer needed. I was devastated, and I wanted to know why. I called the general manager's office, but my phone calls were not returned. After many calls, I finally got a response: I was told that the new coach did not place any value in sport psychology.

I have found that this type of honest and open feedback helps me bring closure to my work with the team and allows me to make adjustments in my approach. Sometimes you may be released, not for doing a bad job, but for things that are totally beyond your control (i.e., the new coach's brother is a sport psychologist). I always tell athletes to learn from their failures, as we have to do the same thing as consultants, but sometimes it is difficult to get the information. I know this is part of consulting work, but at times, it is difficult for me to deal with.

Confidentiality is important if you desire a long-term relationship with an athlete or a team. Once you break confidentiality, you have lost the trust of the people you are working with. As a young practitioner, be patient, and establish a support system to get input from colleagues you respect. In addition, as a consultant, you must learn to bring closure to your work so that you can learn from each consulting experience and continuously refine and develop your approach.

Summary

In this chapter, I have addressed the background to my approach and methods to gain access to working with athletes and teams. I emphasized the importance of increasing the athlete's awareness and the use of practice as a wonderful place to refine and develop the awareness skills. I also have shared some of the lessons I have learned from working in this volatile environment. My approach, techniques, and philosophy have been in a constant state of evolution, and I know that I will continue to grow as a consultant and person as I continue on my journey.

I want to conclude this paper by thanking all of the coaches and athletes who have shared so much with me for so many years. They have allowed me the extraordinary opportunity to learn from them. I just hope the reader can learn a few valuable insights from this article.

References

Dowling, T. (1970). *Coach: A season with Lombardi.* New York: Norton.

Eliot, T.S. (1971). Little Gidding. *Four quartets.* New York: Harcourt, Brace, and Jovanovich.

Gallwey, T. (1974). *The inner game of tennis.* New York: Random House.

Gould, D., Greenleaf, C., Guinan, D., Medbery, R. Strickland, M., Lauer, L., Chung, Y., & Peterson, K., (1998). Factors influencing Atlanta Olympian performance. *Olympic Coach, 8* (4), 9–11.

Halliwell, W., Orlick, T., Ravizza, K., & Rotella, B. (1999). *Consultant's guide to excellence.* Quebec, Canada: Baird, O'Keefe.

Orlick, T. (1996). *In pursuit of excellence.* Champaign, IL: Human Kinetics.

Ravizza, K. (1977). Peak experience in sport. *Journal of Humanisitic Psychology, 17*, 35–40.

Ravizza, K. (1988). Gaining entry with athletic personnel for season long consulting. *The Sport Psychologist, 2,* 243–254.

Ravizza, K. (1990). Sport psych consultation issues in professional baseball. *The Sport Psychologist, 4*, 330–340.

Ravizza, K. (1998). Increasing awareness in sport performance. In J. Williams (Ed.), *Applied sport psychology* (pp. 171–181). Mountain View, CA: Mayfield.

Ravizza, K. (in press). A philosophical construct: A framework for performance enhancement. *International Journal of Sport Psychology.*

Ravizza, K., & Hanson, T. (1994). *Heads-up baseball.* Indianapolis: Masters Press.

Summit, P., & Jenkins, S. (1998). *Reach for the summit.* New York: Broadway Books.

The Provision of Sport Psychology Services During Competition Tours

Jeffrey W. Bond

The AIS Sport Psychology Service Provision Model

The Australian Institute of Sport (AIS) was established by the Australian government in 1981 as a fully resourced elite-athlete residential training center. The AIS sport psychology department (established in 1982, with five current full-time psychologists, one research assistant, and one graduate intern) has developed a comprehensive service provision program containing the following key elements:

1. **Personal Development Training** (includes individual and group workshops in areas such as communication skills, assertiveness training, conflict resolution, leadership training, presentation and media skills)
2. **Lifestyle Management Skills** (includes strategy development and counseling in areas such as time management, relationships, lifestyle balance, career and education planning)
3. **Clinical Interventions** (includes diagnostic assessment and therapeutic interventions in issues such as eating and weight control, depression and suicidal ideation, trauma and early childhood abuse, injury rehabilitation, substance abuse and self-esteem)
4. **Group and Team Dynamics** (includes advice and interventions in organizational issues such as roles and responsibilities, team structure and function, communication hierarchies, cohesion, team culture and image)
5. **Performance-enhancement Training** (includes training and counseling in traditional areas such as goal setting, arousal control, concentration, imagery, performance planning and preparation, peaking/tapering, cognitive skills, emotional control, performance briefing and debriefing and travel skills)
6. **Applied Research** (includes development and implementation of qualitative and quantitative investigations of issues pertinent to individual and group/team performances)
7. **Education** (includes involvement in coach education, graduate internships and placements, university undergraduate and graduate teaching, conference and workshop presentation)

The AIS psychology department staff delivers relevant program elements to:

- AIS residential athlete scholarship holders (performance-based scholarships are renewed annually)
- AIS resident coaches (appointed on 2- to 4-year performance-based contracts)
- national team training camps (typically 2- to 3-week visits)

- designated Olympic Athlete Program athletes and coaches

Full-time appointments to the AIS sport psychology department and day-by-day access to residential athletes and coaches provide an ideal environment for the implementation of ongoing sport-psychology service provision. AIS psychologists consult with athletes and coaches formally and informally on an individual and team basis, provide workshops, and attend training sessions and competitions.

Holistic Sport Psychology and Performance Enhancement

After some 20 years experience as a psychologist working in elite sport, it is the author's view that psychological aspects of performance enhancement are critical to international competition performances (although precisely how much psychological factors contribute, we may never really know). High-level competition performances are a function of many facets of athlete preparation, including technical, physical, and mental aspects. The focus of the AIS sport psychology program is on the holistic psychological development of the athlete and coach. This is achieved through an integration of the service provision program with the coach's training program and within a multidisciplinary framework. This applied, multifaceted psychology program is not simply directed towards the traditional performance-enhancement skills training models promoted in the past primarily by North American universities. The AIS sport psychology program recognizes and reflects the complexity of personal, lifestyle, and sport-related issues that face the aspiring elite athlete who undertakes an intensive international competition preparation program.

The experience of sport psychology practitioners confirms that the initial presenting issue is rarely the underlying core issue. For example, the athlete who presents with a seemingly straightforward concentration or performance anxiety problem may not be assisted effectively with a traditional dose of relaxation training and visualization of effective performance content and outcomes. The core issue may be much more complex. As practitioners, we must constantly be asking, "Why?" Why is the athlete experiencing concentration difficulty? Is it because he or she is having difficulties with an upcoming university examination or some problems in a relationship or at home? Perhaps the athlete is overtrained or still grappling with recovery from an injury. Perhaps the athlete is still in the early stages of learning or consolidating the technical skill. The athlete may carry an excessive fear of failure that has resulted from early experiences in his or her sporting career. In short, there may be many reasons why a particular athlete is experiencing some difficulty or other. The most effective solution will almost certainly not be a short course of relaxation and imagery training. If elite sporting-performance outcomes are the result of the balanced combination of psychological, physical, technical, and management preparation, then why should we assume that an issue confronting an athlete can be quickly resolved through a simplistic relaxation-based performance-enhancement training program?

Experience in the field clearly points to a need for holistic psychological development programs for elite athletes that include lifestyle management, personal development, group and relationship dynamics, clinical interventions, and performance-enhancement training. These programs must be integrated with other sports science and medicine programs and provided in a planned way within the structure and phasing of the coaching program. It is critical, of course, to have the full support of the coaching staff for the inclusion of integrated athlete development programs.

Training in Sport Psychology

To effectively implement a holistic sport psychology program as outlined above, it is essential that service provider training include a combination of

- Psychology (providing a broad theoretical base and developing competence in diagnostic and therapeutic clinical and counseling skills)
- Sports science
- Sport psychology training and experience

Clearly one does not have to be an 8-year trained psychologist to deliver some of the more traditional performance-enhancement training programs. Many nonpsychologist individuals in sport (for example, coaches and trainers) have traditionally provided training in relaxation, visualization, concentration, goal setting, and elements of mental preparation for competition. Personal development and lifestyle management areas are well serviced by many individuals and organizations within the general community who may not often be trained psychologists. It is essential, however, that quality training as a psychologist and a thorough knowledge of the demands of elite sport provide the basis for effective diagnostic and treatment programs in many of the group dynamics, relationships, and critical/clinical intervention areas that are common sources of high stress for athletes in training and competition.

In Australia, all sport psychologists are registered (licensed) psychologists with specialized graduate or postgraduate training in sport psychology. Membership in the Australian Psychological Society's College of Sport Psychologists requires the following:

- Four years of undergraduate training (honors or equivalent) in psychology, including undergraduate courses in sports science

- A 2-year coursework master's degree (courses, supervised placements, and thesis) in sport psychology
- Two years of supervised specialist supervision in sport psychology

This training and supervision model provides an opportunity for sport psychologists to gain the psychological, sports science and practice knowledge and competencies required to provide effective services to elite athletes and coaches.

The National Rowing Team Service Provision Model

National sporting teams in Australia typically appoint a multidisciplinary sports science and medicine team over the 4-year preparation period for the Olympic Games (psychology, physiology, nutrition, medicine, physiotherapy, massage, and biomechanics). These professionals are drawn largely from the national and state sports institute network. These appointments permit the development of ongoing programs as part of a multidisciplinary team in parallel with the coaching program. AIS psychologists are typically appointed to a national team in addition to their AIS team responsibilities. The author currently holds an appointment to the Australian rowing team as team psychologist and as national coordinator of the rowing psychology network.

The Australian rowing team that competed at the 1998 World Championships comprised the head coach, 12 crew coaches, two managers, a sports medicine practitioner, psychologist, physiotherapist, masseur, and 52 rowers in 16 crew categories (including sweep and sculls, men and women, and lightweight and heavyweight categories). The domestic/national rowing season extends from October through April (including the National Championships and two National Selection regattas). The international season extends from May through September (8 to 12 weeks are spent traveling overseas for international competition, including several World Cup regattas and culminating in the World Championships in September).

The team psychologist coordinates a national network of sport psychologists (State sports institute based) that provides ongoing sport psychology assistance over the course of the domestic season (October through April). Most of the elements of the AIS psychology program are available to the elite rowers holding scholarships with each of the state and national sports institutes. At the completion of the final national team selection regatta (April), those rowers selected for the international senior A regatta season are relocated to various intensive training centers within the national sport institute network. Whilst in final preparation for the international competitions, psychology services are delivered by the sport psychology network.

When the team finally assembles for departure, the team psychologist assumes responsibility for the provision of services while on tour. At this time, the range of relevant psychology services includes performance-enhancement training, group and team dynamics, aspects of lifestyle management, and critical interventions. Given the heavy demands for applied psychology services from the touring national team of approximately 70 persons, it has not yet been possible to include an applied research program. A good deal of effort on the part of the team psychologist is directed towards the enhancement of the team working capacities of the coaching staff. National team crew coaches are appointed from various Australian States (each with its own political agenda) and after having completed a domestic season of competition against one another. Throughout the domestic season, the coaches' goals are to place as many rowers on the national team as possible and to se-

cure a coaching appointment to the national team in their preferred boat category. This selection process, combined with the natural competitiveness of the coaches, does not always contribute in a positive way to a cohesive national coaching team.

A Typical Day in the Life of a Touring Team Psychologist

The following actual diary page is taken from a 4-week tour period with the Australian rowing team and is dated 2 weeks prior to the 1998 World Rowing Championships with the activities taking place at a team training venue and the team hotel in Europe.

6.00AM
Rise, breakfast, arrive at training venue (informal discussion with individual athletes/coaches en route)

6.45AM
Attend crew briefing prior to on-water training session

7.00AM
Accompany the crew coach (in coaching boat) observing coach-rower interactions, athlete responses to training and coaching. Also includes specific discussion with the coach about performance issues and general discussion about team and personal issues. Attend postsession debrief and follow up contact with individual rowers (raise issues, reinforce application of psychological skills, etc.)

9.30AM
Return to team accommodation (informal discussion with coach, rowers en route)

10.00AM
Facilitate crew and coach session with different group with focus on discussion/brainstorming ideas for mental aspects of the final 2-week peaking/tapering process.

11.00AM
Meeting with head coach regarding final crew selection process (men's heavyweight

8) and reactions of and strategies for debriefing of two reserves. Further discussion regarding a meeting with all team reserves to clarify roles and contributions

12.00PM

Planning discussion with crew coach regarding upcoming crew sessions over final 2 weeks of competition preparation

1.00PM

Lunch (opportunity to sit with different athlete groups in order to ascertain general progress and status of team "culture")

2.00PM

Individual athlete consultation. Presenting issue is performance anxiety and depression; underlying issue is impending retirement with implications for both individual and remainder of crew

3.00PM

Relaxation/imagery/energizer crew session in preparation for afternoon training (set timed race pieces over 500 and 1000m)

4.00PM

Travel to training venue (discussion with individual rower en route)

4.30–6.15PM

Cycling with coaches along 2-kilometer rowing course as various crews simulate race segments. The 4-kilometer cycle is repeated five times to follow five different crew groupings. Post training analysis of times against prognostic times and significant coach interactions

6.30PM

Return to team accommodation (includes discussion with individual rower en route)

7.00PM

Team dinner (sit with different rower group)

8.00PM

Crew session with emphasis on mental aspects of enhancing the transition to speed/racing workloads. Includes introduction of topic, anecdotes from previous experience, brainstorming of practical strategies and short imagery session reinforcing the concept of an "explosive/powerful/sharp and fast" mental set

9.00PM

Crisis intervention with sweep pair in conflict. Potentially significant as one of the pair does not want to continue rowing with pair partner

10.00PM

Team staff meeting to discuss final travel, accommodation, and competition arrangements for World Championships

10.00PM

Meet with smaller group of coaches for a quiet social drink and discussion of team-related issues

11.30PM–12.00AM

Sleep!!

Touring with a national team is a very challenging and rewarding experience for a team psychologist. It is tiring when one considers a daily regime as outlined above continuing for 7 days each week for 4 weeks (in this case) with no time off and responsibility for maintaining regular professional contact with 16 different crews and individual rowers and coaches within those crews. There is also a need to include ongoing contact with other team staff in the medical and sports science areas, team management and administration, and importantly, maintaining regular contact with the head coach.

In recognition of the stresses associated with the rigors of touring team appointments, the Australian Olympic Committee places a good deal of importance on the comprehensive assessment of the medical and physical fitness of team staff. A touring team or major international competition psychologist position is not for the frail or traditional 9:00AM to 5:00PM worker.

Basic Principles for the Touring Psychologist

I have evolved a set of personal and professional practice principles over some 20 years of national and international service provision with a wide range of elite sporting teams. The following list is not exhaustive, but represents some of the more significant principles that might impact on the effectiveness of applied sport psychology service provision in the context of the touring international team:

1. Team Psychologist Roles and Responsibilities

The psychologist must establish a clear set of position responsibilities, initially with the head coach and subsequently with other team coaches and management staff, other sports science and medicine professionals, and the team athletes. It is essential that the team psychologist understand the expectations and limits placed on his or her professional contribution. Is the psychologist to be restricted to clear performance-enhancement work, or are there to be more expanded responsibilities such as team culture, crew dynamics, mediation, management, or applied research? It is essential that the team psychologist identify to whom he or she is responsible. In a rowing team situation, the psychologist has several "masters," including the individual athlete, crew, crew coach, and head coach. It is not a simple task to identify one person as the exclusive client. This is one of the many balancing acts confronting the team psychologist. In my rowing work, I focus on my responsibility to the head coach, and I respond to his requirements and expectations. I target crew coaches and their crews in accordance with the priorities set by the head coach. I enlist the assistance of the team managers, the team doctor, other medical staff, and the boat builder. I maintain very regular contact with these people so that I can be "ahead of the game," in touch with the team climate, and in a position to make recommendations to the head coach and team manager. I avoid going in with my own agenda, and the feedback I have had from coaches is that they appreciate the loyalty and the capacity to quickly fit in with the needs of the team and to provide appropriate support for the entire team.

2. Integration with the Coaching Program

The work of the team psychologist must be directed through the head coach and specific crew coach. The psychologist position is delicately balanced between the coaches and athletes and between the crew coaches and head coach. There will be some coaches in a large, multidisciplined national team who prefer to take total responsibility for psychological work with their athletes, and others who are secure enough to delegate that work to the team psychologist. It would be unrealistic to expect to work equally amongst each of the 12 coaches on this particular national team. There is one crew coach who comes to mind, who does not permit me to work directly with his rowers, preferring to manage the individual and crew psychological processes himself. I could have taken exception to that situation, but I was aware of this coach's individual needs, cultural background (Eastern bloc), and the type of education that placed the coach in a position of total responsibility for all facets of the athletes' preparation. I have approached this coach from a position where I am an unofficial "adviser" to the coach on matters that he wishes to raise with me.

I have functioned on the premise that when a crew coach seeks comprehensive involvement, effective service provision will have a down trickle-down effect, and other crew coaches will eventually come on board. There is no need to force the issue or to attempt to push the need for servicing too far. A good approach is to wait for the "teachable moment," which, of course, will inevitably occur on a 4- or 6-week tour when the psychologist is on hand every day for extended hours.

3. Client-Practitioner Interactions

The team psychologist is part of at least a three-way client-professional interaction (that is, the psychologist, coach, and athlete). As a member of a multidisciplinary team, the team psychologist will learn that other professionals may also become part of that network. Whilst the team medical practitioner may be held responsible for recommendations regarding the medical status of athletes, and the psychologist for recommendations specifically relevant to psychological status, the appropriate hierarchical team structure places the head coach in the primary/senior position. The head coach holds the ultimate responsibility for team performance. A team psychologist who ignores his or her responsibility to work to the head coach or crew coach will ultimately fail in maintaining an effective position on the team. A sporting team environment is not the place to adopt a lone practitioner role; it is an environment typified by common goals and shared responsibilities. One of my sport psychology colleagues is finding it very tough at the moment because he persists in establishing a profile within the team based on his professional position rather than on his capacity to work across all facets of the team and, more important, within the team framework. He refuses to undertake any duties that are not "psychological" and refuses to work with the team athletes to share information with the coach on a "need-to-know" basis. Because of this stance, he now finds himself isolated. The coaches and athletes don't see him as having a full commitment to the team, and the coaches are suspicious

of a team psychologist who takes the individual athlete confidentiality issue perhaps too far (see below).

4. Comprehensive Needs Analyses

The complexity of the needs analyses required for individual athletes and coaches, groups/crews, and ultimately the entire team cannot be underestimated. The needs at various levels will, of course, vary as the season progresses through different phases of preparation and competition. I use the elements of the AIS service-provision model as the basis for needs analyses at different stages of the season. For example, personal development needs and training would be appropriate during the domestic season, but less important during the competition phase. I choose not to function as a team psychologist with a standardized, prepared set of skills to which I sequentially expose athletes and coaches. I develop a broad framework in consultation with the coach and then adapt the program to contextual situations as they occur. In my experience, flexibility in program planning and implementation is essential.

5. Adopting a Process Focus

The team psychologist must maintain a clear process focus (just as we advise most of our athlete clients to do). There have been numerous examples of psychologists who unfortunately placed their own ego needs and emotional involvement ahead of their professional responsibilities. It is not difficult to imagine a team psychologist who has implemented a long-term program with a team (with all the usual highs and lows) to finally accompany them to a major international competition and then to become emotionally involved in performance outcomes. As professionals, we must be prepared to minimize any transference of our own emotional needs; we must be prepared to work in the background, to be in the "engine room." I have a clear recollection of a team psychologist who implemented an ongoing sport psychology program with a team through a World Championship. Unfortunately, this person became so emotionally involved that he leaped the fence at the end of the final match and ran onto the field to join the athletes in their victory celebrations. A short time later, he turned around to see the head coach slowly walking onto the field with a scowl directed squarely at the psychologist. Clearly, the coach did not think it appropriate that the team psychologist should be the first staff member onto the field demonstrating emotions that might be more appropriate coming from the athletes who were actually on the field winning the tournament. Suffice it to say that that psychologist wasn't invited to work further with that team.

I had a personal experience with a sport psychologist who stated quite categorically: "I want to get a job at the Olympics so I can win a gold medal." I was quick to remind that person that it is not our job to win medals; it is our job to contribute effectively to an environment in which the athletes inevitably win their medals. Sport psychologists work in the "engine room." We are the background contributors who assist the coaches and athletes to create a successful environment. I don't believe that there is any room for a psychologist who transfers his or her personal needs to the performance environment. A somewhat cynical view would state that the psychologist will generally not receive any accolades for successful athlete performances anyway, but should expect to be blamed for contributing to poor athlete or team performances.

6. Competitive Performance Requirements

The mission of elite international athletes and coaches is to perform to their potential and, if possible, to win. The team psychologist must be acutely aware of the competitive performance requirements facing the client group. For a team psychologist to adopt a too-simplistic, a too-theoretical/academic approach or to be the "warm/fuzzy" psychologist at the expense of a clear view of the complex performance requirements would be to make a significant error of judgment. There is a hard edge to the business of winning and competing internationally, and the team psychologist must be an active contributor to that process. A successful team psychologist must adopt a multidimensional and eclectic approach and be very sensitive to the competitive context he or she operates within. A national coach I know sacked a sport psychologist because she believed that the psychologist was not really in touch with the need to be competitive and to win. In her words, the psychologist was sympathetic to the individual concerns of the athletes but not empathetic to the needs of the team, the coach, or the sport. The business of winning is important at all levels of the sport, and the team psychologist must be very sensitive to the need to align with that focus.

7. Preparing for the Worst

It has been my experience that the value of the team psychologist is most often judged by the coaches and ultimately the athletes on the outcomes of the most serious situations (critical interventions) that occur on tour. For example, the psychologist may present excellent preventative/education workshops on tour and have interesting and informative performance-enhancement discussions with coaches and athletes, and these will contribute to an overall team view of the psychologist's contribution. The psychologist may be regarded as a "good" member of the team if he or she interacts well at the interpersonal level with team staff and athletes (the practical, witty, "good" personality vote). However, the psychologist must be able to provide more than this to ultimately gain the final seal of approval/acceptance and professional respect. The team psychologist must be able to be effective in the most difficult crises in assisting the athlete or coach to get back on track or to return to optimal functioning. In cases of serious misconduct, significant interpersonal conflict, serious emotional disturbance, poor early competition form, injury and illness, loss of confidence, etc., the psychologist must be an effective contributor. Experience over the past 20 years of international and domestic touring with teams reinforces the decision taken by the sport psychology community in Australia that all sport psychologists must be legally registered (licensed) psychologists in addition to the more usual sports sciences and specific sport psychology training. We must prepare ourselves to contribute effectively in the most difficult situations. These often occur in close proximity to important competitions when there is considerable pressure for a timely resolution.

I clearly remember a situation from the 1997 rowing tour in which a rower from a quad scull experienced a "breakdown" to the extent that the team doctor prescribed a sedative medication, ordered a blood profile test, and recommended several days away from training. This occurred in the week leading into a major international regatta. Naturally, the coach was extremely concerned for the individual and the impact that this exclusion from training was having on the remaining three crew members. I was asked by the head coach to intervene in what had initially been seen and treated as a "medical" issue. My objective was to get the rower back into the boat so that the crew could finalize their last few days of preparation. In consultation with the head coach, crew coach, and team doctor, it

was decided to take the rower off the sedative drug (the blood profile was normal) and to replace the medication with other forms of relaxation and stress management, some refocusing techniques, and crew and coach support. This was a short-term approach based on the requirement for the crew not only to compete, but also to finish in a reasonable position in the final as part of a confidence-enhancing lead-up to the World Championships several weeks later in the tour. I felt that it was not the time to undertake a comprehensive assessment of the complexities that might have led to the intense fear of failure that I anticipated had led to the breakdown. That would have to wait until a more appropriate time. Two years later, the short-term resolution of that crisis is still talked about amongst the coaches. The importance of having a team psychologist on tour was further strengthened.

8. Confidentiality

Athlete/client confidentiality must be preserved for the intimate detail of personal/clinical interventions, but the culture of elite international teams will recognize and require/demand that more general and performance-enhancement psychological information that is directly relevant to crew/athlete/team performance be shared with the relevant coach. Given the performance-based nature of coaching appointments and the coaches' reliance upon successful performance outcomes for continuation of their career and the livelihood of their families, it is imperative that they be informed on a need-to-know and professional confidence basis about issues that affect performance. For example, an athlete who consults the team psychologist while on tour concerning the presence of significant depression should expect normal confidentiality with regard to the finer detail of the factors contributing to and enhancing the depressed mood state. However, a failure on the part of the team psychologist and athlete to inform the coach and medical staff about a confounding emotional issue that might adversely affect performance would more than likely lead to further problems for the athlete. For example, the coach might not see the need to adjust training loads or to compensate for the emotional state. Perhaps the coach would understandably be sensitive to the fact that the team psychologist did not indicate that there was anything deserving special consideration or additional involvement of the multidisciplinary support team. Normally, one would expect or encourage the athlete to discuss the issue with the coach, but there may be occasions where the athlete might prefer the team psychologist to act as an intermediary.

9. Time and Energy Commitment

In accepting a national team appointment, the psychologist must be prepared to make the necessary time and energy commitment. Psychologists do not necessarily need large amounts of expensive equipment, but we do require ongoing access to our client group; we must be there as it happens. Given the establishment of an effective role within the team, this may require the psychologist being available for consultation and team involvement across varied and, at times, "abnormal" time periods. This applies to availability for team competition travel and while on travel to be available essentially 7 days per week and 24 hours each day. Time commitment for the psychologist is partly a function of the team competition and training calendar, team size, and the agreed roles for the psychologist. It is also partly a function of the psychologist's personal and employment situation. In the rarified atmosphere of elite sport and in supporting the athlete and coach in striving for excellence

in international competition, the psychologist will be expected to make similar personal sacrifices for the athlete and coach. We can never underestimate the seemingly obsessive-compulsive nature of the constant drive towards world-best sporting results. It has been previously proposed that the work of the team psychologist should be complete before the competition takes place and that there is no place for a sport psychologist at the competition. This type of view is usually proposed by those psychologists who either are supreme idealists or are completely ignorant of the psychological demands on the athletes and coaches at major competitions. Perhaps these psychologists are not confident in their own ability to perform effectively at the "front line" when it really counts. It has been my very clear experience that there is a huge role for the team psychologist at every stage of the competition calendar. This is just as true for the "physiological" sports such as rowing and endurance events as it is for other sports that are commonly described as the "mental" sports (such as golf). This type of view is sometimes proposed by some sporting officials who are looking for an excuse to save money on team travel, or who feel that other professionals (interestingly it is usually another medical acquaintance) should take up the available team accreditation. As psychologists, we should be available to the athletes and coaches when they are under the greatest stress. Twenty years' experience has convinced me that the highest levels of athlete and coach stress occur in the final lead-up to and during major international competitions. Would sporting administrators or sports medicine officials consider not including team coaches at a World Championships or Olympics on the basis that they should have completed their preparation work before the event takes place?

10. The Breadth of Commitment Required

The psychologist must be prepared to be involved in a range of nonpsychologist activities as part of the overall commitment to the team. For example, the rowing team psychologist sometimes acts as a coaching boat driver, race segment timer, videotape operator, boat loader, assistant manager, social director, etc. These team-related activities normally would not compromise the quality or frequency of athlete consultations, but do assist in effective team functioning and in team networking. It is always interesting to observe just how often effective interactions and even subtle therapy can occur during these "nonpsychological" involvements. The team psychologist must be vigilant, however, in not using these nonpsychologist activities in place of the effectiveness of professional service provision as the main means to gaining approval from the team. Whilst on the subject of "immersion" in team activities, it is worth emphasizing that the team psychologist should commit to wearing team issue clothing as often as is possible. It is not advisable to wear team clothing from other sports, clothing from nonteam sponsors, or indeed to refer too often to experiences with other sports. My experience with international teams has been that they seek evidence of a strong commitment to the sport and the team on the part of all team staff. Clothing is a small but important part of the issue. As psychologists who might provide services to other teams as well (for example, if employed in a sports institute environment), we must remember that the coaches and athletes are committed to and focused single-mindedly on their sport and their sport alone, and they expect us to be the same.

11. Planned Obsolescence

The psychologist, like the effective coach, must ideally work towards becoming obsolete in the long term. It is probably true to state that some professionals create work for themselves as a form of justification for their position on a team, or simply because their ego feels stronger if they are heavily and constantly involved. Sometimes it is the case that the normally busy professional feels guilty because he or she has quiet or inactive periods on tour. This might occur because the psychologist has done an excellent job in the early stages of a tour, or perhaps it is a function of an effective and well-managed team. There is a delicate balance between being too entrepreneurial and not being proactive enough. Notwithstanding this, it is my view that in an ideal situation, we should ultimately be aiming for obsolescence, just as the coach and athlete aim for perfection (but rarely achieve it). We should be focused on assisting the athlete to become functionally independent in the sporting environment. With this approach in mind, the team psychologist is unlikely to become a crutch for athletes or coaches. Creating dependency and indispensability will, in all certainty, tarnish the respectability and effectiveness of the psychologist. A positive team evaluation based on professional competence is in the final analysis the most satisfying feedback.

12. Maintaining a Professional Relationship

The team psychologist must constantly monitor the basis of his professional relationship with athletes and coaches. It is easy to unknowingly permit social relationships to develop with coaches and athletes that will ultimately prejudice the effectiveness of the professional relationship. The delicacy of the balance between professionalism and friendship cannot be overestimated. This is particularly true in respect of the relationship between psychologist and athlete, but particular attention should also be given to the psychologist-coach relationship. My experience has been that coach acceptance of the consultant as a professional is critical to the psychologist's effectiveness with that coach's athletes. It is a bonus if the coach actually "likes" the psychologist, but this may not necessarily translate to the need for the psychologist and coach to be social friends. While on tour, I will join the coaches for a drink in the late evening, not necessarily for the purpose of cementing or developing a friendship, but as a means to furthering the goals of the psychology service provision program and the team in a relaxed social atmosphere. There have probably been many important breakthroughs with coaches and vice versa made subtly over dinner, a quiet beer, or a glass of wine.

13. The Learning Curve

The psychologist must be prepared to learn the sport (basic physiology, biomechanics, sports medicine, nutrition, nature of injuries, etc.), its selection policies, and the culture of the sport. For example, the psychologist must interact constantly with the individual coaches in order to understand their personal and coaching philosophies. Without specific knowledge of the sport, the psychologist cannot conduct a proper needs analysis or effectively implement performance-enhancement training. In rowing, for example, attentional focusing is dependent on specific knowledge of the structure of the rowing stroke or segmented race plan. Without a clear understanding of the crew coach's training and competition approach, it would be extremely difficult to provide effective sport psychology services. This principle is not to be confused with usurping the coach's role. The psychologist must be very wary of encroaching upon the coaching domain. All team staff are highly motivated to assist the athletes in any way possible, and it is all too easy for a team psychologist to make the mistake of offering technical coaching advice (particu-

larly after having worked with a team for several years and thus gaining a very good understanding of the sport). I know of one sport psychologist who worked on the professional tennis circuit dressed in a tennis outfit with a tennis racquet in hand. This person was even observed out on the court, racquet in hand, while the player and coach were practicing. In my opinion, this type of image is not the one a psychologist should be portraying to coaches or athletes.

14. Inclusiveness

The psychologist must wherever possible include the crew coach in the conduct of performance-enhancement sessions. For example, the crew coach will have more precise technical information for input into relaxation/energizing/imagery sessions. Most of the coaches on the Australian rowing team are happy to and want to be involved in technique, race simulation, and crew-culture imagery sessions. In many cases, the psychologist implements the relaxation sequence and sets the context for the imagery session. The crew coach then delivers the technical or race plan information with the psychologist calling the split times. The psychologist completes the session with a summary and energizer routine. In coxed boats, the coxswain may deliver the race calls according to the appropriate time/segment splits. Some coaches, however, prefer the psychologist to provide the agreed technical input on the basis that they sometimes do not feel confident in doing this as well as the "specialist," or alternatively, they prefer that the athletes hear a different voice (presumably with enhanced impact)

15. Seizing the Moment

The touring psychologist must adopt an opportunistic approach to consultations. One great advantage in touring with a team is the ongoing contact that is possible with the coaches and athletes. This contact provides a wide variety of consultation opportunities and, in many cases, opportunities that are ideal for timely reinforcement, suggestion, or implementation of change strategies. It is not always possible for the team psychologist to have a single room in the team hotel that can double as a consulting room. It may not be possible for the psychologist to have access to any other formal location for consultations. Team finances, competition organizing committee policies, etc. might mean that the psychologist has to share a room with coaching staff or other team staff. This does not mean that effective consultations are impossible. The training/competition venue, transportation to and from venues, meal times, and the casual contact in the laundry all provide such opportunities. The team psychologist must be flexible in these matters and quick to seize on any opportunity for input.

16. The "Hard Yards"

The new touring psychologist should not expect that the image of international "jet setting" held by the normal population to necessarily be true for sporting team travel. Australian national sporting teams usually experience significant budgetary restrictions. Air travel is often via the cheapest seats available and the cheapest routes/airlines available. Seat allocations are made on a group rather than individual basis. Hotel accommodation will be budget level rather than five-star. Food will tend towards the bland rather than exotic, high-energy style, and sharing of accommodation is common. The hours are long, and the work is tiring, and while the psychologist is away, the work at the home office piles up. There is little, if any, chance for time off or investigating any of the tourist attractions while on tour. The team usually only sees the inside of the hotel and the scenery between the hotel and training/competition venue. On government-funded tours (as in Australia), it is not possible for employees to take recreation leave at the end of the tour, so one usually returns home quite exhausted.

In spite of the above, I have found touring with international teams to be very stimulating and satisfying. The competition is intense, the stakes are high, the coaches and team staff are intensely committed, and the athletes are highly trained and prepared. To be part of a professional environment where the objective is to be the best in the world and to squeeze out the last vital percentage point in a performance are positive, challenging, and exciting for a team psychologist.

Summary

My recommendation is that aspiring team psychologists develop their own set of guiding professional practice principles as they might apply in a specific team touring situation. Based on these guidelines or principles, a multifaceted program that attends to the complex needs of elite athletes and coaches can be devised. Implementation whilst on tour or during the preparation phases is part art and part science. Some aspects of implementation cannot be easily learned from the textbook or in a classroom. Sometimes we simply "fly by the seat of our pants." The team psychologist should not expect formal or public acknowledgment for his or her contribution. Rather, as a member of a helping profession, we should receive satisfaction in seeing athletes and coaches successfully apply the skills and strategies we have recommended and facilitated in the high-pressure competitive environment that typifies elite international sport. It is not our job to create champions; rather we should be contributing to an environment in which champions are inevitable.

Sport Psychology Practice in Two Cultures: Similarities and Differences

Boris Blumenstein

In this chapter, I describe my work as a sport psychology consultant in two different countries: the former USSR and Israel. I share my approach, and by doing so, I outline the difficulties and successes that I have experienced in my work.

The model that guides this presentation consists of three main stages, starting with personality evaluation and sport-specific knowledge base, through diagnosing precompetition regulation of arousal and emotion, up to the current self-regulation of performance in competition utilizing biofeedback technologies (see Figure 1). Next, I describe these stages of development in detail.

My "Soviet Area": From Personality Profiles to Prestart Regulation

At the outset, similar to many other sport psychologists in the former Eastern bloc, I provided athletes with personality inventories, such as 16PF, MMPI, STAI, and the like, in order to produce "personality profiles." The idea behind this procedure was to identify general personality dispositions that can be found in all (or at least most) elite athletes. For example, Milman (1983) found that elite athletes from a variety of sport disciplines share a unique C, E, H, and Q_3 characteristics in the 16PF inventory. They were

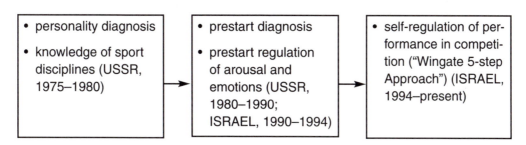

Figure 1.
Stages of my personal development: Specific issues within periods.

found to be more stable, dominant, active, and self-controlled in comparison to nonelite athletes. However, the predictive power of these tests (i.e., in relation to actual behavior) was quite low. Therefore, to improve our ability to make reasonable recommendations to coaches and athletes, we realized that it was necessary to take into account the athlete's sport-specific "environment." We found out that only through the knowledge of "persons in situations" (i.e., athletes with particular personalities participating in specific sports) was a reasonable prediction possible. As a result, we attempted to apply specific psychological tests, such as CSAI, CSAI-2, SCAT, and Milman (1983) SPD (which is a sport-personality test developed in the USSR). For example, the Milman SPD scales indicated that athletic motivation, emotional stability in competition, self-regulation, and confidence were crucial in determining athletes' performances. In addition, that test revealed stress-related factors that distract the

athlete, such as the significance of competition to the athlete and the perceived uncertainty of the outcome. This approach resulted in a series of sport-specific profiles, which included general as well as specific personality dispositions. We designed tests and norms that typically characterized each group of sport disciplines (i.e., combat sports, ball games, speed-power sport disciplines, sprinting, jumping, etc.). These tests and norms were determined by diagnosing the best athletes in each discipline in the USSR (i.e., many Olympic, World, European, and Soviet champions).

The next stage in my "Soviet" period was characterized by "individual regulation styles." Here, we tried to identify individual athletes' styles of self-regulation (e.g., "continuous" vs. "explosive") and cognitive functioning (e.g., orientation of attention—internal vs. external). In this way, we substantially improved our predictions as well as our communication with the coaches out of and in

Table 1. Examples of Personality Profiles of Elite Athletes in Different Sports.

		PROFILES	
Sport discipline	**General**	**Specific**	**Individual regulation styles**
• combat sport: wrestling, boxing, judo, fencing	stable, dominant	high sport motivation high self-regulation	continuous style with external orientation of attention
• ball games: soccer basketball	anxiety not stable extroversion	high sport motivation low self-regulation	explosive style with external orientation of attention
• speed-power sports: sprinting, jumping	stable dominant	high sport motivation low emotional stability	explosive style with internal orientation of attention
weight-lifting	introversion dominant	low emotional stability high sport motivation	explosive style with internal orientation of attention
• aerobic sport: long distance running, swimming	stable high self-control	high emotional stability high sport motivation	continuous style with internal orientation of attention

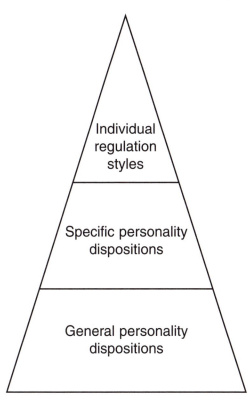

Figure 2.
Hierarchy of athletes' personality characteristics: From the general to the specific.

competition. The first stage in Figure 1 is summarized in Figure 2. It presents in the form of a pyramid the hierarchical nature of the abovementioned development over this period (1975–1980). To illustrate this approach, a list of sport disciplines, profiles, and recommendations is presented in Table 1.

I remember my first official meeting with the chief track and field national coach, who, after speaking with me briefly, permitted me to work with his team (jumping-throwing) at their training camp, which was isolated in a forest, for 3 to 4 weeks of training. There were 2–3 training sessions a day. That afternoon, I entered a room where there were five women seated, fatigued after a hard training session. They were specialists in throwing (discus). The height of these women was between 195 and 200cm and their weight between 100 and 115 kg; my 165cm height was much shorter. I asked them to answer several questionnaires. They were disciplined athletes, and they agreed; I received their completed questionnaires before supper. Throughout the night, I worked on their responses, and in the morning, my recommendations were ready. Before breakfast, I met with the coach, and from our conversation, I learned that he already knew his athletes from his own observations more than the information revealed to me from their questionnaires. The reaction of the athletes was different: They couldn't understand how I was able to recognize certain information about each athlete, and they were surprised at how good I was at understanding sport (they perceived my recommendations as very relevant).

When I asked top athletes and coaches from different sports about their feelings during their successful performances in the Olympic, European, and world events, I realized that the overwhelming majority perceived the competitions as easy; they weren't worried, were concentrated, and were very confident. Moreover, several coaches said that although sometimes they made corrections in the athletes' techniques during competitive stress, it did not always help; apparently, in elite sport, where individual technique is usually stable, there seems to be more of a mental problem than a technical one. Consequently, I learned that an attempt should be made to change and optimize the athlete's mental state before and during competition. I concluded that more attention should be given to diagnostic methods and regulation of the athlete's prestart state in sport disciplines such as track and field, wrestling, soccer, hockey, tennis, sailing, and windsurfing. In these sports, we also measured psychophysiological components, such as HR, GSR, EMG, and respiratory rate and volume, and worked out a cognitive plan as well as self-talk during competition.

From USSR to Israel: Diagnosis and Regulation of Prestart States

In the USSR, I was already aware of the limitations of the "personality profiles" approach, be it general, specific, or individual. For example, this approach enables the sport psychologist to provide recommendations, but does not permit efficient integration of such knowledge into the training process. As a result, I was convinced that athletes must learn to regulate their mental state through psychoregulation methods, and this can be an advantage if they can observe their daily improvement in controlling their mental states. Athletes who are good at mental skills can feel the relaxation states and quickly shift from calm and relaxed states to excitation and vice versa, and they have a clear mind and good concentration; however, in imagery or simulation training, they can be easily activated into training or competition situations. These two different feelings are very clear and under control. For example, many times, after our mental training sessions, athletes

told me, "I remember my best mental state before the competition starts, and I knew what I should do to maintain it. I can regulate it quickly, and I had confidence to apply it under different competitive conditions."

The prestart diagnosis of athletes focused on their motivational state, goals set, and arousal level, as well as on cognitive aspects such as concentration, attention, and focusing. To conduct this diagnosis, we used psychophysiological and/or psychomotor tests and indices, such as reaction time (simple, choice, discrimination, anticipation), physiological measures HR, GSR, EMG, time reproduction, rhythm perception with tapping test, and others.

In general, I believe that the optimal arousal required for maximal performance depends not only on the athlete's personality, but also on the demands of the task to be performed (i.e., the characteristics of the sport discipline) and on the environment or situation in which it is performed. In other words, I became a "transactionalist", even though I didn't realize it at the time; it was only the most practical way. The relationship among these three major classes of performance determinants is illustrated in Figure 3.

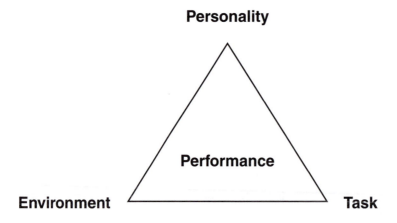

Figure 3.
Performance determinants: A transactional approach to practice.

It should be noted that in the beginning, I applied this basic conception for diagnosing and regulating prestart states; later, however, I also adapted it for conceptualizing self-regulation of performance during competition within the framework of the five-step approach (discussed later).

To illustrate this approach, let me present the following example, applicable to combat sports such as wrestling (an extremely high-level sport in the former USSR). In this sport discipline, prestart state is a period starting from about one week before the competition. This period is usually characterized by a decrease in training load; simultaneously, wrestlers usually feel an increased tension due to the approaching competition and the relatively greater amount of spare time. Thus, I usually filled in the free time of the athletes by strengthening their mental recovery processes and self-confidence towards the upcoming contest. This was done by diagnosing their mental state (using measures such as reaction time—simple, choice, discrimination, anticipation—and time reproduction) in reference to preexisting norms based on tests conducted on hundreds of elite athletes, and using mental techniques such as Jacobson's progressive muscular relaxation, Schultz's autogenic training, and the Alekseev modification-psychomuscular training, and imagery incorporated with music.

For example, a typical well-prepared wrestler in this prestart stage should demonstrate a reaction time (RT) in 15 trials, simple RT—155–160 msec x±10; 2 choices RT in 30 trials—175–180 msec x±10; Discrimination RT in 30 trials (2 stimuli; 1 response)—170–175 msec x±10, and Time reproduction 5sec in 10 trials between 4.90—5.10 sec, etc. Such results would reflect an appropriate mental state, which would provide the wrestler with positive feedback and enhanced self-confidence. In case of an inappropriate state, there is still sufficient time to conduct the necessary corrections. Before traveling to an important competition, such as the Olympic games or World or European championships, top athletes were taken to events presented by the USSR's top entertainment artists (i.e., musicians, pop singers, standup comics, etc.). The artists themselves considered their own participation in such events as a great honor; but even more important, they had a highly positive effect on the athletes' mental state.

During the trip to the contest location (by car, bus, train, or airplane), usually about 2 to 3 days before the start of the competition, wrestlers were kept busy and relaxed by listening to their favorite music, reading books, playing portable games, and engaging in other activities.

The wrestlers were placed in hotel rooms according to their own preferences. Activities during the 2 to 3 days that preceded the competition start included not only training, but also recreational walks through the city. Such walks not only had the function of distracting the athletes from unnecessary tension, but also of getting them physically tired (i.e., to facilitate their night's sleep).

On the night before the competition, I stayed awake until I was completely certain that all the wrestlers were asleep. During the day of competition, I helped the wrestlers increase their concentration and self-confidence during the warm-up. The warm-up was concluded by conducting four imagery fragments: (a) entering the competition hall, (b) standing next to the mattress (reproduce tactical plan), (c) standing on the mattress (concentrating, aggressive), and (d) beginning the match. If, as a result of this process, the wrestler was not in an optimal arousal state (i.e., 8–15 kohm, according to the national USSR wrestlers' GSR norms), other mental preparation techniques were used, such as showing short, concise previously prepared videotapes (which included, for example, the athlete's family members talking to him or her about the upcoming competition), or coaches' or teammates' assertive verbal interventions. It should be noted that after the competition, I insisted on the athletes' achieving mental recovery, which is highly important for future events. It is evident that a similar pattern of prestart preparation was used not only with wrestlers, but also with athletes in other sport disciplines (and included all required sport-specific modifications).

From my experience, cooperation with coaches is extremely important. In the USSR, coaches were highly powerful in the training process; they were completely professional in their sport, and were highly knowledge-able in different sport sciences, such as bio-mechanics, physiology, and theory and methods of sport training. However, they often argued that psychological preparation should follow general training preparation, and they did not understand many of the psychological terms. In general, they always started from principles such as periodization, loads, performance, and recovery; if the sport psychological consultant did not understand sport or athletic performance, the coaches immediately stopped any contact with him or her. Sometimes, mental preparation was neglected entirely; coaches did not always like or want any cooperation with sport psychological consultants. Moreover, if one trained many athletes, one always could select the best, that is, the ones with "a strong character and will-power" (as coaches used to say), and not be afraid to lose one or two weaker ones.

My Israel Experiences: The Wingate 5-Step Approach

In 1990, I immigrated to Israel and confronted several problems (in addition to language). Israel is a small country that was at that time in the initial stages of the development of elite sport (for example, the first two—out of a total of three—Olympic medals were won only in 1992). Sport in Israel was characterized by unique problems such as the absence of large numbers of elite athletes, numerous trips abroad (there was no strong competition in the country itself), low levels of competition in training (because of the small number of athletes), and very hot climatic conditions most of the year. As opposed to the USSR, I had to adapt to working with athletes from different sports, instead of concentrating mainly on many athletes from few sport disciplines.

I started to work with wrestlers (most of them new immigrants from the former USSR; therefore, I could cope with the language better because we spoke Russian). However, after 4 to 5 months, I started giving sport psychological consultations with elite athletes from other sports as well. They understood my "international" language very quickly: the language of psychological preparation for elite sport. Currently, 95% of my athletes are native Israelis, talented young people trying to achieve high sport results. I have met with high-level experts in the area of sport psychology, and I have taken part in several research projects in which my practical East European experience was combined with modern Western research technologies. Our research team at the Wingate Institute has conducted several high-level research projects with biofeedback (BFB) treatments used for mental preparation of athletes; these projects were concluded by the development of the Wingate 5-Step Approach, a mental preparation technique that includes a self-regulation test with BFB apparatus.

More specifically, this mental training program consists of five steps, three conducted in laboratory settings and two under training and competition conditions. In addition to the BFB apparatus, today we use VCR and a video camera (for double-feedback system). The main idea of the five-step approach is to learn various self-regulation techniques to identify and strengthen the athletes' psychoregulation style, not only in the laboratory, but also under training and competition situations, and to obtain optimal regulation in competitive situations. The technique consists of five stages, with flexible time-session limits that can be individualized: (a) introducing mental techniques, (b) determining and strengthening the appropriate BFB modality, (c) BFB training with simulated competitive stress, (d) transforming the mental training to practice, and (e) realizing the technique in competitive situations. A schematic description of the five-step approach appears in Figure 4.

All mental training processes include approximately 75–90 sessions, each of which lasts 40–45 minutes, 2–3 times a week. Before and between each step of the program, the athlete undergoes a self-regulation test (SRT) to indicate his or her individual responses. After recording the athlete's psychophysiological baseline (HR, GSR, EMG) in the laboratory setting, the athlete is asked to imagine him- or herself in resting, tense, and warm states and in a competition situation. Toward the end of each of these imagery phases, each lasting about 2 minutes, the athlete's psychophysiological responses (HR, GSR, EMG) are recorded, in order to indicate the type of alteration in each response modality, as well as its relative intensity.

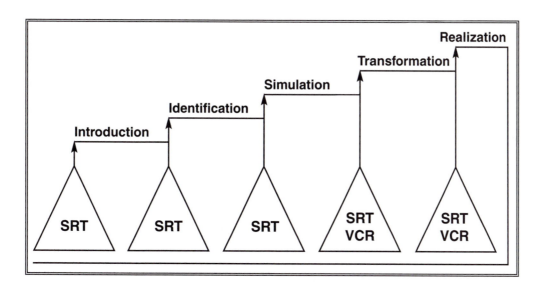

Purpose

Learn self regulation techniques	Identify & strengthen BFB responses	BFB training + simulative stress	Transform from lab to field setting	Attain optimal self regulation in competitions

Location

Laboratory	Laboratory	Laboratory	Field	Competition

Figure 4.
A schematic description of the Wingate 5-Step Approach.

We have carried out several mental programs based on the five-step approach. Each is adapted to the requirements of sports such as swimming (children 12–16 years), sailing, windsurfing, canoeing/kayaking, judo, wrestling, shooting, and taekwondo. We are currently working with soccer and basketball players, and we have developed a series of mental exercises to be performed at home with a portable BFB system, as well as mental exercises with BFB for training and competition that can be used in different situations, such as at sea (on a boat) or in a hall during precompetition preparation and/or between races or matches.

The BFB apparatus enables an athlete to observe his or her positive self-regulation changes and individual improvements in confidence, because it is the athlete's own mental performance that can be seen and felt. In the five-step approach, well-established East European sport psychological experience and Western research technology are integrated. Moreover, in this approach, we simultaneously utilize and combine general (step 1) and specific (steps 2–5) mental training, which evolves from the laboratory conditions to the real world (competitive situations, steps 4–5).

We use the BFB system not only for mental preparation but also for mental recovery. For example, to facilitate facial self-regulation, we carry out a double-biofeedback system with a video camera with which we film athletes' facial expressions. This is crucial not only for the athlete to better control emotional states through regulation of facial expression during competition, but also for competitive purposes, for instance, to deceive the athlete's rival. Moreover, each specific five-step program includes mental homework exercises with a portable GSR-EMG BFB.

To illustrate my experiences using the Wingate 5-Step Approach in different settings, I will present some examples taken from different sport disciplines; each corresponds to a different aspect of the program.

Example 1—Application of the 5-step approach during prestart phase—entire 1-week program. In the following, an example of an approximate precompetition weekly mental training program applied to elite Israeli combat sport athletes is presented, based on steps 4 and 5 of the entire program.

Saturday— Extended relaxation with music accompanied by portable GSR modalities—15 min (homework)

Sunday— Concentration exercises in warm-up with portable EMG-GSR$_{BFB}$ + IM (imagery-excitation & concentration)—1–2 times × 2–3 min

Muscle relaxation and rest between fights —2–3 min

Brief relaxation after training—5 min with portable GSR$_{BFB}$

Monday— Homework with portable GSR$_{BFB}$ and videotapes with competition fights—3–4 times × 5–10 min

Tuesday— Relaxation + Imagery (excitation part) with concentration on concrete competition fight and next relaxation (EMG 0.8–0.9$\gamma\eta$V)

1 × 5 min

1 × 3 min

1 × 1 min ("double feedback")

Mental recovery after training (group)

10–15 min with portable GSR$_{BFB}$

Wednesday— Concentration exercises

1–2 times × 2–3 min

Imagery with portable GSR$_{BFB}$ before fights

2–3 times × 1 min

Relaxation with portable GSR$_{BFB}$

5–10 min

Thursday— BF training with GSR—relaxation-excitation (IM—different competition fragments)

2 times × 5 min

Competition fight—4 IM fragments with GSR:

a) Exit to competition hall
b) I see my opponent (tactical plan)
c) On mattress (concentrate, aggressive)
d) Match (tempo, movement)

3 times × 3 min (with different opponents)

Brief relaxation after training with portable EMG—GSR$_{BFB}$—5 min

Friday— BF training with GSR relaxation-excitation waves

2 times × 1 min

2 times × 2 min

2 times × 3 min

Mental recovery after training EMG-GSR$_{BFB}$—10–15 min

Example 2—Application of the five-step approach during prestart in contest. At the last European taekwondo championship, we waited for our competition matches from 9AM to 5PM. While waiting, we used different BFB exercises, mainly GSR and EMG modalities and mental games with several of the athletes, for optimal regulation in concrete situations. The athletes noted that they had a good mental state during the competition day, an excellent ability to regulate their attention and thoughts from external factors into relevant ones, and a high level of confidence during competition. An athlete can continuously control these states and modify them quickly and accurately. In one of the breaks in competition, one of them said to me, "Boris, don't worry. Today I'm strong. Our BFB test agreed with me."

Example 3—Application of the five-step approach on court during competition. In the last rifle-shooting world cup games, one of Israel's best athletes built his mental performance plan with a time limitation of 28 to 30 seconds, in the following order: (a) concentration and regulation of breathing rhythm, (b) muscle control, (c) direction-correction in line with wind conditions, and (d) firing and shooting.

The rifle-shooter developed this specific order together with me and underwent intensive training of this entire program using the five-step approach in my laboratory. After achieving an extremely successful result (far beyond prior expectations), he indicated to me that a substantial part of his success should be attributed to the fact that for the first time in his career, he was able to accurately regulate his arousal state.

Example 4—Postcompetition recovery using the five-step approach. After wind-surfing races, the athlete—one of the world's best—used to regularly recover by applying portable GSR biofeedback. In addition, one of the computerized elements of the program was used in the boat to achieve an immediate relaxation state, which is essential for efficient recovery. Interestingly enough, other competitors were intrigued by the "funny" apparatus and asked if they could "make an attempt" on this apparatus, which caused a "traffic jam" in the sea. This response made me think seriously about the possibility of establishing a "mental preparation recovery center" in elite athletic contests.

Summary and Conclusions

In this chapter, I have described my work as an applied, practicing sport psychologist in the USSR and Israel. Based on my experience with elite athletes from two different countries, I would like to propose the following common principles:

- It is necessary to thoroughly know and understand sport, including the specific conditions and requirements of each sport discipline.

- It is important to account for athlete's individual peculiarities, including his or her psychophysiological states under different training and competition situations.
- It is often more important to regulate athletes' mental states than to modify their technical parameters, especially in competition.
- We usually apply the same psychological techniques in different countries. It is important to account for cultural differences, various national traditions, and particular sport developments in different countries.

In my opinion, the practicing sport psychologist should always be aware of his or her role as the coaches' and athletes' *helper*; the sport psychologist is never a replacement for a coach or for an athlete's physical or technical-tactical training. We are one team; any medals or victories are first the athlete's and his or her coach's victory; I work for them, not the opposite. At the same time, in case of defeat, I accept the possibility that it may be my failure, because the coach or athlete may complain about low mental readiness, which lies in my own professional area, and for which I should consider taking responsibility.

I am currently working with many athletes from various sports, over long periods, and I am very glad if I can help them in any way. I am sure that after another 25 years of practicing sport psychology, I will have new experiences to tell and lessons to share, and many of the above mentioned basic principles will still be valid for future generations of coaches, athletes and sport psychologists.

Reference

Milman, V.E. (1983). Stress and personality constructs in the control of sports activity. In: Y. Hanin (Ed.), *Stress and anxiety in sport.* Moscow: Physical Culture and Sport Publishers.

Consulting With the Equestrian: The Unique Challenges of Working With the Horse and Rider Team

Grace M. H. Pretty

Abstract

The sport psychologist confronts special challenges when working with the equestrian because of the additional dynamic of the horse and rider relationship. This paper describes some of the mental problems that riders face when working toward a more effective partnership with their horses. Fundamental information is presented to assist the psychologist in understanding the nature of horse and human relationships and how this affects the rider's physical and mental skills in training and competition. Cases illustrate various assessment and intervention strategies that incorporate the psychology of the horse and rider dyad in attaining better performance outcomes.

Tom, a coach, thought Paul had lost his nerve for cross-country competition. As a result, Paul's new horse was not performing as well as it could.

Susan complained that no matter what strategies she tried, her horse knocked rails in triple combination jumps. Susan was starting to get tense approaching them and was losing confidence in her show jumping.

Jamie, a dressage rider, and Mitchel, her coach, could not understand why Jamie's horse had begun anticipating movements since they started competing at Prix St George level competitions. Jamie was losing patience, and her stress was affecting her concentration.

Most sport psychologists can readily identify the psychological aspects of these problems, that is, Paul's anxiety and fear, Susan's loss of confidence and concentration, and Jamie's performance stress. The sport psychologist can help the equestrian to resolve such mental aspects of his or her performance difficulties. However, as is evident in the above examples, it is often the horse that is identified by the rider as the source of the problems. Hence, some of the psychological problems riders experience arise out of unresolved issues between themselves and the horse. The interpersonal dynamics between horse and rider are not unlike those between athletes in other sports involving pair competitions, where one blames the other for hampering their performance. The sport psychologist can facilitate the resolution of such relationship issues. However, accomplishing this with the two members of an equestrian team takes some ingenuity. Although the horse attends to the rider's verbal and nonverbal communication, the horse does not respond using human language.

The sport psychologist must understand how the relationship between horse and rider is established through mutual sensitivity to messages transmitted by touch and feel, vocal utterances, and body gestures. The psychological state of the rider determines his or her behavior toward the horse, affecting the content and tone of the rider's messages to the horse. Similarly, the psychological state of the horse affects its behavior toward the rider. Hence, the mental condition of each member of the equestrian team inevitably affects the other's performance. In short, the rider's thoughts and feelings can either enhance or compromise the individual's riding technique. If the rider's communication with the horse, through use of the reins, leg, and seat, is not correct, precise, and consistent, the horse becomes confused and loses confidence. Its ability to do the job in the competition arena is then compromised because the horse is unsure of what is expected of him. Similarly, the state of anxiety or calmness in the horse can influence the rider's ability to use his or her skills effectively in training and competition. Anyone who has braved the occasional trail ride knows that horse-rider reactivity is reciprocal.

The challenge for the sport psychologist is that having a rider as a client effectively means having a horse as a client. Our psychological work to improve the riding skills of the human athlete will inevitably affect the equine athlete's performance. Ultimately, it is the horse's athleticism that defines success in the equestrian sport. Our goal is to help the rider develop and support his equine partner to perform consistently and reach his potential. Indeed, some equestrians go as far as to insist that the real athlete on the team is the horse and that the human is literally just along for the ride. Therefore, the sport psychologist's model of equestrian consultation must accommodate the psychology of the horse-rider relationship, even if one of the pair never sits, or stands, in the consulting room.

My experience has led me to the following conclusion. We cannot be effective with equestrians if we do not appreciate the psychological attributes of the equine athlete, as well as the human athlete. This is supported by other psychologists who have worked with equestrians, as well as by feedback from riders and their coaches that the psychologist's client is "the pair." Together, it is the combination of horse and rider's motivation, commitment, discipline, and trust that produces performance legends.

The purpose of this chapter is to present a model of equestrian consultation that appreciates the psychology of the horse and rider dyad and incorporates this dynamic in assessment and intervention methods. The chapter will be helpful particularly to those who have the opportunity to assist equestrians but have not had the pleasure and challenge of working with horses.

I begin by exploring the "intelligence" of the horse. This helps in appreciating just how sensitive he can be to the physical, cognitive, and affective dimensions of the rider's behavior. It is also central to understanding how the rider's problems in these areas can result in serious communication and relationship difficulties with the horse and undermine training and performance. Examples from cross-country, show jumping, and dressage riders will illustrate some of the psychological issues faced by equestrians. They will also indicate how sport psychologists can help to keep the mind and body of horse and rider working together in harmony.

A Little Horse Sense

Watching the precision of a show jumping duo, the elegance of the dressage pair, or the daring of a cross-country team, we see how much the horse and rider must be in sync for elite performance. The achievement of such exceptional teamwork is even more remarkable when we recognize that one member is an animal. Unfortunately, this is sometimes forgotten by the rider, who starts to react to and have expectations of the horse as if it were human. These expectations can then become a source of the rider's performance distress.

A survey of state-level cross-country and dressage competitors indicates how much riders endow their horses with human traits and abilities (Pretty, 2000). This is further illustrated in the comments made by the elite Australian equestrian Prue Barrett, who said of her horse, Wendela Jackamon, "He's a vain horse . . . he doesn't like to embarrass himself" (Holden Equestriad Series, 1998). Indeed, this kind of anthropomorphizing is well documented throughout centuries of literature that celebrated horses. It is understandable why riders develop these notions. Such feelings are inherent in attachment formed between long-time partners who share mutual commitment and trust. The use of humanized discourses is also the only way riders can express the characteristics of the relationship they have with their horse. However, although these human attributions serve to express the affection between horse and rider, they can become problematic when they are embraced as unchangeable "truths." They can become the basis for a rider's irrational reactions and expectations, and consequently result in disruptive emotional states while training and competing.

Equestrians often make attributions about their performances, both successes and failures, based on their "truths" about the states and traits of their horses. To understand which states and traits are and are not possible, I have found it useful to know some-

thing of how horses "perceive" human behavior and how they learn to respond to it in ways that affect the rider's performance objectives. The following case is an example.

John, a show jumper, was not performing as expected on a recently acquired horse. The young rider showed elite potential and had moved up a class beyond the physical capabilities of his older horse. This necessitated the acquisition of a new mount. The coach suspected the performance problems were caused by John's attitude. John always complained that the horse's refusals at the jumps and the knocked rails were the horse's fault. John insisted that he and the new horse had a mutual dislike. Although a simple solution might have been to find another horse for John, several coaches thought the pair well suited if they could learn to work together.

I found that, as is often the case in initial interviews with equestrians, John was determined that counseling him about his attitude would not result in either he or his horse improving their performance. Therefore, before assessing the psychological aspects of John's attitude problem, it was necessary to remind him of the connection between his mental state, his physical interaction with his horse, and the horse's performance response. This is where it is beneficial for the psychologist to have some knowledge of horse psychology and the physical mechanics and "feel" required for effective riding technique.

In this case, where the rider had a negative attitude about the horse, I started my assessment by asking John to describe how training sessions usually started, beginning with grooming and tacking up. I find that what happens between horse and rider when both are on the ground is a good predictor of what happens when the rider is in the saddle. John described problems starting in the stable and continuing when they got on the course. The horse threw its head and fidgeted while being groomed, tried to bite while being girthed, moved off while being mounted, and ran out on jumps at the slightest opportunity. John claimed that he had to keep anticipating the horse's behavior so he could discipline the mount at the slightest indication of disobedience. This vigilance was affecting John's ability to focus on the jumping course. He insisted that no matter what strategies he used, the horse would not be obedient for him.

This case illustrates a common pattern of complaints for equestrians: frustration from trying to change a horse's behavior and not getting results and losing confidence in the horse, in themselves as a rider, and in the team effort. This mental state then leads to poor performance and loss of previous training gains. When, as in this case, a coach insists the horse's problems are rooted in a rider's attitude, then the sport psychologist has to appreciate rider-horse relationship dynamics. This is essential in assessing the source of the problem and in planning interventions to change attitude, boost motivation, increase confidence, etc.

John needed to be reminded that his equine partner was a herd animal. Ethologists, researchers who study the social behavior of animals in their own natural habitats, say that horses' behavior toward humans is indicative of perceiving the human as a herd member (Kiley-Worthington, 1987). Horses are ever attentive to visual and auditory signals from herd members. They rely on such signals to tell them if they are safe or in impending danger. These signals are the basis of social communication within the herd. Hence, horses are attentive to human signals of safety or harm. Obviously, horses will not be obedient or perform well if they are "told" that they are in harm's way.

In John's case, it was necessary for him to understand that his horse could "perceive" that John did not "like" him. That is, the horse attended to the signals of dominance and threat that the rider was displaying. Research indicates that horses attend to and "read" human signals transmitting threat or friendship and learn to respond accordingly through classical conditioning (Fraser, 1992; Williams, 1976), for example, the pairing of an angry tone of voice with the use of a crop, or the grip on a rein with a bit tearing at the sensitive part of the mouth, or an aggressive stance (such as arms waving or marching into the horse's space), or while bridling in an aggressive way.

Horses communicate their response to threat by using physical gestures. An aggressive "I won't submit to you" response is indicated by pinning ears back, baring teeth, extending and swinging the neck, turning hind quarters, flicking the tail, and raising a hoof. Lowering the head below the withers indicates a compliant attitude. Although John knew all of this, he had not applied his knowledge to rationally analyzing the grooming and tacking misbehavior. For the psychologist, making sense of the horse-rider communication dynamics with the rider is no different than explaining to a marriage partner how his or her discontent is the result of how that person's behavior was perceived and responded to by the other partner, producing a cycle of offensive action and defensive reaction.

So, why don't equestrians who have much "horse sense" perceive the link between their behavior and that of their horse? We know as psychologists that when there is heightened emotional arousal, one's cognitive abilities to rationally examine the situation are decreased. With equestrians, because of their emotional connection to their horse, they sometimes cannot recognize that some of the horse's misbehavior is not "personal." Rather, the biting, kicking, and other "disobedience" are automatic responses that have evolved to help the horse survive threatening situations. The equestrian must appreciate how the rider is part of the environment and the circumstances within which the horse has learned to adapt and react. When a rider changes his or her behavior toward the horse, the horse will change its perceptions of the rider from being a threat to being a herd member who can be trusted. The horse then learns to relax around the rider and to attend to his job as an athletic team member.

Here, the sport psychologist is working with principles of learning. He or she explains how the rider's behavior, the result of the rider's thoughts and feelings, has established conditioned and habitual responses in his horse. Horses' "intelligence," defined as their ability to learn new tasks, has not been found to rank very high. They take many trials to learn experimental tasks and are poor at problem solving (McCall, 1990). However, horses are extremely adept at making associations; once they do learn something, they have exceptional memories; and they do "learn to learn." That is, they can generalize from one task to a similar one requiring the same strategies (Fiske, 1979). Hence, the rider working with a new horse should realize the importance of the "first impressions" the horse has of him or her and how these early associations of rider as "threat" or "trusted partner" will affect the horse's willingness to perform.

Although the notion that horses have "personalities" is questionable, there is no doubt that they have different temperaments related to their early imprinting and place in the pecking order of the herd (Budiansky, 1997; Kiley-Worthington, 1987). These experiences affect how they respond to dominance and submission signals from humans, whether they challenge these signals with "disobedience" or accept them with compliance. Under these circumstances, the human's dominant position is not guaranteed and is always up

for challenge. Resolution of a disagreement one week does not preempt another conflict the following week.

I am not suggesting here that the sport psychologist should be a horse psychologist in order to work with equestrians. Indeed, sport psychologists can consult with many talented horse trainers to assist in work with coaches and riders addressing discipline and behavior problems. Moreover, I am not suggesting that all behavior problems stem from how the client is interacting with the horse at the time, as many clients inherit previous owners' poor management. However, it is good for the sport psychologist to understand how a negative attitude between rider and horse can become a self-fulfilling prophecy of poor performance, as in human relationships, when assumptions, perceptions, and expectations are left unchallenged.

Getting the Mind and Body Together in the Saddle

The example of John focused on the importance of understanding the interaction between horse and rider on the ground. It illustrates how diagnosis of the rider's mental state begins with analyzing thoughts, feelings, and behavior associated with the horse while out of the saddle. Next, we consider how the behavioral mechanics of riding techniques are linked closely to the rider's cognitions and subsequent emotive states.

When an observer watches an elite dressage rider, it appears as if the horse "knows" what to do and as if the rider is just sitting there. In fact, the rider is in constant contact with the horse. She directs him through use of what are called riding "aids": slight hand movements adjusting the reins, subtle leg and foot adjustments positioning them in relation to the girth, and fine modifications of the placement of seat bones, shifting position and balance in the saddle. It is this complex combination of hand, leg, and seat aids that guide a horse through intricate dressage movements, direct a horse through difficult show jumping courses, and pace a horse across demanding cross-country fields.

In brief, all aids must be precise and consistently used; they are the basis of the touch and feel communication system between horse and rider. The hands must be steady and "giving" to the horse's mouth; the legs must be precise in their position relative to the girth, and firm and consistent in pressure to the horse's side; the seat must balance the upper body and be positioned properly for the walk, trot, canter, and gallop paces and movements. The concern of the coach is the technical skill of the rider's hands, legs, and seat. The rider's mind, which I maintain should be considered the fourth riding aid, is the domain of the sport psychologist.

There comes a point in many riders' careers where mastery of these technical skills does not seem to be enough to progress to the next level of competition. There are times when the coach's instructions and the rider's own self-directives are not transmitted to the rider's mind to effect the required riding aids. The rider hears coaches' admonishments to loosen the reins, apply a stronger leg, look up over a jump, or relax the lower back, but something impedes the riding aid from being engaged. This is commonly referred to as a mental block, and it can cause talented horses and riders to be "put out to pasture" before reaching their potential. The sport psychologist can help the rider get past this block, and it helps to have an understanding of the connection between the rider's thoughts and feelings and the physical riding aids.

Many equestrians are acquainted with the psychological aspects of general performance issues such as motivation, goal setting, and performance anxiety. However, they are often unaware of how less obvious

obtrusive thoughts and feelings can influence their riding aids and, hence, their horses' performance.

To continue with John's case, in addition to his aggressive ground manner, he also had very aggressive riding aids. He pulled unnecessarily hard on the reins, used his spurs excessively, and sat heavily on the horse's back. The coach showed John videotapes of his jumping practices. From these, John started to recognize how hard he was being on the horse. Altering John's riding behavior required more than technical adjustments; it also required changing the cognitive and affective sources of his aggressiveness.

Through explanations using learning principles, John accepted the connection between his behavior and the horse's disobedience. We next discussed his feelings toward his new partner. Sometimes this meant using anthropomorphizing language to talk about the horse's psychology, his motivation and behavior, to cue John's own intuitive sense of his horse. A narrative approach to counseling, letting John tell his story of his horses, revealed that John was not convinced that it had been necessary to give up his long-time mount with whom he had had a rewarding relationship since pony club. He had misgivings about separating from his horse that had carried him up to the elite squad level. Because he attributed much of his success to his old horse's talent, he doubted whether he could make it to the next level of competition without his old partner. Further use of cognitive structuring techniques indicated that he had cognitively structured changing horses as abandoning his old faithful mate. This interpretation of events produced much guilt for him.

John's guilt culminated in anger, resentment, and self-doubt, all of which was displaced behaviorally onto the new horse. John communicated his anger and resentment to the horse through his behavior on the ground and in the saddle. The horse's reactions were understandable, as he was defending himself with instinctive behavioral responses to threat. These aggressive actions and reactions between rider and horse did not build the mutual trust and respect required to jump five-foot fences; nor did it facilitate John's riding skills.

When sitting in a consulting room, it is sometimes difficult to help a rider become conscious of how his or her body reacts to thoughts and feelings when the rider is in the saddle and, furthermore, how these impede riding technique. When possible, I work with the rider in the riding arena. Here I use body-focusing techniques to raise awareness of how the body is feeling, of what hand, leg, and seat aids are doing. If this is not possible, I use video-assisted imagery. The rider watches his or her performance to access thoughts, feelings, and physical memory of how the body felt riding the competition. Another technique that helps the rider's awareness is recalling earlier competitions when there was little performance pressure and competition was purely for fun or noncompetitive experiences such as having a relaxing ride in the country. In preparing for these sessions, it can be helpful if the client brings pictures of these events or of a favorite horse. Using physical memory to make comparisons of how the body felt when riding relaxed versus how it felt when riding with tension can raise the rider's sensitivity to the link between mental states and effective execution of riding aids. A review of these techniques can be found in a valuable sport psychology text by Edgette (1996).

In John's case, he felt differences in, for example, how tightly his hands gripped the reins, how relaxed his arms, shoulders, and back were, how confidently he applied pressure from his legs, and how deeply he sat in the saddle. He uncovered the tenseness in his body resulting from his anger and resentment about riding this horse and his lack of trust in this horse. He realized that as he rode with these thoughts and feelings, his body reacted accordingly with tight-fisted, un-giving hands, rigid arms and shoulders, and stiff posture. Psychologically and physically, John was positioned for a fight with his horse, and that is what he usually got. Watching videotapes together, we saw how his rigid riding aids prevented the horse from having adequate reach at the point of take-off and the proper balance to land safely. John's behavior was inhibiting this sensitive, well-schooled elite horse from jumping correctly and safely, so the horse was running out from the fences. An important point here is that the rider was unaware that his usual, competent jumping techniques were so compromised by his attitude toward the horse. The horse had been trying to "tell" him, by running out, that they were not in the correct position to manage the fences safely. The mistrust between rider and horse was mutual.

Once John experienced the relationship between his mental state and his partner's performance, he willingly engaged in the work necessary to change his attitude and improve their relationship. This required cognitively and emotionally letting go of his previous horse. We watched tapes of their competitions and acknowledged both the talent of his horse and of himself. These observations became the basis for self-affirmations of the skills and talent John brought to the new partnership. They also provided data for John to dispute his irrational self-talk that he was not elite squad material. We made lists of similarities between his two horses, noting some of the problems his old horse had had and how John managed to work them out. John's recall of his skills and abilities, and those of his new partner, became part of his routine training and competition preparation. John learned to "tack up his mind" with them while he tacked up his horse. In time, he and his horse relaxed and came to trust each other. At that point, the horse stopped running out on fences.

When Fear and Anxiety Are Reasonable Responses

This above example is one in which the coach elicited the assistance of the sport psychologist. Other equestrians find their way to a sport psychologist out of self-awareness. The most common emotions prompting equestrians to seek assistance are the anxiety and fear surrounding jumping. In addressing this, the sport psychologist must again consider the nature of the rider-horse relationship, particularly the dimensions of trust and responsibility. The horse has to rely on the rider for safe approaches and take-off spots. Because of the nature of the horse's vision, he does not get to see the fence too far before he jumps it. Shane Rose, an Australian World Equestrian Games competitor, says that

> horses learn to trust you . . . if you can put them in the right spot . . . the odd occasion you might miss and get to the wrong spot to take off they will help you out . . . where the combination comes into it is they learn to trust you and help you out as much as you help them. (Holden Equestriad Series, 1998)

Anyone who has watched advanced levels of cross-country and show jumping can understand how rational anxiety and fear are for these athletes. The elements of personal risk are obvious. This is especially true of cross-country riding where the obstacles are fixed, allowing little flexibility for errors in approach, take-off, or speed.

Acknowledging that some levels of anxiety are normal and expected, the psychologist has several choices in methods to help a rider through *debilitating* anxiety and fear. Before choosing an approach, it is advisable to consult the coach as to the rider's level of skill. Anxiety founded on the rider's belief that she or he is jumping above the rider's technical knowledge and skill needs to be dealt with differently from anxiety originating from other thoughts. Riders are particularly vulnerable to these thoughts when they move up to the next class where the jumps are higher and the course requires more technical knowledge. In equestrian sport, a rider often advances not because the rider or the coach *decides* that the rider is ready, but because the rider has won particular competitions at the current level. The rider is, therefore, excluded from further competitions at that level and must move up to continue competing. For these clients, careful assessment of how they are coping with the riding anxiety is important, as physical symptoms of anxiety can jeopardize not only their use of effective riding aids, but also the very safety of the rider and horse. "If a horse is confident in the rider and the rider is confident in the horse and they know each other then they will get away with things that horses who don't trust their riders don't get away with" (Craig Barrett, Australian International 3-day eventer, Holden Equestriad Series, 1998).

The case of Susan illustrates these points. She was having problems riding triple (three-fence) combination jumps once she had advanced to a higher competition level. Invariably, she would ride the first fence, but then miss the second and third. It was evident from her tapes that she "stopped riding" once she started her take-off. That is, her leg aids relaxed, and she released the reins and shifted from her forward seat. In our first session, I used deep relaxation and guided imagery to take her around the course. I encouraged her to listen to her inner dialogue as she rode. Eventually, she became aware of the change in her self-talk indicating less confidence as she came onto the line approaching the triple combination. As she sat in the chair, I saw her shoulders tense as she held her breath, just as we had seen on the tape. She then realized that she used to shut her eyes and let her horse manage the rest of the combination as best he could. She indicated that her "mind left the saddle." As a result, her communication to her horse ceased. He responded to her lack of direction by losing impulsion. Hence, he knocked rails as he tried to get through the fences. She discovered she opened her eyes and took a breath only after she felt the final landing. Her immediate response to this awareness was that she was lucky her horse took care of her, but she realized that the course at her new level of competition was getting too much for the horse to handle on his own and that he needed her to "stay in the saddle" and navigate.

In our next session, we walked a jumping course together, and Susan described her strategies and preparations for each jump, except the triple combination. She admitted she avoided walking the strides between the fences because it made her too anxious. My intervention for this was to treat it as if it were a simple phobia. We developed a desensitization hierarchy of fence heights and difficult approaches. Gradually, she was able to walk the course and mentally ride the jumps, keeping her focus and attention through the triple combination. As she consciously and purposefully acknowledged her abilities to guide her horse through the combination fences, Susan's anxiety decreased. She progressed to actually riding the course, and she was able to use her aids effectively. Her horse stopped dropping the second and third rails of combinations.

When working with jumping phobias, I suggest to riders that, like all adversaries, once we become acquainted with feared obstacles, they lose some of their threat. I have riders spend time in the presence of their most feared ditches and fences. They walk around courses and approach all sides of their adversaries. When possible, they dismantle and rebuild them. This gives them a physical sense of their dimensions, which, in some cases, are only a few centimeters higher or wider than nonthreatening jumps. One rider has found it helpful to talk *to* the jumps, much to the worry of her coach and fellow riders. When she misses a jump, she tells it she will be back and will get it next time. She finds that this motivates her next time as she has already "engaged the enemy."

Another traditional approach to managing anxiety is to teach the rider to engage the physiologically competing response of relaxation when anxiety cues are present. Personally, I have had limited success with this. Although use of progressive muscle relaxation and imagery work well during mental rehearsal, I find its effects do not generalize once the rider is on the horse. This may be for several reasons. Relaxation of the upper body is important, especially in dressage. However, to engage effective aids, the rider must have a disciplined posture that can compete with the usual progressive muscle relaxation procedures. A second reason why the rider's relaxation response often fails once on the horse is that the horse is a reactive being who does not always give warning before panicking. Even the most calm and obedient horses will at times revert to instinctive flight behavior when faced with an unsuspected or unknown "spook." Hence, when the rider is waiting to start a competition, or is actually on course, part of his or her psyche is consciously or unconsciously preparing for the unexpected. For example, consider the dressage rider who was in the middle of her test when a skydiver, who had been blown off course, sailed into the arena. Other riders tell me that relaxing themselves is not as important as relaxing their horse. If the horse is tense, no relaxation technique will completely offset the rider's stress, for it seems, riders and their horses soak up each other's anxiety by processes of osmosis. Relaxation to the competing equestrian is more a matter of remembering to breathe and using thought-stopping techniques to keep catastrophizing under control, so the mind can focus. These two techniques I have found to be most beneficial.

Other traditional anxiety-management techniques of dissociation and distraction can be useful as long as there is trust between horse and rider. If the rider does not trust that the horse will be "honest" in his attempts to do what the rider asks of him, then cognitive techniques will have limited success. For, without this trust, the rider faces the reality that his or her well-being is precarious whenever in the saddle. In this instance, anxiety can be adaptive for the rider as it keeps him or her vigilant to possible problems. I always ask riders to be honest with themselves and with their coach if they do not trust a horse. Many are reluctant to do this, as implicit in the code of conduct for equestrian sport is the "show no fear" commandment, especially amongst cross-country riders. The shame of admitting fear and lack of control over a horse to other equestrians is often considered far worse than the anxiety itself. The sport psychologist must be sensitive to this and give the rider support to express dreads and worries.

A final source of riding anxiety to which the sport psychologist must be perceptive is that stemming from previous unresolved accident trauma. The sudden and unreasonable development of fears and anxiety around a particular jump, obstacle, or competition venue can indicate previous trauma being cued by association.

For example, Jane, a very bold and successful cross-country rider, started to have what she described as "sick" sensations whenever she came up to a rail fence with a big ditch underneath it. Because this started suddenly after she had advanced up a level of competition, we initially thought it was due to a lack of confidence to handle the additional height and width of the jump. However, other methods, as described above, did not help her. Her distress increased, and she began to have nightmares about jumping the ditches. The physical sensations and the nightmares led me to suspect that she had an earlier unresolved trauma that had a strong emotive cue. We did some work to explore her past riding experiences. We first worked with imagery to create a safe psychological environment for her in her mind. Using guided regression techniques, she went back and visited with other horses she had ridden. She had brought a photo album with her to assist in engaging her memory. Using guided imagery took her back to her earlier years of riding in the paddock and jumping logs and ditches. It was not long before her eyes became tearful. She described an accident on one of her first horses. Despite warnings not to go galloping over unfamiliar obstacles, she had gone for a fast gallop one day and had taken her horse over a ditch that had a log fallen across it. The horse missed its take-off for the jump and hung its back leg over the log. The leg broke, and she had to get a neighbor to put the horse down. Jane watched him do this and helped him bury the horse that afternoon. She never cried about it with anyone as she felt it was her fault. She always felt guilty. Now she wondered whether she had the judgment necessary to take her horse over the demanding cross-country ditches. She worried that she would make a mistake resulting in his fatal injury.

Here again we see the power of the bond between horse and rider. Although many observers worry about the safety of the rider, the equestrians themselves are often more worried about keeping their horses from harm. Riders are ultimately responsible for the well-being of their teammates, taking care of their food, shelter, and physical health. This dependency is reciprocal, and the rider is aware of the responsibility the horse takes for seeing the rider safely through training and competition.

In instances where riders have to recover from the ghosts of other injured horses, or from flashbacks of their own injuries and, sometimes, near-death experiences, the sport psychologist must follow protocols for working through post-traumatic stress disorder. In Jane's case, she gradually recalled the event and was able to restructure her memory of it so that she was able to understand and forgive herself for being a spirited young girl. She was then able to identify how she had grown in skills and knowledge of cross-country riding. She learned to use such affirmation statements to dispute intrusive thoughts suggesting that her carelessness would damage another horse. Part of her recovery from her repressed guilt and grief involved her visiting the site where her horse had been buried. She told him of her sorrow and said her goodbyes. After that visit, she felt she was able to let go of the memory of the accident and associated fears that it would happen again.

The Psychology of Creating Harmony Between Horse and Rider

Most of the above examples illustrate the application of sport psychology principles within the more dramatic equestrian sports of show jumping and cross-country. Similar examples can be found amongst riders in polo, western, and endurance events. However, the more sedate equestrian discipline of dressage also requires a particular mental state to be successful.

The characteristics we see in the champion dressage horse are the result of its natural physical talents and years of disciplined training. However, these are evident in the competition arena only when the rider is able to engage the horse in a partnership reminiscent of two dancers. The graceful appearance of dressage movement is produced by the horse's flexibility and suppleness, balance, rhythm, and impulsion. The apparent effortlessness comes from the horse's attention and focus on the rider's subtle communication through the riding aids. The dressage test requires the duo to exhibit this while performing specific movements (halt, circle, passage) using specific paces (walk, trot, canter, counter-canter) at markers (letters) around the dressage arena. The horse-rider team receives points not only for executing the right movements in the right sequences, but also for the quality of these movements. The rider is afforded points for technical work in addition to those awarded to the horse for his obedience.

Accomplishing this level of precision and discipline puts intense mental and physical training demands on a dressage horse. It is important that the rider rewards the horse consistently and nurtures a positive attitude from him. Without such a positive relationship, the calm and obedient, yet energized, persona essential in a dressage horse is not possible. I find that my dressage clients present the biggest challenges in terms of keeping stress under control. Little stress can be tolerated if the mind is to maintain its focus on the intricacies of the dressage test, and if the body is to maintain its elegant but disciplined posture to enable the precision of subtle riding aids. There is little time in a dressage test for the slightest loss of attention or delay in the use of riding aids.

Most of my approaches with dressage riders involve riding the dressage tests while using mental rehearsal. The difficulties a rider exhibits in maintaining focus throughout the mental rehearsal of a test is very predictive of similar problems when in the dressage arena. For example, Jamie started to have "discipline" problems with her horse when she began to ride the pirouette. This movement requires the rider to maintain the horse's momentum as he turns in a circle off his hindquarters. Her horse would only complete three quarters of the turn before he "fell out" of the movement. Her coach kept instructing her, and Jamie thought she was using her aids accordingly. However, mental rehearsal indicated that she anticipated the next movement before the pirouette was completed. She discovered that she didn't finish the aids for the last quarter of the pirouette, as her attention moved on to the rest of the test. Hence, her horse was following her instructions. This is not an uncommon problem for dressage riders who have concerns about particular movements. They often unconsciously rush to get the anxiety-provoking movement in the test completed. This mental anticipation is evident in the horse's rushing and loss of consistent rhythm, and his apparent lack of attention to the movement at hand.

Another example of this problem is seen in the horse that does not do a complete halt at the beginning of the test when asked. During mental rehearsal, riders often identify that they themselves have not halted mentally, but have proceeded on up the center line to the first movement of the test. Similarly, dressage horses who seem to lack impulsion (not going forward freely) are often ridden by riders who also lack mental impulsion. Their mental rehearsal indicates lack of confidence, and sometimes motivation, to ride the dressage test with energy and enthusiasm. In all of these examples, the sport psychologist can assist riders to expand their attention and improve their focus while riding the dressage test, one movement at a time.

The harmony one sees in a dressage team is possible only when there is a calm and relaxed relationship between horse and rider. This requires the rider to be able to relinquish the stress and distress from her or his daily routine before training and competing. As the case of John illustrated, carrying anger, frustration, and other emotions while riding impedes the use of the riding aids and, hence, the horse's performance. I have found it beneficial to teach riders to use thought-stopping techniques or other imagery techniques, such as locking their worries from the day in their tack box, before getting into the saddle. This has resulted in enhancing the calm and relaxed attitude required of the dressage rider and horse.

Conclusion

All of these cases indicate that equestrians need to be given understanding and support to work emotively with their horses as if they were their best friends, which sometimes they are. Without this kind of empathy, the psychologist will not form the therapeutic alliance necessary for successful outcomes. The use of behavioral, CBT, and RET approaches, imagery and mental rehearsal, physical focusing, and relaxation methods can instruct the client as to how to change the mental aspects of his or her riding (Edgette, 1996). However, riders' motivation to engage in these will only extend as far as they feel understood by the psychologist. In addition, there is no understanding between sport psychologist and equestrian if the psyche's of the horse and rider are treated as separate. It has become apparent to me that such a separation is not only undesirable, but also is impossible. This is the challenge to the sport psychologist.

Author's Note: The author wishes to thank the riders and coaches who have given permission for their stories to be shared in this article.

References

Budiansky, S. (1997). *The nature of horses: Their evolution, intelligence and behavior.* London: Phoenix.

Edgette, J. S. (1996). *Heads up: Practical sports psychology for riders, their families and their trainers.* New York: Doubleday.

Fiske, J. C. (1979). *How horses learn.* Wistaston, UK: Stephen Green.

Fraser, A. F. (1992). *The behavior of horses.* Wallingford, UK: CAB International.

Holden Equestriad Series. (1998). Peter Machin (Series Editor). Michael Williams (Chief of Production). Gabrielle Dorley (Production Manager). Nine Network Australia.

Kiley-Worthington, M. (1987). *The behavior of horses in relation to management and training.* London: J. A. Allen.

McCall, C. A. (1990). A review of learning behavior in horses and application in horse training. *Journal of Animal Science, 68,* 75–81.

Pretty, G. H. (2000). Understanding the enmeshment in equine and human relationships: How riders think about the horse in their attributions of performance success. The Abstracts of the 34th Annual Conference of the Australian Psychological Society, *Australian Journal of Psychology Supplement,* 107.

Williams, M. (1976). *Horse psychology.* London: J. A. Allen.

Professional Practice in Sport Psychology: Developing Programs With Golfers and Orienteers

Patrick R. Thomas

My involvement in sport psychology came about when my university commenced planning a new undergraduate degree in sport sciences and I was asked to coordinate the sport psychology strand. To do this effectively, I visited a number of prominent sport psychologists in the United States in 1990 and observed many of their interactions with athletes, before spending 2 months in the psychology department at the US Olympic Training Center in Colorado Springs. Toward the end of this period, I developed the conceptual framework shown in Figure 1 that extended existing models of performance enhancement and described the processes I had observed. This framework has been presented and described fully elsewhere (Morris & Thomas, 1995; P. R. Thomas, 1991). It has also been used by Hardy, Jones, and Gould (1996) to explain how consultants and coaches can develop a psychological skills training (PST) program.

Rather than describe each of the phases again, my intention here is to use the conceptual framework to structure reflections on some aspects of my own professional practice with athletes, particularly golfers. That practice is conducted as a full-time academic staff member in an Australian university. Although that may initially seem un-

usual, it is my impression that many practicing sport psychologists in the United States and United Kingdom also hold positions within universities. In Australia, approximately 40% of members of the College of Sport Psychologists currently hold university appointments. That proportion will decrease as more sport psychology graduates enter employment and establish their own practices. However, very few practicing psychologists in this country work solely with athletes; those who do are generally employed in institutes or academies of sport.

The Initial Program

For the past 8 years, I have been asked to conduct PST programs for elite golf squads from which state-representative teams are chosen to play in the national championships. Each team has a manager and a professional golf coach who has overall responsibility for the preparation program. In addition to the sport psychology sessions, the players work with a physical trainer to improve their health and fitness. The overall program thus addresses psychological, biomechanical, and physiological issues crucial in golf performance. Although we each have specific responsibilities in these areas, our activities often overlap, and I need to know

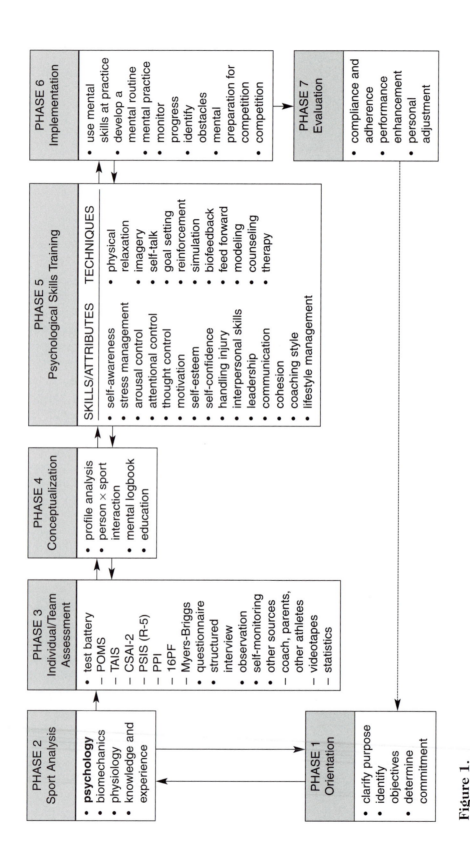

Figure 1.

An overview of performance-enhancement processes in applied sport psychology. From "Approaches to Applied Sport Psychology," by T. Morris and P. R. Thomas, 1995, in Sport Psychology: Theory, Applications and Current Issues, edited by T. Morris and J. Summers (p. 238). Copyright 1995 by Jacaranda Wiley Ltd. Reproduced by permission of Jacaranda Wiley Ltd.

what initiatives my colleagues are taking. The interventions are usually more effective when the psychologist and coach work together. For example, players who are performing poorly because their confidence is low can often be helped if they combine biomechanical feedback from the coach with the use of positive self-talk and imagery techniques to rehearse the correct execution of a skill. It also helps me to understand a player's lack of confidence if I know he or she is making a swing change. The psychological, biomechanical, and physiological demands of an activity are more likely to be understood by a consultant who has undertaken a multidisciplinary training program.

The sport psychology consultant also needs knowledge and experience of the specific sport, particularly when working with advanced players. Ravizza (1988) identified lack of sport-specific knowledge as a major barrier to gaining entry with athletes and outlined some of the steps he took to become familiar with the demands faced by his clients. When the consultant plays the sport, advice and illustrations can be readily contextualized, but detailed accounts from others, who are either high achievers themselves or able to provide a unique perspective in a sport, can also be used very effectively. For example, I have found that players can easily relate to professional golfers' comments on mental factors in golf (McCaffrey & Orlick, 1989). Elite athletes do not expect a consultant to perform at their level. However, increasing numbers of elite athletes are studying sport sciences, and some will make very effective consultants because their knowledge and personal experience are highly developed. Sport psychology consultants are likely to become increasingly specialized, both with respect to working in particular sports and to handling particular types of problems or issues.

The orientation session is of paramount importance, both in terms of content and process. I often begin a program by asking athletes how important mental factors are in their sport. Most athletes acknowledge these factors are very important, accounting for at least 50%, and probably more like 80% to 90%, of performance. In my experience, elite athletes attribute more importance to mental skills than other athletes do. These skills may also be more important in some sports such as golf than in other sports (Weinberg & Gould, 1995). Despite their importance, athletes typically spend little time practicing psychological skills. A recent sample of 231 athletes across diverse sports reported an average training time of 11.25 hrs per week, of which 8 hrs were spent on physical skills, 2.3 hrs on technical skills, and only 0.9 hrs on psychological skills training (Jackson, Thomas, Marsh, & Smethurst, in press). Drawing athletes' attention to this anomaly often strengthens their commitment to a PST program.

It is important that consultants tailor PST programs to their clients' needs. That is relatively straightforward when working with an individual client, but it can be a challenge when the consultant is working with a group. In the first year that I worked with the state golf squads, I asked them to nominate the skills that should be targeted in the training program. The topics nominated most frequently were stress management, self-confidence, and emotional control, followed by relaxation techniques, thought control, and attentional control. I then devised training activities to develop skills in each of these areas as well as visualization/imagery, which was nominated less frequently. The program consisted of eight 1-1½ hr sessions conducted in the 11 weeks prior to the 1992 national championships.

The players' psychological skills were assessed in the initial session using the Golf Performance Survey (P. R. Thomas & Over, 1994). Of particular interest were their scores on Concentration, Negative Emotions and Cognitions, and Mental Preparation subscales. Other subscales measured their tactics, psychomotor skills, and commitment to golf. Players received their skills profiles in the second session, together with feedback on team averages for each subscale and comparative averages for high- and low-handicap club golfers. Players verified the results before training commenced. Research with the sample of club golfers had shown that simply providing feedback on psychological skills profiles produced little improvement in those skills and had no significant effects on performance (P. R. Thomas, 1993). Psychological skills training was necessary if the intervention program was to be effective (P. R. Thomas & Fogarty, 1997).

Various source materials were adapted for use in the training sessions. For example, material from the South Australian Sports Institute (SASI) psychology program (Winter & Martin, 1991) was used to develop the players' concentration skills. Because of the nature of the sport, most golfers find it helpful to switch their attention on and off rather than concentrating deeply throughout a round. This requires consistent use of an effective preshot routine. Players were helped to use shifts in the direction and width of attention to build their own preshot routines (Nideffer, 1985). After starting with a broad external focus to assess salient features in the situation, attention shifts to a broad internal focus to analyze the information, select the appropriate club, and visualize the shot. A narrow internal focus is then adopted to prepare for the shot by adjusting tension and developing feel. Finally, there is a narrow external focus of attention on the target and ball as the player acts in executing the swing. In July 1992, Nick Faldo won the Open golf championship at Muirfield. His second shot to the 15th green had a significant bearing on his scores and the ultimate outcome. His

preshot routine provided a superb illustration of what was being recommended to the players, who asked on several subsequent occasions to see that shot again.

To address the players' need for stress-management strategies, we began by examining sport psychology literature on the relationship between arousal and performance. Drive theory's proposition that the relationship is linear once a skill has been acquired was rejected in favor of a curvilinear relationship (Oxendine, 1970; Yerkes & Dodson, 1908). The players agreed that the arousal dimension might have multiple components, both positive and negative (Martens, 1987). The zone of optimal performance was then characterized by high levels of energy, activation, and positive emotion and low levels of stress and negative emotion. In the sport of golf, however, "playing in the zone" does not demand maximum levels of activation and minimum levels of stress as might be implied from Martens. Players typically reported playing their best golf with an activation rating of 7/10 and stress rating of 2/10 or 3/10. They readily acknowledged that some stress was beneficial for performance, as recognized in the concept of eustress, and understanding this relationship helped them manage some of the symptoms of stress commonly experienced before a championship round. Players also examined catastrophe theory's model of the relationships among physiological arousal, cognitive anxiety, and performance (Hardy, 1990). Although the relationships are complex, players' attention was drawn to the proposition that cognitive anxiety can benefit performance providing physiological arousal is minimal. Finally, players found some aspects of Csikszentmihalyi's (1990) theory of flow helpful in understanding the psychology of optimal performance, particularly the notion that they were more likely to experience flow if their perceived ability matched the demands of the situation.

Physical relaxation techniques were taught to help players regulate their arousal levels, beginning with active progressive muscle relaxation so they would recognize the difference between tension and relaxation in the various muscle groups throughout their body. They also learned to use centering techniques to help them relax and focus during a round (Nideffer, 1985). Both techniques incorporate diaphragmatic breathing, producing relaxation on exhalation. Faldo's preshot routine, referred to earlier, included not only contraction of the muscles in the left hand, but also a deep breath and audible sigh on exhalation, both timed optimally to produce a relaxed state for a crucial shot. Later in the program, players learned to use deep relaxation/self-hypnosis techniques (Nideffer, 1992) in mental preparation for the championships.

In addition to relaxation techniques, players learned to manage stress by controlling their emotional reactions. Much of what happens on the course is beyond the players' control, but they can control how they react to the situation. A cognitive-behavior theory framework was presented to players, suggesting that it was their thoughts and feelings about a situation, not just the situation itself, that determined how they reacted and performed. They learned to use thought-stopping techniques to avoid or change negative cognitions that led to counterproductive emotional reactions. Players used cue words, as outlined by Crace and Hardy (1989), to focus or refocus their thoughts, feelings, and attention and to recreate a mental set for optimal performance. Players reflected on the time, place, and characteristics of their previous best performance in selecting their cue words, which they then used on the course in combination with a deep centering breath.

This focus on cognitive processes was maintained in the following session, which aimed to develop the players' self-confi-dence. As suggested in the SASI psychology program (Winter & Martin, 1991), players were asked to write affirmation statements identifying strengths in their attitude and mental approach to sport and life in general; skills, technique, and knowledge of sport; and physical fitness. Some players found it difficult to express these thoughts on paper, and few would have been comfortable sharing their statements with other players on the team. They were encouraged, however, to keep a record of their affirmations and refer to it regularly, particularly if they experienced a performance slump. Players also identified situations where their thoughts and emotions were negative and discussed alternative interpretations that would benefit performance. For example, instead of worrying about how their nerves would affect performance on the first tee, players learned to recognize and interpret their nerves as a sign their body was ready to perform.

Imagery training began with the demonstration of imagined movement using a ring suspended above a circle with marked diagonals (Martens, 1987; Vealey, 1986). Players then watched the video, *What You See is What You Get* (Botterill, 1987) and discussed how they could implement the guidelines presented by Terry Orlick. Gaining the feel for a shot was considered a crucial component of their preshot routine. Players agreed that imagery could be used to rehearse the correct execution of skills, establish and rehearse a game plan, develop concentration, and enable participation or foster a positive attitude when they were recovering from injury. To develop vividness and controllability in their images, players relaxed and completed training exercises adapted from Vealey. Players were asked to imagine themselves on the first tee of their course under various conditions; imagine the feel of their putter and of using their putter on a green; imagine, in all of the senses, a flawless swing using a 5 iron; and imagine performing correctly a particular shot they found difficult. Players also imagined competition situations that negatively affected their performance, developing strategies to deal with the negative cues, and using those strategies successfully. This exercise thus reinforced the cognitive-behavioral framework presented earlier.

The final session in the program was aimed at completing the players' mental preparation for the championships. Players reflected on their thoughts, feelings, and attentional focus during their best and worst performances in developing competition plans as described by Orlick (1986). They also discussed ways in which team spirit and harmony could be promoted to improve performance (Orlick, 1990). For many of the players, golf had been an individual sport. They had participated in pennant competitions for their clubs and had experienced the benefits of strong support from other team members, but these competitions only provided individual match-play experience. The national championships also involved foursome competitions, and players needed to develop psychological and tactical skills specific to that format. Interpersonal skills were also needed in handling travel, accommodation, dining, practice, and administrative arrangements made for the team. Players familiarized themselves with the championship venues by discussing descriptions of the courses and studying yardage charts. The final session concluded with a deep relaxation exercise coupled with a brief review of the program's main points and a guided visualization of the players competing at their best in the championships, recovering well from difficult situations, and finishing strongly.

Players competed successfully in the national championships after the initial offering of this program, winning one of the team competitions for only the second time in 8 years as well as an individual match-play title. One month after the championships, they completed the Golf Performance Survey a second time and rated each of the topics addressed in the sessions for its interest, usefulness, and whether it should be followed up the next year. The players were also invited to comment on the overall benefits and weaknesses of the PST program and suggest improvements or new areas that should be included.

Analysis of the Golf Performance Survey responses revealed significant improvement in concentration skills and a significant reduction in negative emotions and cognitions after completing the program. Players also reported better mental preparation although the improvement was not statistically significant. All of these areas were targeted in the training sessions whereas other subscales showed very little change. There was general agreement by the players that all components of the program were both interesting and useful. Players were most interested in the topic of building confidence and positive thinking, and they showed strong interest in the Golf Performance Survey profile, relaxation training, and the preshot routine. The players' ratings identified the preshot routine, confidence and positive thinking, visualization training, and mental preparation for competition as the most useful topics. Although players agreed an audiotape on concentration skills was interesting and useful, it received the lowest ratings. Players agreed that all of the topics were worth following up the next year, particularly those dealing with relaxation and visualization training, confidence and positive thinking, and the preshot routine.

Some of the players' open-ended comments and suggestions for improving the program were particularly helpful. For example, when asked to identify the main benefits of the PST program, players wrote:

I thought one of the major benefits I got out of the program was with the visualization and relaxation exercises. I found these very helpful when out on the course, especially when not hitting it the best. I also think the program brought us together more as a team.

In different situations I could call upon different skills in order to escape a situation or put myself into a situation. The relaxation skills, I found, were the biggest help because I always had a routine and a particular style of play but not a controlled direction of play or speed of play.

Reading other material on other people's approaches where they actually work—made you confident that it would work for you. Learning to refocus after a rough trot using my two-word performance cue.

Several players stated there were no problems or weaknesses in the PST program. One or two indicated that a few of the topics were "a little too deep and hard to comprehend" and expressed difficulty in being able to learn the skills or put them into practice. One comment about the duration of the training program was particularly interesting:

The only problem that the program had was that we were not exposed to these learning processes early enough. I felt that because we were only together for a short while, these skills were not well enough known for that kind of extreme pressure.

Various suggestions were made about new areas that should be included or how the program might be improved the following year. Players were keen to study golf videotapes in order to "pick out the major points like preshot routines and mental approaches to each shot" or "put concentration skills into practice." One nominated "more physical practice of concentration or imagery—within groups." Another suggested:

We should have more personal or group involvement, whether it be involvement between different sporting codes or groups in the same sport to get an in-depth view of others' ideas which could in turn aid us in the way we view certain ideas.

Two other comments emphasized the need for individual attention. One player suggested that I "pull aside each individual and find their strengths and weaknesses and personally try to strengthen each person"; the other requested that I "walk around with them (the players) during the round."

In the first half of the following year, the sport psychology training was again combined with fitness training and coaching in a similar program for the junior boys' golf squad. The seven players selected to represent their state achieved outstanding results in their national championships, not only winning the interstate teams event, but also finishing 1st, 2nd, 3rd, 5th, 6th, and 7th in the individual title, which attracted a field of more than 200 players. These results were considerably better than those achieved in the years before the program commenced, and although that standard is almost impossible to match, an excellent record has been maintained in subsequent years. All of these players were under 18 years old and were clearly ready to benefit at that age from psychological skills training.

Extending the Program

As the initial training program was well received and the players had performed successfully, I was invited back the following year but immediately faced some new challenges. About 80% of the players selected for the state squads that year had participated in the initial program. They would not have benefited greatly from a repetition of the same training activities. The new players, on the other hand, had received little, if any, prior psychological skills training, and their needs had to be met. One option was to conduct separate sessions for the different subgroups. Like the players' suggestion for individual consultations, this option would have been more expensive for the golf organization, and the sessions would have been less effective in building team spirit. Resolving this dilemma effectively is an issue that must confront many sport psychologists who conduct ongoing programs with teams. It is an issue that deserves careful consideration and planning.

My initial response to this problem was to run whole group sessions that addressed core topics from the initial program in a different way, added some new topic areas, incorporated suggestions made by players the previous year, and helped individuals determine their strengths and weaknesses. The first of the five sessions introduced the sport psychology program by showing how athletes in another sport, Australian Rules football, were benefiting from mental skills training (National Australian Football Council, 1990). In this video, coaches and players clearly endorsed the value of such training and explained how psychological techniques were used to enhance performance, facilitate injury rehabilitation, and improve communication and motivation. The second session followed up the video's focus on goal-setting techniques. Elite professional golfers' comments on the importance of goal setting were considered, and players were provided with worksheets for recording their long- and short-term goals as well as their strategies for achieving those goals. Players were encouraged to set technical, psychological, and physical goals each week (Winter & Martin,

1991) and set goals for their daily practice sessions after determining their strengths and weaknesses in shotmaking skills (Bann, 1993). Worksheets were also provided so that players could keep systematic records of their performance statistics (drives on fairway, greens in regulation, sand saves, putts), as well as their ratings on selected psychological skills before and during competitions. Players found it particularly instructive to compare their own performance statistics with those published for the US PGA Tour.

The third session in the second year of the program focused on peak performance in golf, extending the earlier material on the zone of optimal performance and the experience of flow by considering comments from elite professional golfers (e.g., McCaffrey & Orlick, 1989) and the findings from Cohn's (1991) research. The earlier procedures for developing an effective performance cue (Crace & Hardy, 1989) were supplemented by consideration of Nideffer's (1992) list of physical and psychological feelings typically reported by athletes when playing in the zone, and the contrasting feelings associated with choking. The fourth session also extended earlier training based on cognitive-behavior theory. It consisted of workshop activities focusing on the use of self-talk to build confidence (Bunker, Williams, & Zinsser, 1993; Owens & Bunker, 1992). Players completed a series of exercises showing how thought-stopping, substituting, countering, reframing, and affirmation techniques could be used in golf.

Opportunities were taken to walk with players during practice rounds to observe their preshot routines and address course-management issues. As in the initial program, the final session was used to help the players prepare mentally for the championships. They were encouraged wherever possible to maintain their normal routines at the championships when developing their precompetition plans (Orlick, 1986, 1990). Players discussed course layouts and the playing conditions expected in a climate very different from their own, and they visualized their performance and goal achievements.

The players again provided useful feedback after this program. They clearly benefited from training in goal setting and indicated a strong preference for group discussion sessions:

The most useful components this year for me included mental preparation before a game and setting goals for yourself to achieve so you are not just playing to get something out of a game only if you win. Using goals, you're always trying to achieve something attainable.

The discussions when everybody airs their fears, their goals, how they think in the morning, before, during and after those important games. Goal setting was the best session for me—getting information on what the good guys do.

I found the program this year a lot better when everyone was sitting around together. There seemed to be a lot more interaction with this format rather than just one person out in front talking, a lot like a lecture format.

Working With Orienteers

Soon after completing this program, I was asked to work with a small group of elite orienteers who were preparing for international championships. Having very little knowledge or experience in this sport, I began with a literature review that yielded material that not only developed my understanding of the specific demands on these athletes, but could also be incorporated effectively in training

sessions (e.g., Gal-Or, Tenenbaum, & Shimrony, 1986; Seiler, 1990). I then learned that several of these elite athletes were teachers or tertiary educators who closely monitored sport science literature in their sport. After considering the feedback from the golf program, the lack of a suitable test instrument specific to orienteering, my own inexperience in this sport, and the expertise present in this group of athletes, I chose to adopt a different approach in this program. I wanted the sessions to reflect more of a bottom-up approach, which drew from the wealth of experience shared by the athletes, than a top-down approach, which presented them with material that others, including myself deemed important. Interactive discussions were therefore favored over other presentation formats. I was keen for the athletes to develop a sense of ownership of the program. With that ownership came responsibility for determining the topics to be discussed. As the program was tailored to meet athletes' specific needs, they were also largely responsible for determining the psychological skills or techniques for which training was provided.

Performance-Profiling Techniques

An essential component of this new approach was the use of performance-profiling techniques as advocated by Butler and Hardy (1992) and illustrated by Jones (1993), and Butler, Smith, and Irwin (1993). In order to identify individual strengths and weaknesses, the athletes were asked to nominate the skills, strategies, or characteristics they would need to perform at their best in the international orienteering championships. Suggestions were initially pooled, but one of the group suggested they classify the skills into three categories. *Physical skills* included cardio-respiratory endurance, fitness that was course related, leg strength, speed in different terrains, agility, flexibility, and vision. *Practical skills* included mobile map reading/interpretation, map memory, terrain interpretation, relocation skills, compass skills, distance estimation, and equipment handling. Finally, the list of *psychological skills* included decision making (speed, accuracy, flexibility), concentration (maintaining external awareness, map contact, implementing routines), motivation, self-awareness (physical state), relaxation, precompetition preparation (mental set, focused, confidence, controlling anxiety), self-regulation in competition (controlling negative thoughts and feelings, recovering from mistakes, confidence), organization (planning ahead in competition), and visualization (imaging optimal performance).

Each of the athletes then selected the skills he or she most needed to develop in order to perform at the best in the championships. They used a 10-point scale to report their current rating on those skills, their rating at the time of their previous best performance (which served to remind and reassure some that improvement was possible), and the target rating they could realistically achieve by the time of the championships. The current and target ratings were then plotted on radar charts for the athletes so they had a record of the goals they were targeting across a range of salient skills. These graphs set individual training agendas for each athlete in the lead-up to the championships. They also informed me of the skills and techniques the athletes wanted addressed in our sessions.

I had no hesitation in again adopting the performance-profiling approach when working with the state junior boys' golf squad early the following year. In identifying the skills needed to perform at their best, these players found it helpful to consider Bann's (1993) account of the skills needed in elite golf, as well as the classification framework developed by the orienteers. Four categories of skills were identified: *physical skills* (such as endurance, strength, flexibility), *life skills* (diet and nutrition, sleep, consideration and, support for others in the team), *technical skills* (sound repetitive swing, technically accurate, short game, putting), and *psychological skills* (temperament, concentration, mental preparation, desire, attitude, confidence).

Each subsequent golf squad has benefited from use of performance-profiling techniques in the initial session of the sport psychology program. These sessions typically review what worked well and what problems were encountered during the national championships the previous year. Ideally, consultants should conduct debriefing sessions soon after athletes compete, but that has not been done with the golfers because of logistical difficulties. Although that is a weakness in the program, it usually ensures a full exchange of views and information in the initial session each year that benefits not only those who were previously involved, but also new players in the squads. Figure 2 shows the list of skills that players this year identified as necessary for peak performance in golf. A fifth category, *tactical skills*, has been added to the four developed initially with the juniors. These skills include planning and preparation that ensure individuals and teams are ready to play at their best, gain an early advantage in their matches, and use strategies to maintain a competitive edge over their opponents. There may be some debate as to whether a particular skill should be classified in one category or another. The preshot routine, for example, was originally classified by the players as a technical skill, although it could just as easily be grouped along with other routines as a tactical skill. The players, coaches, and team managers like to discuss such issues and are comfortable with the classifications in Figure 2, but perhaps researchers will now relocate and even extend the lists of skills shown.

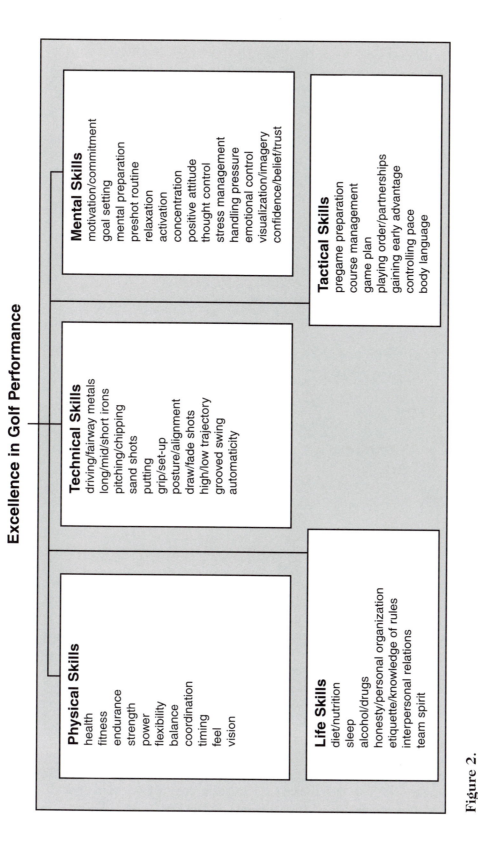

Excellence in Golf Performance

Physical Skills
health
fitness
endurance
strength
power
flexibility
balance
coordination
timing
feel
vision

Technical Skills
driving/fairway metals
long/mid/short irons
pitching/chipping
sand shots
putting
grip/set-up
posture/alignment
draw/fade shots
high/low trajectory
grooved swing
automaticity

Mental Skills
motivation/commitment
goal setting
mental preparation
preshot routine
relaxation
activation
concentration
positive attitude
thought control
stress management
handling pressure
emotional control
visualization/imagery
confidence/belief/trust

Life Skills
diet/nutrition
sleep
alcohol/drugs
honesty/personal organization
etiquette/knowledge of rules
interpersonal relations
team spirit

Tactical Skills
pregame preparation
course management
game plan
playing order/partnerships
gaining early advantage
controlling pace
body language

Figure 2.
Skills needed by golfers to perform at their peak.

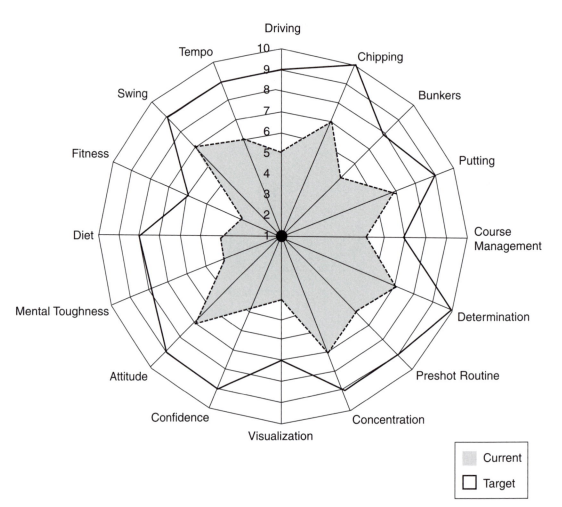

Figure 3.
Performance profile of an elite amateur golfer.

Figure 3 shows a recent example of a performance profile constructed from a player's current and target ratings. Players use the 10-point scale differently even though anchor labels such as *very poor* and *excellent* are suggested. That does not cause a problem unless the players exchange or compare profiles that may prove embarrassing for some who were relatively harsh in their self-ratings. I have found that players are honest in their appraisals and use the feedback in exactly the way it is intended—to guide their training in preparation for the championships. They are cautioned against setting unrealistic target ratings. It may, for instance, be unrealistic to expect driving to improve from a rating of 5 to 9 over the course of 10 weeks, but that improvement is possible if gains in other skills (e.g., swing, tempo, preshot routine, concentration, confidence) are achieved. A change in equipment may also bring immediate benefit. Large short-term gains may be more unrealistic in some other areas. The profile in Figure 3 generally shows high but not unrealistic or idealistic targets given current ratings. Current ratings for fitness and diet are clearly a cause for concern, but the player is being honest in setting only moderate targets in these areas given the timeframe.

Players are encouraged to discuss their profiles with their coaches or others who have a significant role in their preparation, such as the physical trainer. Coaches can often provide useful feedback by indicating how they would rate the players on selected skills. Players are also encouraged to revisit their profiles regularly and note the gains they have made. In using these profiles at the start of the program, the initial focus is often on individual weaknesses, but that shifts to the gains that have been achieved with training, and the ultimate focus at the time of the championships is on individual strengths. Finally, I ask the players to sign their profiles on the line provided as a contract with themselves that they will commit to achieving their target goals. They each do that in front of their teammates, a strategy that not only increases motivation and determination to expend effort, but also builds team spirit and camaraderie among the players.

Test of Performance Strategies

In addition to using performance-profiling techniques, the Test of Performance Strategies (TOPS; P. R. Thomas, Murphy, & Hardy, 1999) has been administered to players since 1994. The TOPS is not golf specific but has been readily accepted by the players. This 64-item test measures athletes' use of psychological skills and techniques at practice and in competition. Eight subscales measure activation, relaxation, goal setting, attentional control, self-talk, imagery, emotional control, and automaticity at practice. Eight other subscales measure these skills in competition except that attentional control is replaced by items tapping negative thinking. After completing the TOPS, players receive their individual profiles as well as the golf squad averages for each subscale, along with a description of the skills and techniques being measured.

The players have benefited from discussion of the group averages when the TOPS feedback is provided in the second session of the program. Discussion about ideal levels of activation and relaxation for golf may lead to further consideration of the relationships between arousal and performance, commitment to developing techniques to regulate arousal, and a greater awareness of individual differences within the team. It soon became evident that players were much less likely to set goals for practice than for competition, but this was quickly addressed through use of a training diary. Anomalies in some results have also prompted useful discussion. For example, players would normally be expected to focus on swing mechanics and to consciously control skill movements more at practice than in competition where they need to trust in their swing. This was not evident in the automaticity subscale scores. Some players subsequently attributed significant improvements in their performance to placing greater trust in their swing during competitions.

In many respects, the TOPS complements the use of performance-profiling techniques. The TOPS provides a comprehensive measure of skills and techniques that warrant the players' attention in preparing for competition. The numeric rating scales make it easy to track individual or group changes over time and enable players to compare their individual ratings with those of the larger group. Performance-profiling techniques, on the other hand, permit the players to determine which skills they will target in their preparation. These techniques are particularly effective when working with groups of players at different levels of psychological skill development as the athletes can each set their own training agenda. The empowerment of athletes implicit in these techniques increases their commitment to training and decreases their dependence on others, including the consultant psychologist.

New Developments

New topics, methods, and resources are continually incorporated into the program. Players have gained new insights into sport psychology concepts and techniques from videos such as *Mind over Golf* (1993) and *Winning with Sports Psychology* (1994). *The Nearly Men* (1994) has been used effectively to help players cope with a setback, and a highlight video such as *My Greatest Golf Shot* (1993) can have positive effects on players just before a major competition. I recall being greatly impressed by the players' rich knowledge of the history of golf as they accurately predicted details of the events portrayed in these videos. Players obviously gain much from watching and discussing spectacular shot making in golf tournament telecasts. But we have also had memorable training sessions that have been scheduled so that live telecasts of Olympic Games events of special interest to the players can be watched and enjoyed by the group as a whole.

Other sources of new material are perhaps less obvious. New workshop activities on intensity, motivation, imagery, and confidence were adapted for golfers from materials I developed for performers in another domain, dance. In the second year, I worked with groups of highly talented dancers in a specialist high-school program; I obtained a copy of Taylor and Taylor's (1995) book. Their ideas were not only useful in extending the dance psychology program, but were also helpful in developing new workshop materials for the golfers. Papers presented at the World Scientific Congress of Golf have also interested players, particularly F. W. Thomas's (1994) analysis of golf performance standards, and Pelz's (1994) findings in relation to putting. Players have derived

benefit from Rotella's (1995) advice on a range of topics. They have also responded very favorably when asked to read and discuss Feinstein's (1996) account of Ryder Cup matches. His two chapters provide an excellent description of team dynamics and how players responded to pressure when representing their countries in different match-play formats.

To strengthen the bond and increase understanding between foursomes partners, I have conducted workshop activities where squad members swap completed worksheets with their playing partners. In this way, players learn, for example, how their partners feel when they play their best golf, the signs that indicate their intensity levels are too high or too low, and what they do to lower or raise their intensity levels. With this information, players are more able to help their partners achieve their ideal playing state and perform at their best.

Some players are reluctant to disclose information in a group setting or discuss the difficulties they are experiencing. To address this issue, group members have been invited to identify the main problem or challenge they face individually or as a team in preparing for the national championships; they have also learned strategies for solving this problem or meeting this challenge. This is done anonymously, and the written responses are collected. We have then considered these problems/challenges collectively and identified additional strategies for dealing with them effectively. Similarly, we have engaged in "What if . . ." planning, considering various scenarios at the championships and finding solutions in advance so they can be dealt with easily if they occur.

The effectiveness of these group discussions in dealing with issues depends on the extent to which players can trust that their contributions will be handled ethically and confidentially. That trust has built up over the years, and the sessions are characterized by an honest exchange of information and excellent rapport among those involved. Care has been taken not to breach that trust in writing this chapter. There are fewer group sessions now than there were initially as most of the players have participated in the program for several years. Indeed, one player participated for 7 consecutive years. Additional individual consultations are provided for those new to the teams or requesting specific assistance. Some sport psychologists advise athletes that anything they discuss may be relayed to the coach. I have not been asked to do this by coaches or managers and can see some situations where such a practice would be problematic. Consultants may need to clarify such stakeholder expectations before commencing work with athletes.

It has been pleasing to see quite a few elite amateur golfers make the transition to professional ranks. I have heard them say they needed to learn new skills to be successful in their new careers. For example, one recently stated that amateur golf taught him how to swing the club effectively. As a professional, he needed to learn how to get himself into a position to win tournaments, but some professional golfers find it difficult to focus on the processes needed to achieve a successful outcome. They know from their training to set process and performance goals rather than just outcome goals, but become preoccupied with their final score rather than building that score one hole or shot at a time. Whereas some tend to get too far ahead, others have difficulty putting the past behind them. We have consequently needed to work on developing posthole routines so that a bad mistake on a putting green does not carry forward to the next tee.

In reflecting on the development of my professional practice with golfers, it is apparent that my approach has changed over the years. The overview presented in Figure

1 is helpful in understanding performance-enhancement processes and provides a systematic approach to work. It enabled me to develop psychological skills training activities that were well received by participants who subsequently recorded excellent performances. At the beginning of my consultancy, I think I needed to work in this way. Nevertheless, a fundamental shift occurred with the decision to draw more on the players' wealth of experience, to encourage them to take ownership of the program and tailor its contents to their needs. The decision to adopt performance-profiling techniques was central to this change of approach. Personalizing the content and increasing player involvement made the program much more meaningful, enjoyable, and effective for all concerned. Hardy et al. (1996) discussed alternatives to the professional practice approach described in Figure 1. Morris and Thomas (1995) also addressed this issue, drawing on Berliner's (1988) theory of the development of expertise.

Future Directions

New training materials are continually needed by sport psychology consultants, particularly those seeing the same athletes over extended periods of time. Not all athletes like reading instructional texts. It is possible to develop effective workshop activities from books, but other media should also be used. Videos are often well received providing the athletes can relate to the content, but we also need to explore the use of computer technology. I expect that highly effective training materials developed over the next 5 years will make much greater use of interactive CD-ROM technology and internet delivery facilities. Consultants will need to stay abreast of those developments and accommodate them in their practice.

Those involved in the preparation of sport psychologists acknowledge that some graduates will have difficulty gaining employment with athletes (e.g., Kirkby, 1995). The athletes most in need of help are often least able to afford psychological services. It is most unlikely that graduates will work with elite athletes until after they have demonstrated their effectiveness elsewhere. The program outlined in this chapter had its origins in psychological skills training sessions conducted for youngsters in the Greg Norman Junior Golf Foundation. That work led to a request from my golf club to work with its pennant teams, which was soon followed by requests from other clubs. Those opportunities need to be taken by new graduates when they arise.

Yet our graduates should look beyond the current boundaries of sport psychology in their quest for suitable work. Many of the psychological skills and techniques used by athletes to achieve optimal performance under pressure are transferable to other domains. These same skills are also needed by businesspeople, those pursuing excellence in the performing arts, and many others in the wider community. Some sport psychologists are already servicing these needs (Clay, 1996; Danish & Nellen, 1997; Murphy, 1996), and the demand for personal development programs and executive coaching is growing strongly (Clay, 1998). Those prepared to look beyond sport and focus on performance psychology will benefit now and in the years ahead.

References

Bann, S. (1993, February). A strategy for elite golfers. *Australian Golf Digest*, 62–67.

Berliner, D. (1988, February). *The development of expertise in pedagogy*. Charles W. Hunt Memorial Lecture at the Annual Meeting of the American Association of Colleges for Teacher Education, New Orleans, LA.

Botterill, C. (1987). *Visualization: What you see is what you get* [Videotape]. Ottawa, Ontario: Coaching Association of Canada.

Bunker, L., Williams, J.M., & Zinsser, N. (1993). Cognitive techniques for improving performance and building confidence. In J.M. Williams (Ed.), *Applied sport psychology* (2nd ed., pp. 225–242). Palo Alto, CA: Mayfield.

Butler, R.J., & Hardy, L. (1992). The performance profile: Theory and application. *The Sport Psychologist, 6*, 253–264.

Butler, R.J., Smith, M., & Irwin, I. (1993). The performance profile in practice. *Journal of Applied Sport Psychology, 5*, 48–63.

Cattell, R. (Producer). (1994). *Winning with sports psychology* [Videotape]. Sydney: ICC Entertainment.

Clay, R.A. (1996, July). Ideals of sport psychology can also work off the field. *American Psychological Association Monitor, 27(7)*, 26.

Clay, R.A. (1998, July). More clinical psychologists move into organizational consulting realm. *American Psychological Association Monitor, 29(7)*, 28.

Cohn, P.J. (1991). An exploratory study on peak performance in golf. *The Sport Psychologist, 5*, 1–14.

Crace, R.K., & Hardy, C.J. (1989). Developing your mental pacemaker. *Sport Psychology Training Bulletin, 1(2)*, 1–6.

Csikszentmihalyi, M. (1990). *Flow: The psychology of optimal experience*. New York: Harper Perennial.

Danish, S.J., & Nellen, V.C. (1997). New roles for sport psychologists: Teaching life skills through sport to at-risk youth. *Quest, 49*, 100–113.

Feinstein, J. (1996). *A good walk spoiled*. Boston: Little, Brown.

Foulser, J. (Producer). (1993). *My greatest golf shot* [Videotape]. Sunset & Vine/Polygram Video International.

Gal-Or, Y., Tenenbaum, G., & Shimrony, S. (1986). Cognitive behavioral strategies and anxiety in elite orienteers. *Journal of Sports Sciences, 4*, 39–48.

Hardy, L. (1990). A catastrophe model of performance in sport. In G. Jones & L. Hardy (Eds.), *Stress and performance in sport* (pp. 81–106). Chichester: Wiley.

Hardy, L., Jones, G., & Gould, D. (1996). *Understanding psychological preparation for sport*. Chichester: Wiley.

Jackson, D.M. (Producer). (1993). *Mind over golf*. [Videotape]. London: BBC Enterprises.

Jackson, S.A., Thomas, P.R., Marsh, H.W., & Smethurst, C.J. (in press). Relationships between flow, self-concept, psychological skills, and performance. *Journal of Applied Sport Psychology*.

Jones, G. (1993). The role of performance profiling in cognitive behavioral interventions in sport. *The Sport Psychologist, 7*, 160–172.

Kirkby, R. (1995). Sport psychology in Australia: Past myths and future directions. *Australian Psychologist, 30*, 75–77.

Martens, R. (1987). *Coaches' guide to sport psychology*. Champaign, IL: Human Kinetics.

McCaffrey, N., & Orlick, T. (1989). Mental factors related to excellence among top professional golfers. *International Journal of Sport Psychology, 20*, 256–278.

Morris, T., & Thomas, P.R. (1995). Approaches to applied sport psychology. In T. Morris & J. Summers (Eds.), *Sport psychology: Theory, applications and current issues* (pp. 215–258). Brisbane: Jacaranda Wiley.

Murphy, S.M. (1996). *The achievement zone*. New York: Putnam.

National Australian Football Council (Producer). (1990). *Psychology and motivation in football* [Videotape]. Melbourne: National Australian Football Council.

Nideffer, R.M. (1985). *Athletes' guide to mental training*. Champaign, IL: Human Kinetics.

Nideffer, R.M. (1992). *Psyched to win*. Champaign, IL: Leisure Press.

Orlick, T. (1986). *Psyching for sport: Mental training for athletes*. Champaign, IL: Leisure Press.

Orlick, T. (1990). *In pursuit of excellence* (2nd ed.). Champaign, IL: Leisure Press.

Owens, D., & Bunker, L.K. (1992). *Advanced golf: Steps to success*. Champaign, IL: Leisure Press.

Oxendine, J.B. (1970). Emotional arousal and motor performance. *Quest, 13*, 23–32.

Pelz, D. (1994). A study of golfers' abilities to read greens. In A.J. Cochran & M.R. Farrally (Eds.), *Science and golf II: Proceedings of the World Scientific Congress of Golf* (pp. 180–185). London: E & F.N. Spon.

Ravizza, K. (1988). Gaining entry with athletic personnel for season-long consulting. *The Sport Psychologist, 2*, 243–254.

Rotella, R. (1995). *Golf is not a game of perfect*. New York: Simon & Schuster.

Seiler, R. (1990). Decision making processes in orienteering: An action theoretical investigation. *International Journal of Sport Psychology, 21*, 36–45.

Taylor, J., & Taylor, C. (1995). *Psychology of dance*. Champaign, IL: Human Kinetics.

Thomas, F.W. (1994). The state of the game, equipment and science. In A.J. Cochran & M.R. Farrally (Eds.), *Science and golf II: Proceedings of the World Scientific Congress of Golf* (pp. 237–246). London: E & F.N. Spon.

Thomas, P.R. (1991, November). *An overview of performance enhancement processes in applied sport psychology.* Paper presented at the Asian South Pacific Association of Sports Psychology 1st International Congress, Melbourne.

Thomas, P.R. (1993). Psychological skills profiles of athletes: The effects of feedback. *European Journal for High Ability, 4*, 161–170.

Thomas, P.R., & Fogarty, G.J. (1997). Psychological skills training in golf: The role of individual differences in cognitive preferences. *The Sport Psychologist, 11*, 86–106.

Thomas, P.R., Murphy, S.M., & Hardy, L. (1999). Test of Performance Strategies: Development and preliminary validation of a comprehensive measure of athletes' psychological skills. *Journal of Sports Sciences, 17*, 697–711.

Thomas, P.R., & Over, R. (1994). Psychological and psychomotor skills associated with performance in golf. *The Sport Psychologist, 8*, 73–86.

Thomas, R. (Producer). (1994). *The nearly men* [Videotape]. Quadrant Video/Festival Records.

Vealey, R.S. (1986). Imagery training for performance enhancement. In J.M. Williams (Ed.), *Applied sport psychology* (pp. 209–234). Palo Alto, CA: Mayfield.

Weinberg, R.S., & Gould, D. (1995). *Foundations of sport and exercise psychology*. Champaign, IL: Human Kinetics.

Winter, G., & Martin, C. (1991). *Sport psychology basic training program* (2nd ed.). Adelaide: South Australian Sports Institute.

Yerkes, R.M., & Dodson, J.D. (1908). The relation of strength of stimulus to rapidity of habit formation. *Journal of Comparative and Neurological Psychology, 18*, 459–482.

From St. Kilda to Kings Cross: Planning Your Specialist Training in Sport Psychology

Steven Christensen

This chapter explores how one becomes a sport psychologist.[1] It provides directions about how someone with undergraduate training in psychology and sport science[2] can plan and manage their specialist training in sport psychology. Although the information is drawn from the author's experiences in Australia, the ideas are applicable to specialist training in sport psychology in other countries.

The chapter employs the metaphor of a journey. The catchy phrase "from St. Kilda to Kings Cross" was selected to help readers keep the image of a journey in mind as they read. This phrase is from a song by Australian popular singer, Paul Kelly (1985). Kelly's journey begins on a sunny St. Kilda beach (Melbourne, Australia) and finishes as he arrives in bustling Kings Cross (Sydney, Australia). As the song describes ". . . from St. Kilda to Kings Cross—it's 14 hours on a bus." Aspiring sport psychologists start their journeys from the location of their current skills, knowledge, and experience in sport psychology. Their final destination is the acquisition of the skills, knowledge, and values of the professional sport psychologist.[3] Like Paul Kelly, the aspiring sport psychologist begins his or her journey with a suitcase full of dreams, ambitions, and skills, and sets off with a degree of apprehension and uncertainty about what lies ahead. The journey from current skills and knowledge to the professional competencies required of an accredited sport psychologist is more abstract than Paul Kelly's journey from St. Kilda to Kings Cross. Just as a map was useful for Paul Kelly, this chapter is intended to be something of a conceptual map for aspiring sport psychologists to plan and manage their specialist training.

This chapter has been written in three parts:

1. The first section, *Planning the Journey: Where Am I Now?*, provides aspiring sport

---

1. In this chapter, a sport psychologist is defined as someone who has undertaken advanced professional training in sport psychology and who spends the majority of working time engaged in teaching, research, and/or consulting in sport psychology.

2. The author recognizes the ongoing debate in the profession about the level of psychology and sport science training that is needed to practice sport psychology. This chapter endorses the position that the aspiring sport psychologist should have undergraduate level training in psychology and sport science.

3. The accreditation needed to practice sport psychology and the registration and licensing required to use the title sport psychologist differ among countries, states, and provinces. In this chapter, the term professional sport psychologist refers to a sport psychologist (see Footnote 1), who is appropriately accredited and licensed in the country, state, or province in which he or she is working.

psychologists with some direction about planning their journey by examining their current skills, knowledge, and abilities. This section aims to help aspirants determine their present location.

2. The second section, *Planning the Destination: Where Do I Want to Go?*, aims to help aspiring sport psychologists determine the skills, knowledge, and values that need to be developed during their specialist training in sport psychology. This section provides some direction about how to determine what skills, knowledge, and values are important in sport psychology. In addition, the section offers some comments about alternative ways of understanding and acquiring these specialist competencies.

3. The third section, *Planning the Route: How Do I Get There?*, provides aspiring sport psychologists with some direction about how they can conduct their specialist training in sport psychology. This section introduces three pathways for specialist training in sport psychology: university-based training, mentor-mentee-based training, and a program of training and retraining involving short courses and other structured experiences.

The author adopts an informal style and outlines the main conclusions at this point because some of the arguments are complex and do not reach conclusions until very late in the chapter. The chapter argues for the importance of developing personal and professional competence during specialized training in sport psychology. While the professional competencies are developed during a specialist training program, it is the author's view that personal competencies should begin developing the moment the individual decides to become a sport psychologist. Personal competencies are defined as the abilities of planning for life, being self-

reliant, and seeking resources from others (Danish, D'Augelli, & Ginsberg, 1984; Danish, Petitpas, & Hale, 1995). These skills are highly valued in sport and are fundamental to many sport psychology practices (Danish et al., 1995).

Planning professional training in sport psychology is a rich opportunity for aspirants to identify, set, and attain their specialist training goals. It is a chance to develop interpersonal and intrapersonal skills, and to experience the empowerment and self-efficacy that sport psychologists believe are so important to foster in athletes, coaches, teams, and sporting organizations. Aspirants must make informed decisions about their professional training. The chapter describes a student-initiated approach to specialist training in sport psychology, which is one pathway for developing the competencies of the professional sport psychologist.

Planning the Journey: Where Am I Now?

For Paul Kelly (1985), "Where am I now?" was a geographical question. Before beginning his journey, Kelly was the lonely figure walking along a windswept St. Kilda beach. For aspiring sport psychologists, it is a question about skills, knowledge, and abilities. It asks whether aspirants are *capable* of planning their journey and *capable* of independently traveling their chosen routes. The question is explored by considering the skills, knowledge, and abilities needed to plan and manage specialist training in sport psychology. In addition, this section considers a strategy that students may use to determine their standing on these competencies.

Firstly, what skills, knowledge, and abilities do aspiring sport psychologists need to plan and manage their specialist training in sport psychology? Initially, an aspirant must have completed undergraduate training in psychology and sport science, which will usually result in having been awarded an undergraduate degree from a university or similarly accredited institution. In most cases, the undergraduate degree will provide opportunities to develop a thorough understanding of the basic scientific principles of psychology and sport science. An aspiring sport psychologist can be expected to have a solid grounding in the generic knowledge base and basic research skills of psychology and sport science. In some cases, the undergraduate program may introduce the aspirant to some applied skills in psychology and sport science that are useful in sport, exercise, health, or rehabilitation settings.

The undergraduate degree provides opportunities to develop other skills that are important for planning and managing specialist training. In a recent Australian survey, Chubb (1992) found that academics placed a high value on developing the intellectual autonomy of their students. Chubb reported that Australian academics aim to develop a range of generic competencies, personal attributes, and values. The generic competencies include critical thinking; intellectual curiosity; problem solving; logical and independent thought; effective communication; and related skills in identifying, accessing, and managing information. Further personal attributes, such as intellectual rigor, creativity, and imagination, and values, such as ethical practice, integrity, and tolerance, were also encouraged.

In a complementary survey, the Australian Business/Higher Education Round Table (1992) explored what graduate employee characteristics are highly valued by Australian academic, business, government, and union representatives. The findings stressed a mixture of generic competencies and work-related skills, such as communication skills, the capacity to learn new skills and procedures, the capacity for cooperation and teamwork, the capacity to make decisions and solve problems, the capability to apply knowledge to the workplace, and the capacity to work with minimum supervision.

With the above in mind, contemporary Western academic careers are often seen as flexible and mobile. It is not uncommon for a Western academic to work in several universities and in different countries during his or her academic career. It is assumed that the knowledge and skills that the academic possesses are transferable across institutions, states, provinces, and countries. It is also assumed that the personal attributes and values that academics hold for tertiary education are common across institutions in different geographical locations. Therefore, it can be reasonably assumed that academics and institutions in other parts of the world generally support the generic competencies, personal attributes, and values rated highly by Australian academics.

During my eight years of training sport psychology graduates in Australia and from comments made to me by Australian and overseas colleagues, there appears to be general agreement on the competencies needed for success in postgraduate university studies. These include communication and other work-related skills (Business/Higher Education Round Table, 1992), a solid grounding in the knowledge and research of the discipline of the study, and the ability to demonstrate intellectual autonomy (Chubb, 1992). In my experience, these are also the important competencies needed by trainees to *competently plan, effectively manage, and complete* their specialist training in sport psychology.

So how does the aspiring sport psychologist determine his or her standing on these important competencies? The following strategy is one approach that aspirants may use to audit their competency. The strategy involves three steps.

Aspirants determine their standing on the generic competencies and work-related skills as identified in the Business/Higher Education Round Table report (1992). This involves self-assessment of these attributes, together with asking a peer, an academic adviser, and an older personal or family friend to also rate the aspirant on the six attributes.

Aspirants test their intellectual autonomy by undertaking a problem-solving task. For example, uncovering the competencies that are highly valued in the experienced sport psychologist would be a challenging project that would test intellectual autonomy, communication, and other work-related skills of any aspiring sport psychologist. This project would include tasks such as framing the research question; collecting and assembling the data, findings, and interpretations; validating the findings through discussions with academic advisers and others; and presenting the findings in the form of recommendations for specialist training in sport psychology. This project would provide two important sources of information. Firstly, objective evidence about intellectual autonomy abilities. A second outcome of the project would be useful information about the skills, knowledge, and values that need to be developed during specialist training in sport psychology.

Aspirants examine the information gathered from steps one and two with assistance from an older trusted friend or family member. The ratings of the aspirant's communication and other work-related skills offered by a peer, an academic adviser, an older personal or family friend, and the aspirant himself or herself is a rich source of information. Initially, the aspirant and a trusted friend sit together to review what this information says about the aspiring sport psychologist. Following this, the pair review the level of intellectual autonomy demonstrated by the student during the self-initiated competency project. This review helps uncover the aspirant's current strengths and weaknesses, as well as understand them in relation to impor-

tant sport psychology competencies. Together the aspirant and an older friend can examine the self-reports, referee's reports, and the process and output of the project to triangulate and confirm evidence about the aspirant's competencies.

This process allows the prospective trainee to determine his or her current location in a skills, knowledge, and abilities sense for a future career in sport psychology. Knowing where you begin is important to planning specialist training in sport psychology.

This section explored the question, "Where am I now?" To return to the Paul Kelly metaphor, this section could have been used by Kelly to determine if he was starting at St. Kilda or still had to reach the beach at St. Kilda. The next section considers where the aspiring sport psychologist wants to go.

Planning the Destination: "Where Do I Want to Go?"

For Paul Kelly, "Where do I want to go?" was another geographical question. His dreams were to be found in Kings Cross. He was in St. Kilda but his destination was Kings Cross. For the aspiring sport psychologist this is a competency question. It asks the aspirant to understand the skills, knowledge, and values of the professional sport psychologist. Like Kelly, aspirants need to know not only where they are now, but also where they wish to go. They need to know what competencies they currently have *and* what competencies they need to achieve.

This section explores the question of professional competencies. The approach taken here is not to answer this using a competency-based definition of professionalism because this approach is problematic for several reasons. While the aspirant might prefer such a deterministic position, the approach here is to discuss the processes at work in planning specialist training in sport psychology. The aim of this chapter is to encourage the aspiring sport psychologist to take *responsibility* for his or her professional development rather than rely on packaged training programs and ready-made answers.

This section will not give an extensive list of the employment-related competencies of the professional sport psychologist in response to the question, "Where do I want to go?" Such an approach would be contrary to intentions and would be tantamount to imposing the author's destination on the aspiring sport psychologist. It would miss the chance for the aspirant to develop personal competencies to supplement their professional competencies. Further, such a list of employment-related competencies would be based on assumptions about the definition and practice of sport psychology. These assumptions may not be appropriate in all contexts, be they cross-national or cross-cultural. At best, such a deterministic solution would be a rough approximation. Such a general destination is not an ideal career goal for an aspiring sport psychologist. Therefore, I will resist providing a narrow and deterministic definition of the competencies of the professional sport psychologist.

This section uses a systems approach to understanding the skills, knowledge, and values of the professional sport psychologist. Bandura (1978) and Lazarus and Folkman (1984) recommend using a systems approach for understanding complex and interrelated phenomena. A systems approach investigates phenomena that are an organized whole rather than a set of isolated units or separate components. The skills, knowledge, and values of the professional sport psychologist may or may not be complex; each aspirant can determine his or her position on this issue. However, these professional competencies are interrelated and a systems approach offers a better understanding of these competencies as an organized whole. The reader is encouraged to see rela-

tions among the competencies discussed in this section, albeit that sport psychology skills, knowledge, and values are presented separately. This separate layout offers easier reading but detracts from gaining an integrated understanding. Nevertheless, it is hoped that the common structure and common-sense recommendations running through each segment will afford opportunities to see mutual interactions among knowledge, skills, and values. Additionally, it is hoped that the reader will look beyond the repetitive structure in this section and begin to see coordinative structures and collaborative processes for planning specialist training in sport psychology.

The author asks three questions of each competency on behalf of the aspiring sport psychologist:

- What are the important features of this dimension?
- In what form do I need to understand these important features?
- And finally, how do I develop such an understanding of these important features?

Sport Psychology Knowledge

Discipline knowledge includes the data, information, knowledge, and wisdom about sport psychology that are used to understand the behavior, cognition, emotion, and motivation of athletes and their teams and sporting organizations.

Four beliefs underpin the author's approach to discussing the knowledge base of sport psychology. Three are drawn from Rainer Martens's (1987) discussion about the relationship among science, knowledge, and sport psychology. Firstly, Martens argues that any schism between academic sport psychology and practicing sport psychology is harmful to developing a trustworthy knowledge base for sport psychology teaching, research, and consulting. Secondly, orthodox methods of science limit the understanding, description, and prediction of sporting behavior. Thirdly, Martens argued that the knowledge base of sport psychology should be equally relevant to both academic and applied activity. The fourth belief holds that sport psychology research and theory building needs to demonstrate trustworthiness or rigor (Lincoln & Guba, 1985) so that sport psychologists can be confident about the knowledge base of their profession.

The immediate question is, "What information and content is important in sport psychology?" Sport psychology, like most professions, describes its discipline knowledge in both formal and informal ways. There are several formal sources of information for describing the sport psychology knowledge base that are useful to the aspiring sport psychologist. For example, the content of undergraduate and postgraduate courses in sport psychology describes the information considered important for sport psychology students. Often, the course rationale and syllabus are distributed to students at the beginning of a course. This information is submitted to University Academic Boards so that courses and university degrees gain university approval and accreditation.

Other formal sources include the criteria that professional associations use to recognize university qualifications and determine professional membership. Additionally, state and national professional registration boards in some countries use criteria that include descriptions of the sport psychology knowledge base to license individual practitioners. While the university accreditation documents are usually not readily available to an aspirant, access can be gained to the other sources of information. For example, information on a course rationale and syllabus, professional membership, and licensing criteria can be obtained by contacting the academic advisers, professional associations representing sport psychology, and relevant registration boards.

Unfortunately, some sources of information may not be available in particular locations because of the way the sport psychology profession is structured alongside other human service, medical, and sport science professions. Therefore, some lines of inquiry may not be successful. However, it is important to remember that the purpose of this reconnaissance is to gain information for describing sport psychology knowledge that is relevant to where the aspirant wishes to eventually work. In some cases it might be useful to collect formal information from countries that have well established peak industry bodies and professional organizations representing sport psychology. This may be a useful supplement to more readily available information or may be relevant should the aspiring sport psychologist consider studying or working interstate or in another country.

There are also informal sources of information describing sport psychology that may be useful. For example, the content pages of undergraduate and postgraduate textbooks usually represent important areas of knowledge. Additionally, sport psychology journals and the proceedings of sport psychology conferences are rich sources of information. Therefore, aspirants can supplement the formal sources of information that are available to them with descriptions that have been collected from these informal sources.

However, there is an interesting second question about sport psychology that is relevant to the aspirant: "In what form does the aspiring sport psychologist need to know the sport psychology knowledge base?" This question moves the issue beyond considering, "What do I need to know?" and considers, "How do I need to know it?"

Rainer Martens (1987) has argued for an alternative form of knowing sport psychology that integrates psychological theory, research, and practice. Martens recognizes four forms of knowledge: *data, information, knowledge*, and *wisdom* that are related in a hierarchical way. *Data* are undigested observations and unvarnished facts, and *information* is organized data. *Knowledge* is organized information that is internalized and integrated into a person's existing knowledge structure. It is useful for guiding action and making decisions within a discipline or domain. *Wisdom* is integrated knowledge that is linked across several disciplines, domains, or specializations.

Martens (1987) has argued for an alternative form of knowing sport psychology that is based on a heuristic philosophy of knowledge (Polanyi, 1958, 1966, cited in Martens, 1987). He encourages sport psychologists to set themselves the goal of developing wisdom *about* sport psychology. This wisdom exists as a form of knowing called *tacit integration*. Tacit integration is a skill. It involves recognizing meaningful patterns in random data, information, and knowledge about a problem by using intuition and insight developed from an integrated understanding of knowledge across disciplines and domains. This differs from conventional approaches to problem solving in sport psychology where solutions to sport problems are determined by relating the data to a single sport psychology theory. Martens points out that the skill of tacit integration enables the sport psychologist to work with the raw clues yet see meaningful patterns in this random data that often other people are unable to see. This form of knowing involves a more holistic approach to understanding the relationship between problems and apparently random data. The reader is directed to Martens's article (1987) for further discussion of this topic.

The obvious question then: "How do I develop a tacit understanding of the sport psy-chology knowledge base?" One approach is to view it as a skill and to use the principles of skill acquisition to develop this competency. In the first step of this approach, aspirants determine whether they wish to understand this form of knowing sport psychology. They are encouraged to talk about tacit knowledge with an academic adviser or professional mentor, and to decide whether to pursue this learning goal. Additionally, the adviser or mentor can assist by modeling this skill and directing the trainee to further examples of tacit integration in sport psychology teaching, research, and consulting. This book, for instance, provides examples of tactic integration. It presents the practice of sport psychology with athletes, coaches, teams, and sporting organizations through the experiences of leading practitioners. The various chapters describe how experienced sport psychologists understand the relationship between particular sporting problems and the sources of data and other information contained in the sporting environment. This is tactic integration in action. Although the chapters do not actually describe how the sport psychologist comes to see such meaningful patterns or establish such forms of knowing, they do provide rich illustrations of Martens's (1987) heuristic form of knowing sport psychology. Clearly then, the skill of tacit integration needs to become an objective of professional training if sport psychology wisdom is to be developed.

A second step is to provide aspirants with ample opportunities to practice this skill under the guidance of an adviser or mentor. The familiar teaching and coaching adage to *provide plenty of perfect practice under play-like conditions with ph(f)requent and pertinent ph(f)eedback* (anonymous), reminds us that this practice should be under favorable conditions until it can be performed skillfully and spontaneously. The final step involves arranging for successful experiences, particularly for the trainee's initial efforts. This, together with opportunities for feedback from peers and more senior colleagues and for critical reflection about decisions and actions, provides an environment that is conducive to developing tacit understanding.

Martens (1979) provides some direction in how this form of knowing can be developed. He argues that sport psychologists should be simultaneously active in the field and in the academy. This means being involved in sport psychology experiences in the field and being required to bring data drawn from the field into the classroom and laboratory for critique and analysis. It also means being involved in sport psychology experiences in the academy and bringing data drawn from the laboratory and classroom into the field for similar critique and analysis.

This process of moving between academy and field settings, and the efforts to understand in a way that is independent of the context, provides rich opportunities for developing tacit integration. Essentially, it engages the aspiring sport psychologist in a recursive process of establishing and re-establishing meaning from random data. As the data is drawn from both settings, the task of assigning meaning is somewhat more complex than would be necessary if only laboratory-based or field-based data was being processed. Although difficult, the nature of the data helps the trainee to resist the temptation of foreclosing on an incomplete understanding of the problem and subsequent solution by simply applying a scientific or common-sense sport psychology theory to the data.

A second process provides the aspiring sport psychologist with opportunities to gain insight into the steps taken to integrate data, information, and knowledge into a process of intuition. Polanyi (1958, 1966, cited in Martens, 1987) and Gelwick (1979, cited in Martens, 1987) explain that tacit knowledge

is a subsidiary awareness. It is not readily accessible to the individual, as it is difficult to be simultaneously solving a sporting problem and monitoring how intuition and insight is being used to solve the problem. The second process aims to raise to conscious awareness the intuitions and insight that an aspirant has used to give meaning to data and solve a sport problem. It involves arranging for opportunities to talk about the problem and the data with other aspiring sport psychologists and more senior colleagues.

However, the role played by these other people is quite specific and differs from the usual debriefing and sharing of experiences that most graduate students and colleagues engage in. Instead, those assisting the trainee use their professional interviewing skills to probe the aspirant for information, knowledge, and the relations between both that have led to recognizing meaning in the data. These interviews aim to help the trainee to develop insight into the cognitive processes that have been used to construct their understanding of the data. In this way the trainee is probed for insight and intuition, and given opportunities for critical self-reflection. This probing helps to make tacit integration more visible to the sport psychology trainee.

The academic adviser or professional mentor has the important role of providing feedback and support to the aspiring sport psychologist. This is a more familiar process to many university staff and postgraduate students. It involves the adviser or mentor providing feedback on the aspirant's efforts to help them better understand and address sporting problems that have been explored in the field, laboratory, and classroom. The adviser or mentor may also provide some collegial support that helps the aspirant through the difficult and demanding experience of learning this form of the sport psychology knowledge base.

Sport Psychology Skills and Practices

Skills and practices relate to the applied dimension of sport psychology. This dimension describes several competencies relating to the practice of sport psychology, including adding to the knowledge base about the science and practice of sport psychology; conducting systematic assessment and evaluation; delivering psychological interventions; establishing and maintaining professional relationships; and communicating effectively with clients, psychologists, other professionals, and members of the public.

Three beliefs have influenced the approach taken by the author to discuss the skills and practices that are important in sport psychology. The first belief is that any schism between academic sport psychology and practicing sport psychology is harmful to further development of the sport psychology profession (Martens, 1987). Martens advocates for a single perspective of sport psychology practice that encompasses teaching, research, and consulting. Martens values the contribution that each sport psychology dimension makes to the profession and recognizes that sport psychology teaching, research, and consulting require different skills, practices, and competencies.

Secondly, interventions and strategies are determined according to the needs of the client and nature of the teaching, research, or consulting problem. Furthermore, these selected skills and practices are implemented in a competent manner that provides clients with the best chance of achieving positive outcomes from the intervention. Lazarus (1989) advocates for a systems perspective of assessment, intervention, and evaluation. He argues that in order to understand the client's problem, it is important to assess the client's needs, personal characteristics, and functioning as well as the physical and social characteristics of the natural environment. Lazarus argues for the need to determine and deliver intervention strategies that match the client's problem in maintaining integrated and optimal functioning.

The final assumption acknowledges the diverse approaches to practicing sport psychology. This view acknowledges the nature of recent discussions about the skills and practices that are important in applied sport psychology and have been held in some countries. This has been an emotional topic of discussion because of its proximity to the debates about what constitutes professional training in sport psychology and accreditation of the professional sport psychologist. The approach here has been modeled on the approach used by Danish, Petitpas, and Hale (1995). While acknowledging that different beliefs about sport psychology practice and training exist, Danish and colleagues focus on whether the aspiring sport psychologist has the necessary skills to implement the chosen intervention, understands the potential consequences of this intervention, and understands behavior, emotion, cognition, and motivation within the client's social, biological, and psychological context.

Notwithstanding the earlier discussion, the immediate question is "What skills and practices are important in sport psychology?" As with comments that have been made earlier in this chapter, sport psychology describes its skills and practice in both formal and informal ways. Given the diverse approaches to practicing sport psychology, it is important for the aspirant to do some reconnaissance and research into the skills and practices considered important. This research involves three steps: collecting formal and informal sources of information about important sport psychology skills and practices; reading this information and assembling it into a concise and reliable summary; and aiming to understand the array of skills and practices for teaching, research, and consulting in sport psychology with reference to discussions about practice, training, and certification.

McCullagh and Noble (1996), Morris and Summers (1995), Murphy (1995), and Zaichkowsky and Perna (1996) summarize some of the recent discussions about sport psychology practice, training, and certification. Aspiring sport psychologists are encouraged to discuss their understanding of these issues with local academic advisers and professional mentors in order to determine the sport psychology skills and practices that are considered important in their country.

There are several formal sources of information for describing the important sport psychology skills and practices that may be useful. For example, the syllabi of various undergraduate and postgraduate courses describe the skills and practices that are considered important. In many cases, the syllabi describe the research skills and professional skills that are the focus of the course but may inadvertently neglect to describe important presentation, communication, and interpersonal skills. After reviewing course materials, the aspirant is encouraged to talk with university lecturers about how they conduct and assess their courses in order to gain a better understanding of the range of skills and practices that are being covered and the depth to which they are being developed.

Aspirants are also encouraged to collect information relating to both undergraduate and postgraduate units. In recent times, there has been a trend in Australian universities to focus on developing discipline knowledge, research, and communication skills in undergraduate psychology degrees and on developing professional consulting and advanced research skills in postgraduate psychology degrees. If this trend is being followed in other countries, it may be important for aspirants to collect information that allows them to understand both the range

and depth of skills training available from university courses.

In addition, there are two other useful sources of information for describing the important sport psychology skills and practices. The criteria that professional associations use to recognize university qualifications and determine professional membership are one useful source of information. In some geographical centers, professional associations in psychology, sport science, or physical education have chapters or divisions representing sport psychology. These various professional associations are useful sources of information. Additionally, in some locations, state or national professional registration boards use criteria that include descriptions of the important skills and practices to license individual sport psychology practitioners. These registration boards, together with some National Olympic Committees, are useful formal sources of information. Information about course rationale and syllabi, professional membership, and licensing and certification criteria can be obtained from academic advisers, professional associations representing sport psychology, national and state registration boards, and National Olympic Committees.

As mentioned earlier, some sources of information may not be available in particular areas because of the way that the sport psychology profession is structured and constructed alongside other human services, medical, and sport science professions. Therefore, some inquiries might not be successful. Nevertheless, the purpose of this reconnaissance is to gain information describing the sport psychology skills and practices that are considered important in the particular country, state, or province in which the aspiring sport psychologist wishes to eventually work. In some cases, it might be useful to collect formal information from countries that have well-established peak industry bodies and professional organizations representing sport psychology. This information might be a useful supplement to more readily available information or may be relevant if the aspirant intends studying or working in another state, province, or country.

In addition there are several informal sources of information describing frequently used sport psychology skills and practices that may be useful. For example, undergraduate and postgraduate textbooks in sport psychology often describe important and highly regarded skills and practices. This book is an example. Sport psychology journals and conference proceedings are additional sources of this information. Therefore, the aspirant could supplement the formal sources of information that are available to them with information collected from these informal sources.

An important part of this process of determining the skills and practices of sport psychology involves aspirants discussing their understanding and views with experienced sport psychologists. Sport psychologists are valuable sources of information about the practice of sport psychology. However, because their time is often limited and discussions about sport psychology practice, training, and certification may become complex, aspirants are encouraged to summarize relevant information and consolidate their views prior to meeting with an experienced sport psychologist. In this way aspirants can maximize the benefits of talking with an experienced sport psychologist. In addition, aspirants are encouraged to speak with several sport psychologists who are predominantly engaged in different dimensions of sport psychology practice.

There is an interesting second question relating to skills and practices that is relevant to the aspirant: "In what form does the aspiring sport psychologist need to be able to understand and demonstrate these skills and practices?" This question is not directed at determining the skills and practices that the author believes are important, or describing the level of proficiency that trainees need to be able to demonstrate in a particular skill or range of practices. Considerations such as these do not help given the national, provincial, regional, and institutional differences in sport psychology practice, training, and certification. Instead, the question considers the process of matching interventions with client problems.

Richard Lazarus (1989) has argued for an alternative form of matching therapeutic strategies to client problems. This argument originally focused on clinical psychology practice and explored the processes of determining psychotherapy and other therapeutic strategies that were appropriate for various mental health problems. However, the argument is relevant to the process of matching interventions with problems experienced by athletes, coaches, teams, and sporting organizations.

A key function that is relevant across the teaching, research, and consulting dimensions of sport psychology practice is the skill of conceptualizing the problem or formulating the case. The words *conceptualize* and *formulate* are frequently associated with clinical psychology practice. However, the process of using data, information, and knowledge drawn from psychological, pedagogical, or sport science assessments to determine a concise description and rationale about a problem is equally relevant to high standards of sport psychology practice. Determining an appropriate intervention program and evaluation strategy for this problem or case is an important skill that complements case formulation skills. Notwithstanding that sport psychology practice can be characterized by educational, counseling, and clinical approaches, determining an intervention program and evaluation program that matches the conceptualized problem or formulated case is an important skill of the professional sport psychologist.

Lazarus (1989) distinguishes two approaches to the concept of strategy-problem-fit that has been adapted by the author in this chapter. The process of fitting intervention strategies to a conceptualized problem or formulated case characterizes the first approach. Within this approach Lazarus recognized two alternative forms of this strategy-problem-fit approach: the restricted treatment model and the restricted problem model. The restricted treatment model endorses a *flexible* style of fitting intervention strategies to problems. Herein, a limited range of interventions or strategies are understood by the sport psychologist who is skilled at adapting these interventions and transferring them to a variety of teaching, research, and consulting problems. The restricted problem model endorses a *narrow* style of fitting interventions to problems. Here, a limited range of interventions or strategies are understood by the sport psychologist who specializes in dealing only with certain kinds of teaching, research, or consulting problems.

The process of matching problems or cases to particular intervention strategies characterizes the second approach. Within a sport psychology context, there are two alternative forms of this approach. The first is an application of the Life Development Intervention model (Danish, Petitpas, & Hale, 1995; Danish, Smyer, & Nowak, 1980) to Lazarus's (1989) argument. Although not discussed by Lazarus, this form considers the temporal location of various sport psychology problems, along with other characteristics. In this form of problem-strategy-fit approach, problems are matched to particular interventions according to the timing of the onset of the problem. That is, whether the objectives of the intervention are to help the client encounter the event or problem, con-

tend with the event or problem, or cope with the event or problem following its occurrence. Applying this problem-strategy-fit approach to sport psychology involves two steps. Firstly, the *temporal* location and other features about the nature of the problem must be determined. Secondly, the *efficacy* of particular interventions to deal with the problem that is distinguished according to its temporal nature, as conceptualized in relation to a Life Development Intervention model, must be determined. The problem is then matched to an effective intervention strategy.

The alternative form proposed by Lazarus (1989) is based on his cognitive and relational theory of emotion and adaptation (Lazarus & Folkman, 1984). This form considers a systems analysis of emotion and adaptation in which the nature of the problem can be located at different causal locations in the system. These include the antecedent beliefs, motives, and commitment; person-environment fit; primary appraisal; secondary appraisal; and coping skills that are held by the coach, athlete, team, or sporting organization. Applying this form of the problem-strategy-fit approach to sport psychology practice involves two steps. Firstly, the *causal* location and other features about the nature of the problem must be determined. Secondly, the *efficacy* of particular interventions must be determined in terms of their ability to deal with a problem that is distinguished according to its causal nature, as conceptualized in relation to emotion, adaptation, and coping. The problem is then matched to an effective intervention strategy.

There has not been widespread discussion about this topic in the sport psychology literature in recent times. In some ways the topic may be viewed as being overly academic or not sufficiently grounded in the day-to-day practice of sport psychology. This is a judgment for the aspiring sport psychologist to make. However, aspirants who are interested in this issue might consider the following exercise. It involves reading about the experiences of leading sport psychologists that are contained in this book and trying to understand the strategy-problem *fitting* or *matching* styles that these experienced sport psychologists have used in their respective teaching, research, and consulting work.

Consistent with the framework used earlier in this chapter, the obvious question is "How do I develop such a form of strategy-problem *fitting* or problem-strategy *matching* for sport psychology practice?" The first step involves determining whether they wish to develop a particular form of conceptualizing a problem and selecting an appropriate intervention and evaluation strategy for their sport psychology practice. The aspirant is encouraged to talk about this issue with an academic adviser or professional mentor and make a decision about whether to pursue learning this skill. The outcome of the strategy-problem *fitting* or *matching* style exercise may be a helpful starting point to stimulate conversation between the pair. It may also be useful for the adviser or mentor to model some of the approaches described earlier, and to direct the aspirant to other instances of strategy-problem-fit in the sport psychology literature.

In some settings there may not be opportunities, resources, or advisers with sufficient expertise to train aspirants in particular approaches to case formulation, intervention, and evaluation strategies. If the trainee is interested in developing a strategy-problem fitting or problem-strategy matching style, and if there are available resources to support this professional training, then it needs to become an objective of their professional training. This form or style of sport psychology practice can then be viewed as a skill, and skill learning principles and practices used to develop it.

A program will need to be developed by the aspirant with assistance from his or her adviser or mentor to provide opportunities to learn this professional skill. Such a program should aim to provide aspiring sport psychologists with many opportunities to rehearse this skill during their professional training. Furthermore, it should aim for skill rehearsal under favorable conditions and accompanied by opportunities for feedback from peers and more senior colleagues, initial experiences of success, and periods of critical reflection about the trainee's decisions and actions. Goal setting (Burton, 1989; Gould, 1992; Weinberg, 1996) or learning contracts (Anderson, Boud, & Sampson, 1996) may be helpful for planning and implementing activities to develop these skills and practices.

Sport Psychology Values

Sport psychology values influence ethical and professional conduct. Values relate to the moral dimension of sport psychology and describe the nature of the relationship between the sport psychologist and their profession, professional organizations, colleagues, clients, students, participants, and oneself. This section is influenced by the author's eight years' experience of training sport psychologists in Australia, and draws upon ethical and professional issues that graduates have presented during this time.

The view of ethical and professional conduct in sport psychology as a moral responsibility rather than as a legal obligation has been adopted in this section. Adopting a moral rather than a legal frame of reference on ethical and professional sport psychology practice argues for conduct being undertaken because of a genuine concern about the wider interests of others. In contrast, a legal perspective is oriented towards determining minimum standards of professional conduct and can foster the impulse to protect the interests of the sport psychology lecturer, researcher, or practitioner. Therefore, the question of what ethical and professional conduct is important in sport psychology needs to be examined.

Like other professions, sport psychology describes its legal and professional conduct in both formal and informal ways. There are several formal sources of information for describing ethical and professional sport psychology practice that are useful to the aspiring sport psychologist. For example, the content of postgraduate courses on ethics and professional practice, and on research methods are useful sources of information about ethical and professional conduct. In addition, university and departmental ethics committees that review ethical and professional aspects of research proposals are usually guided by written codes of conduct.

Other formal sources include the standards of ethical practice that professional associations use to inform and manage their members. Additionally, where state or national professional registration boards in psychology, teaching, or sport science are responsible for licensing individual sport psychology practitioners, codes of conduct are used to maintain standards of professional practice.

In some countries, the National Olympic Committee acts to accredit sport psychologists to work with their national and Olympic coaches and athletes. In such instances, both the registration boards and the National Olympic Committees have established standards of ethical practice that are used to guide the conduct of accredited sport psychologists. Therefore, formal information about ethical and professional conduct in sport psychology can be obtained from academic advisers and professional mentors; professional associations representing sport psychology; the state, provincial, or national registration or licensing boards; and some National Olympic Committees.

As acknowledged previously, some sources of information may not be available in particular locations because of the way the sport psychology profession is structured. Therefore, some lines of inquiry may not be successful. However, it is important to remember that the purpose of this search is to gain information for describing the ethical and professional conduct in sport psychology that is relevant to the country, state, or province that the aspiring sport psychologist wishes to work in. As suggested earlier, in some cases it might be useful for an aspirant to collect formal information from countries that have well-established peak industry bodies and professional organizations representing sport psychology. This information may usefully supplement more readily available information or may be relevant to the aspiring sport psychologist who is considering studying or working overseas.

There are also several informal sources of information describing ethical and professional conduct in sport psychology that may be useful to the aspiring sport psychologist, like, for example, specific chapters on ethical practice in sport psychology textbooks. Additionally, sport psychology journals are rich sources of information. The aspirant can supplement the formal sources of information with descriptions that have been collected from these informal sources.

There is a second question about ethical and professional conduct that may interest the aspirant: "In what form does the aspiring sport psychologist need to know about ethical and professional sport psychology practice?" The question moves the issue of ethics beyond considering the rules and procedures the trainee needs to know to considering *how* the trainee needs to know about ethical and professional practice.

Approaching ethical and professional conduct from a moral framework allows this dimension of sport psychology to be viewed as a skill in professional decision-making and judgment, rather than as adherence to a set of regulations that direct the profession. In Australia, the codes of professional conduct provided by the major professional associations representing sport psychology, state registration boards, and university and departmental research ethics committees often have insufficient detail to direct conduct across the range of circumstances that might be encountered. Instead, they are viewed as a set of guiding principles for ethical and professional conduct in sport psychology teaching, research, and consulting. Given the relative infancy of sport psychology as an independent profession, this may also be the case in other countries.

This moral perspective influences the form of understanding ethical and professional sport psychology practice; additionally, the aspiring sport psychologist may consider learning about ethical and professional conduct in this form. Ethical and professional practice in sport psychology is about making sound decisions from the best evidence and knowledge that is available at the time. These decisions are made in the best interests of our students, participants, and clients, and draw upon the guiding principles of ethical and professional conduct that are outlined in the various codes of conduct. This form of understanding and practicing ethical and professional conduct aims to help the professional sport psychologist act in a respectful manner to his or her profession, professional associations, other colleagues, students, participants, clients, and of course, himself or herself.

Given the above, the aspiring sport psychologist may question how to develop an understanding of ethical and professional practice that leads to sound, responsible, and respectful decisions. One approach is to view the decision-making as a skill or competency of the professional sport psycholo-

gist and to use the principles of skill learning and acquisition to develop this skill. The first step in this approach involves aspirants determining whether they wish to understand this form of ethical and professional sport psychology practice. Each aspirant is encouraged to talk about this view of ethics with an academic adviser or professional mentor. The adviser or mentor may introduce personal experiences and other familiar anecdotes into the conversation to demonstrate how values influence teaching, research, and consulting practice. If the trainee is interested in developing a moral decision-making approach to ethical sport psychology practice, then this skill should become an objective of their professional training.

An approach to learning sound and ethical decision-making involves providing the aspiring sport psychologist with many opportunities to rehearse this skill during their professional training. The professional development program can stimulate and direct the development of professional values by using modeling, behavior rehearsal, and social reinforcement processes to train decision-making behaviors. This involves surrounding the trainee with decision-making opportunities in the classroom, laboratory, and field; it also involves providing modeling, guidance, reward consequences, and initial favorable conditions to shape initial success and subsequent decision-making behavior. Because of the more subjective nature of this dimension of sport psychology, it is important to surround the trainee with opportunities to discuss their decision-making and receive feedback from peers and more senior colleagues. In addition, encouraging trainees to critically reflect about the sources of ethical and professional information, the processes that are being used, and the nature of their decisions and actions produces favorable results.

Since ethical and professional conduct occurs in teaching, research, and consulting settings, following Martens's (1979) suggestion that sport psychologists be simultaneously active in the field and in the academy may enhance learning. This means involving trainees in fieldwork and encouraging them to bring information about their professional conduct drawn from the field into the classroom and laboratory for discussion and analysis. Similarly, involving trainees in teaching and research experiences in the academy and encouraging them to bring information about this professional conduct into the field setting for discussion and analysis. This process of moving between the academy and the field, coupled with efforts to understand the values and processes underlying decision-making that is independent of the context, provides rich opportunities for developing skills in ethical and professional conduct.

A valuable adjunct to this process is to provide aspirants with opportunities to talk with other aspiring sport psychologists and more senior colleagues about the processes, outcomes, and consequences of ethical decision-making. These discussions help aspirants to gain insight into how they have come to make sound decisions in sport psychology practice. In this instance it would be useful for colleagues to focus on the decision-making process, rather than the actual decision itself. Colleagues would use their interviewing skills to help trainees gain insight into the information and processes used to come to a decision. In some instances, it may be helpful for some more senior colleagues to provide feedback on the outcome of a decision, and to support any subsequent consequences it may have for future sport psychology practice. When conducted in a sensitive and professional manner, this process reminds aspirants that developing professional values is about getting better at the skill of professional decision-making, rather than always getting it right. This approach can empower trainees to accept that making and learning from mistakes is an important part of the professional development process.

Planning the Route: "How Do I Get There?"

The final step of the planning phase is for aspiring sport psychologists to determine a pathway for acquiring the competencies of the professional sport psychologist. Prior to this step, they have identified personal strengths and weaknesses that will influence their decisions about a type of specialist training. This information has come from an assessment of skills, knowledge, and abilities. Additionally, they have identified some preferred specialist training priorities that will also influence their decision.

There are three considerations in determining the specialist training program in sport psychology that is most beneficial to an aspiring sport psychologist:

- Firstly, considering what form the sport psychology training will take;
- Secondly, the route or pathway that will permit the aspirant to maximize their specialist training in sport psychology;
- Thirdly, the expectations of self and others who are traveling a similar journey during their specialist training in sport psychology.

There are several different forms or vehicles for the aspirant to reach his or her professional training destination, much like there are several vehicles for traveling from St. Kilda to Kings Cross. For example, Paul Kelly chose an interstate bus, but he could have traveled to Kings Cross by foot, car, train, plane, or boat. Specialist training in sport psychology can be undertaken in three basic forms or vehicles:

- A postgraduate university degree in sport psychology;

- Working and training alongside an experienced sport psychologist in a mentor-mentee relationship;
- Participation in a structured program of short training courses, field experiences, and other activities that teach new skills and transfer existing professional skills to a sport psychology context.

Some aspiring sport psychologists may be able to select from all three forms of specialist training. If there are several forms of specialist training to choose from, aspirants are encouraged to determine the merits and shortcomings of each available form. They are encouraged to make an informed decision about the specialist training that maximizes their training opportunities and to devise an action plan to reduce the impact of any shortcomings that are associated with this training route.

Some forms of specialist training may not be available in some parts of the world. For example, in some countries, specialized sport psychology training may not be available through a recognized postgraduate degree. If it does exist, it may be prohibitive to aspiring sport psychologists because of financial or other considerations. In such instances, prospective students are encouraged to explore alternative pathways for achieving their specialist training, rather than compromise their professional training goals. In each case, aspirants are encouraged to select a form of specialist training that will satisfy their training goals and career aspirations for working as sport psychologist in their chosen region, state, or country.

It is important for aspirants to check that their preferred form of specialist training will be recognized by potential employers, professional associations representing sport psychology, registration or licensing boards, and National Olympic Committees. It is meaningless, not to mention financially unwise, for aspirants to determine a form of specialist training that may be regarded as insufficient.

Like the journey from St. Kilda to Kings Cross, once prospective trainees have determined their preferred form or vehicle for specialist training, the next decision concerns the route or pathway to travel. Paul Kelly chose a bus that traveled along the Prince Highway—the main coastal highway between Melbourne and Sydney; however, he could have traveled by an alternate route. Similarly, having decided on a postgraduate university degree, mentor-mentee relationship, or course training-retraining vehicle, the next consideration involves which university, mentor, or program of professional courses to take.

In instances where they have several pathways available, this decision-making process involves researching alternative pathways to determine the strengths and weaknesses that are associated with each route. The final decision should maximize the potential for training opportunities and minimize any shortcomings associated with this path. Prospective trainees are encouraged to develop a contingency plan to minimize the influence of any obstacles and roadblocks associated with their preferred university, mentor, or program of professional courses. An important part of determining the strengths and weaknesses of each route is gaining information about academic advisers, professional mentors, and training or field experiences that are associated with each route.

Trainees who are currently engaged in this form of specialist training may also be very useful sources of information about this specialist-training route. It can be very helpful to speak with current in-training sport psychologists, recent graduates, and other professional sport psychologists who have successfully used this specialist-training pathway. Clearly, once a professional training destination has been identified, the form of professional training decided, and the preferred route(s) determined, the aspirant should do everything possible to be selected for this university degree, mentor relationship, or program of professional courses. The overall planning activity has been futile if, after having developed such an elaborate plan of action, the aspirant fails to turn intentions into action.

Finally, "What can aspiring sport psychologists expect of themselves and others who are traveling a similar journey during their specialist training?" The metaphor of a journey between St. Kilda and Kings Cross has been useful for considering the process of professional training in sport psychology. However, there is an important departure from the metaphor. Paul Kelly's role as a passenger on the interstate bus was largely passive. He settled into his seat and aimed to stay as comfortable as possible for the 14-hour trip. Aspiring sport psychologists *do not* have a passive role in their specialist training. They often can expect to be on the edge of their professional and personal comfort zones throughout the duration of their professional training program.

Successful trainees are very active during their professional training journey, both in learning from academic advisers and professional mentors and in learning from field and other experiences. The professional training process that has been described in this chapter has emphasized *the responsibility of the aspiring sport psychologist for planning and conducting their professional training experience.* This responsibility is similar regardless of the form and route chosen by the aspirant. No form or route is necessarily easier or requires less personal investment. Instead they should be viewed as requiring equivalent levels of commitment and investment of personal resources, albeit they are different pathways to largely the same professional destination. The approach of this chapter has

been *to emphasize the student's autonomy and responsibility to learn, and to de-emphasize the teacher's responsibility to teach.* Goal setting (Burton, 1989; Gould, 1992; Weinberg, 1996) or learning contracts (Anderson, Boud, & Sampson, 1996) may be helpful for structuring learning opportunities and experiences, but *essentially, the aspiring sport psychologist is responsible for his or her professional training.*

There are two other roles that are important in this learning process. The first is that of the other trainees who are undertaking similar professional development at approximately the same time. These fellow travelers are important sources of social and professional support for the aspiring sport psychologist. They are also likely to be future professional colleagues; therefore, the development of close professional and personal relationships for mutual benefit is strongly encouraged. Many of these people will continue to be the aspirant's professional colleagues throughout his or her sport psychology career.

Secondly, the academic adviser or professional mentor fulfills an important role for aspiring sport psychologists. This academic adviser or professional mentor provides a great deal of practical, theoretical, and personal support needed by the aspirant to achieve his or her professional training goals. It would be tempting to see the adviser or mentor in the role of the bus driver or ship's captain for the specialist-training journey. However, this would convey a false notion as the adviser or mentor is simply responsible for ensuring a safe and rewarding passage.

While the adviser or mentor oversees the trainee's personal and professional safety and overall progress, it is the aspiring sport psychologist who is responsible for the successful or unsuccessful passage to the professional training destination. It would be better to cast the aspiring sport psychologist as the driver of the chosen vehicle and the academic adviser or professional mentor as a more experienced companion who travels alongside the trainee throughout the professional training journey. In this metaphor, other sport psychologists-in-training can be cast as traveling companions. They sit alongside and behind the aspirant for part of the journey and occasionally may do some of the driving to allow for rest, reflection, and a chance to recharge taxed batteries. These companions may join in with the professional conversations that the aspiring sport psychologist and the adviser or mentor have while traveling the journey, or they may initiate professional conversations and light-hearted banter to help some of the more tedious parts of the journey to pass without incident.

Conclusion

This chapter is written to provide some direction to individuals who are currently training or considering becoming professional sport psychologists. The approach has been to encourage the aspiring sport psychologist to recognize that both personal and professional competencies are important for high standards of sport psychology teaching, research, and consulting practice. Furthermore, it is the view of the author that developing personal competencies, such as the ability to plan for life, be self-reliant, and seek resources from others, can be developed from the moment that the individual decides he or she wishes to become a sport psychologist. While the professional competencies are developed during the specialist-training program, it is the author's view that the aspirant should be given the autonomy and responsibility for achieving his or her professional training objectives. Finally, the roles played by the academic adviser, the professional mentor, and the other sport psychologists-in-training are important for the aspirant, who can receive from them practical, theoretical, and social support during the exciting but challenging period of professional development.

It is also hoped that this information will encourage aspiring sport psychologists to look differently at the experiences that prominent sport psychologists have described throughout this book. It is hoped that this information will encourage students to seek to extract the wisdom contained within these sport psychology experiences.

The chapter is also intended to be helpful to experienced sport psychologists who act as academic advisers and professional mentors. The aim has been to provide some information, ideas, and suggestions that may encourage them to empower trainees to play an active role in their specialist training in sport psychology. It is hoped that this chapter leads the experienced to reminisce about their own professional training and their early professional practice, and to share these memories, anecdotes, and stories as valuable sources of information for aspirants.

Finally, this chapter uses the metaphor of a journey from St. Kilda to Kings Cross in order to frame a discussion of how to become a sport psychologist. It is hoped that this metaphor has helped the aspiring sport psychologist to appreciate that specialist training in sport psychology is somewhat akin to a journey from the aspirant's current skills, knowledge, and abilities to the competencies required of a professional sport psychologist. This chapter is something of a conceptual map for the aspiring sport psychologist to use to plan and manage specialist training in sport psychology. Let the journey begin.

References

Anderson, G., Boud, D., & Sampson, J. (1996). *Learning contracts*. London: Kogan Page.

Bandura, A. (1978). The self-system in reciprocal determinism. *American Psychologist, 37*, 334–348.

Burton, D. (1989). The Jekyll/Hyde nature of goals: Reconceptualizing goal setting in sport. In T. Horn (Ed.),

Advances in sport psychology (pp. 267–297). Champaign, IL: Human Kinetics.

Business/Higher Education Round Table. (1992). Educating for excellence: Business/Higher Education Round Table 1992 education surveys, commissioned report No.2. Melbourne: Author.

Chubb, I. (Chair). (1992). Higher education: Achieving quality (Report of Higher Education Council, National Board of Employment, Education and Training). Canberra: Australian Government Publishing Service.

Danish, S. J., D'Augelli, A. R., & Ginsberg, M. (1984). Life development intervention: Promotion of mental health through the development of competence. In S. Brown & R. Lent (Eds.), *Handbook of counseling psychology* (pp. 520–544). New York: Wiley.

Danish, S. J., Petitpas, A. J., & Hale, B. D. (1995). Psychological interventions: A life development model. In S. M. Murphy (Ed.), *Sport psychology interventions* (pp. 19–38). Champaign, IL: Human Kinetics.

Danish, S. J., Smyer, M. A., & Nowak, C. A. (1980). Developmental intervention: Enhancing life-event processes. In P. B. Baltes & O. G. Brim, Jr. (Eds.), *Life-span development and behavior* (Vol. 3, pp. 339–366). New York: Academic Press.

Gould, D. (1992). Goal setting for peak performance. In J. Williams (Ed.), *Applied sport psychology: Personal growth to peak performance* (2nd ed., pp. 158–169). Mountain View, CA: Mayfield.

Kelly, P. (1985). From St. Kilda to Kings Cross. On Post [Record]. Sydney: Mushroom Records.

Lazarus, R. S. (1989). Constructs of the mind in mental health and psychotherapy. In A. Freeman, K. M. Simon, L. E. Beutler, & H. Arkowitz (Eds.), *Comprehensive handbook of cognitive therapy* (pp. 100–121). New York: Plenum.

Lazarus, R. S., & Folkman, S. (1984). *Stress, appraisal and coping.* New York: Springer.

Lincoln, Y., & Guba, E. (1985). *Naturalistic inquiry.* Newbury Park, CA: Sage.

Martens, R. (1979). From smocks to jocks: A new adventure for sport psychologists. In P. Klavora & J. V. Daniel (Eds.), *Coach, athlete, and the sport psychologist* (pp. 56–62). Champaign, IL: Human Kinetics.

Martens, R. (1987). Science, knowledge, and sport psychology. *The Sport Psychologist, 1*, 29–55.

McCullagh, P., & Noble, J. M. (1996). Education and training in sport and exercise psychology. In J. L. Van Raalte & B. W. Brewer (Eds.), *Exploring sport and exercise psychology* (pp. 377–394). Washington, DC: American Psychological Association.

Morris, T., & Summers, J. (1995). Introduction. In T. Morris & J. Summers (Eds.), *Sport psychology: Theory, applications and issues* (pp. xxiii–xxxiv). Brisbane: John Wiley.

Murphy, S. M. (1995). Introduction to sport psychology interventions. In S. M. Murphy (Ed.), *Sport psychology interventions* (pp. 1–16). Champaign, IL: Human Kinetics.

Weinberg, R. S. (1996). Goal setting in sport and exercise psychology: Research to practice. In J. L. Van Raalte & B. W. Brewer (Eds.), *Exploring sport and exercise psychology* (pp. 3–24). Washington, DC: American Psychological Association.

Zaichkowsky, L., & Perna, F. (1996). Certification in sport and exercise psychology. In J. L. Van Raalte & B. W. Brewer (Eds.), *Exploring sport and exercise psychology* (pp. 395–412). Washington, DC: American Psychological Association.

Index

The Editor

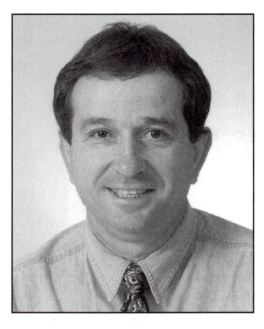

Gershon Tenenbaum

Gershon Tenenbaum is a professor at Florida State University. He is a former Head of the Centre of Research and Sport Medicine Sciences at the Wingate Institute in Israel (1982–1994) and the coordinator of the graduate program in sport and exercise psychology at the University of Southern Queensland in Australia (1994–1999). Gershon is the current president of the *International Society of Sport Psychology* (1997–2001), the editor of the International Journal of Sport Psychology and the ISSP's Newsletter. Gershon's areas of interest are in psychometrics, expertise (decision-making), and exertion tolerance. He has an extensive list of publications in journals and books, and is a board member and reviewer for twelve scientific journals. He is a member of the Australia Psychological Society, College of Sport Psychology, New York Academy of Science, The American Society for the Advancement of Applied Science, North American Society of Sport and Physical Activity, The International Statistical Institute, and others. He received the ISSP Honor Award (1997), the USQ Researcher of the year (1997/1998), and the 1987 Meritorious Contribution to Education through Research by the Journal of Educational Research. He was the captain of the Israel National Team Handball and Maccabi Tel-Aviv. He is married and has three children.

The Chapter Authors

Boris Blumenstein

Boris Blumenstein is the Head of the Sport Psychology and Biofeedback Laboratory at the Ribstein Center for Sport Medicine Sciences and Research at the Wingate Institute, Netanya, Israel. He received his Ph.D. in sport psychology in 1980 from the All Union Institute for Research in Sport in Moscow, Russia (former USSR). Dr. Blumenstein's publications in English, Hebrew, and Russian include about 50 refereed journal articles and book chapters, mainly in the area of sport and exercise psychology (including biofeedback, music, and other mental techniques for elite athlete preparation for competition). In addition to his research activities, Dr. Blumenstein has been intensively engaged in applied work. From 1978–1990 he was the sport psychologist for the Soviet National and Olympic teams (Moscow, 1980; Seoul, 1988). Since 1990 he has been a sport psychologist advisor/consultant to the Israeli National and Olympic teams (including the delegation to Atlanta in 1996). He has also lectured and conducted numerous workshops, mainly in the area of applied sport and exercise psychology. Since 1996 Dr. Blumenstein has been the representative of the Israeli Society for Sport Psychology and Sociology within FEPSAC.

Jeffrey Bond

Jeffrey Bond is the chief psychologist at the Australian Institute for Sport in Canberra and has held that position since the Institute opened in 1983. As the chief psychologist at the AIS, Mr. Bond is responsible for the coordination and development of psychological services provided by the Institute. Far from being simply an administrator, he is also responsible for the day-to-day provision of services to the individual athletes, coaches, and teams that live and train at the institute. He travels extensively, accompanying various teams to the world championships, commonwealth games, and the Olympic games.

Steven Christensen

Steven Christensen is a lecturer in the master of psychology (sport and exercise) degree program at the University of Southern Queensland, Toowoomba, Australia. Steven is a registered psychologist in Queensland and a member of the Australian Psychological Society College of Sport Psychologists. He conducted his professional training in sport psychology under the guidance of the late Professor Denis Glencross at the Curtin University of Technology. More recently, he has maintained his ongoing professional development under the guidance of professor Gershon Tenenbaum and associate professor Grace Pretty. Steven enjoys teaching, research, and consulting in sport psychology, and has been fortunate to have worked with numerous dedicated coaches and athletes involved in regional, state, national, and international competition for many years.

Noam Eyal

Noam Eyal was born in Tel Aviv, Israel, in 1959. In 1986 he graduated in psychology and political studies at Bar Ilan University in Ramat Gan. In 1992 he completed his masters degree in clinical psychology at Ben Gurion University in Beer Sheva. Today, he is working as an expert and consulting clinical psychologist at the Wingate Institute and in his private clinic. He heads the services in the Elite Sports Unit of the Israel Olympic Committee, the unit for gifted young athletes, and the National School Coaches at the Wingate Institute. Noam was a high-level competitive athlete in his younger days and is an enthusiastic believer in the importance and contribution of physical activity to mental health and well being.

Sandy Gordon

Dr. Sandy Gordon is a senior lecturer in sport and exercise psychology in the Department of Human Movement and Exercise Science at the University of Western Australia in Perth Australia. He is a full member of both the Australian Psychological Society (APS) and APS College of Sport Psychology, and is also a registered sport psychologist in Western Australia. He has consulted with various sporting groups and athletes from many sports in the UK, Canada, and Hong Kong. However, since 1987 when he arrived in Perth, his main interests and experiences have been in professional golf and cricket. During this time, he has assisted several Western Australian State amateur and professional teams and individuals, and continues to serve the PGA as consultant. In cricket he has been part of eight national titles with the "Western Warriors" and just recently, as the first sport psychologist appointed to the National Australian teams, the 1999 World Cup title. His services, as consultant, also continue to both Western Australian Cricket Association (WACA) and the Australian Cricket Board (ACB).

Daniel Gould

Dan Gould is an Excellence Professor in the Department of Exercise and Sport Science at the University of North Carolina at Greensboro where he specializes in applied sport psychology. Dr. Gould's teaching efforts over the last 20 years have focused on sport and exercise psychology, applied sport psychology, the psychology of coaching, and children in sport. His research efforts have centered on practical issues such as the stress-performance relationship, sources of athletic stress, mental preparation, athlete motivation, and sport psychological skills training use and effectiveness. Dr. Gould has made over 500 sport psychology coaching clinic presentations and written over 150 research and practice articles in sport psychology. Dan has consulted with Olympic and World champion athletes and their coaches from a variety of sports, professional athletes, and novice young athletes. Currently, Dan serves as co-chair of the USOC Science and Technology Committee and from 1984–1996 was an active member of the USOC Coaching Development Committee. He is a former President of the Association for the Advancement of Applied Sport Psychology (AAASP), a certified AAASP consultant, and a fellow in the same organization.

Dieter Hackfort

Dieter Hackfort received his Ph.D. at the German Sport University in Cologne, Germany, in 1985. In 1985–1986 he was a visiting professor at the Center for Behavioral Medicine and Health Psychology in the University of South Florida, USA. In 1986–1991 he was a professor of sport sciences at the University of Heidelberg and since 1991 he has been a professor of sport psychology at the University of Munich and heads the Institute for Sport Science and Sports. His main areas of investigation are action theory, emotions, self presentation, and health and exercise. He was awarded the most distinguished prize for his research in Germany. Dieter is a past president of the ASP, officer in the ISSP–MC and is the sport psychologist at the Olympic Center in Munich, and a counselor of various national and Olympic teams and world-class athletes. Dieter was an invited speaker in many congresses and wrote and edited many books.

Keith Henschen

Keith P. Henschen, P.E.D., is a professor in the Exercise and Sport Science Department at the University of Utah (USA). He received his P.E.D. from Indiana University in 1971. Dr Henschen has 29 years of professional experience in the field of applied sport psychology. He has published more than 200 articles and 20 book chapters, co-authored three books and seven monographs, and has made over 350 presentations on sport psychology. He has worked with numerous national governing bodies of sport and with many world-class and professional athletes. He has been a member of the American Psychology Association and the Association for the Advancement of Applied Sport Psychology, and was until 2000 a vice president of the International Society of Sport Psychology. Dr Henschen was also President of the American Alliance for Health Physical Education, Recreation and Dance.

Barry Kerr

Barry Kerr began practice as a sport psychologist with surf lifesaving clubs from the resort area of the Sunshine Coast in Queensland, Australia. He was a member of the state junior and senior surf teams as well as the Australian team from 1983–1986. He has worked with Olympic athletes as well as elite athletes at a local and district level. His interests have been in children and sport and in being involved in coach accreditation programs with weightlifting, swimming, rugby league, and equestrians. As well, he has lectured to the local branch of the Australian Sport Medicine Federation and the Queensland Academy of Sport. In 1999, he was appointed as an associate to the faculty of psychology at the University of Southern Queensland.

Trisha Leahy

Trisha Leahy, M.A., M.Phil., is a psychologist at the Australian Institute of Sport where she has been providing psychological services for elite sports personnel since 1996. Trisha previously spent 12 years in Hong Kong, during which time she was the Unit Head of the Psychology Department at the Hong Kong Sports Institute. Trisha has provided psychological services to athletes and coaches at major international competitions, including Olympic Games and World Championships, and is currently working with the Australian national sailing team in their preparation for the Sydney 2000 Olympics. A fluent Chinese speaker, she has extensive experience in crosscultural counseling and in trauma recovery with elite athletes and general populations. She is currently combining her main interests in elite sport and trauma issues in a Ph.D. research program at the University of Southern Queensland, supervised by associate professor Grace Pretty and associate professor Gershon Tenenbaum.

Mark Lowry

Mark Lowry is a clinical psychologist who spent eight years in the military as a major, helping in the selection and training of elite special operations units. Now a full-time member of the Enhanced Performance Systems team, Dr. Lowry still consults with the DEA, SWAT units, and special operations units, and brings his assessment, team-building, and leadership-training skills to the corporate arena as well.